Do You
Really Need
Back Surgery?

Do You Really Need Back Surgery?

A Surgeon's Guide to Neck and Back Pain
and How to Choose Your Treatment

Second Edition

Aaron G. Filler, MD, PhD, FRCS

OXFORD
UNIVERSITY PRESS

OXFORD

UNIVERSITY PRESS

Oxford University Press is a department of the University of Oxford. It furthers the
University's objective of excellence in research, scholarship, and education by publishing
worldwide.

Oxford   New York
Auckland   Cape Town   Dar es Salaam   Hong Kong   Karachi
Kuala Lumpur   Madrid   Melbourne   Mexico City   Nairobi
New Delhi   Shanghai   Taipei   Toronto

With   offices in
Argentina   Austria   Brazil   Chile   Czech Republic   France   Greece
Guatemala   Hungary   Italy   Japan   Poland   Portugal   Singapore
South Korea   Switzerland   Thailand   Turkey   Ukraine   Vietnam

© 2013 by Oxford University Press

Published in the United States of America by
Oxford University Press
198 Madison Avenue, New York, NY 10016,
United States of America
www.oup.com

Library of Congress Cataloging-in-Publication Data
Filler, Aaron G., 1956–
Do you really need back surgery? : a surgeon's guide to neck and back pain and how to
choose your treatment / Aaron G. Filler. — 2nd ed.
    p.—cm.
Includes bibliographical references and index.
ISBN 978–0–19–989551–9 (pbk. : alk. paper)
1. Spine—Diseases—Treatment.   2. Spine—Wounds and injuries—Treatment.
3. Neck—Diseases—Treatment.   4. Patient education. I. Title.
RD768.F54 2012
617.4'71044—dc23
2012011932

9 8 7 6 5 4 3 2 1
Printed in the United States of America
on acid-free paper

» Contents «

» Foreword «

J. Patrick Johnson, MD
Director, Institute for Spinal Disorders,
Cedars Sinai Medical Center

I am delighted and honored to write the foreword for Dr. Aaron Filler's latest work, *Do You Really Need Back Surgery? A Surgeon's Guide to Back and Neck Pain and How to Choose Your Treatment*. Dr. Filler has been both a talented friend and colleague for more than a decade and has developed his talents as a leading surgeon and scientist, particularly within the realm of spine and nerve disorders. He has pioneered previously unobtainable nerve imaging techniques by using magnetic resonance imaging and thereby established the new, unique specialty of MR Neurography.

The understanding of spinal disorders has vastly improved with the precision imaging of digital X-rays; spiral computerized tomography (CT), with the benefit of minimal radiation to the patient; and the exquisite detail of magnetic resonance imaging (MRI), which involves no radiation exposure. Other recent advances in functional imaging now provide video studies of body fluids, including blood flow, cerebrospinal fluid flow, and metabolic activity of tissues in normal and diseased states that were previously unobtainable or obtained only with invasive procedures. These detailed imaging studies can now be shared with expert colleagues in consultation around the world through digital transmission of huge data sets from desktop computers.

The treatment of spinal disorders has evolved with computerized rehabilitation technology for the nonsurgical patient to avoid and prevent surgery or to optimally rehabilitate the patient who requires a surgical procedure. A variety of new medications have been developed for the treatment of pain, inflammation, and degenerative diseases. The surgical treatment of spinal disorders has changed dramatically, especially in the past decade with "macro" surgery being transformed into "micro" or minimally invasive surgery with the ability to achieve comparable outcomes. Many spinal surgeries are now being performed in an outpatient surgery setting by using microsurgery and endoscopy; patients are going home in less than one day. Even comparably larger reconstructive surgeries are now being performed with short hospital stays. Traditional surgical procedures are now greatly enhanced by computerized image guided surgery, which enables the surgeon to visualize the anatomy inside a patient where we previously could not see beyond the tissue surfaces.

High-speed digital monitoring provides more than just the basic vital signs; now nerve and spinal cord monitoring are also commonplace. A new era in intraoperative imaging with CT and MRI scanning in the operating room, combined with innovative technologies, will make surgery even safer, more accurate, and faster. New technologies of artificial disc replacement and molecular biology to regenerate and heal tissues are currently areas of intense research and hold promise for new breakthroughs in the treatment of many spinal problems in the future.

The entire discipline of spinal disorders has seen a remarkable expansion in recent years paralleling the exponential growth that has occurred in the computer and information industry. Dr. Filler's book is a comprehensive and insightful treatise reviewing the diverse and frequently mysterious aspects of spinal disorders while providing a fresh perspective in an easily readable format that the layperson will enjoy. Part I: Spine Health has insightful chapters on anatomy, sources of pain, diagnostics, and nonsurgical treatment. Part II: Spine Surgery has very informative chapters on the surgical treatment of many spinal disorders that range from simple to complex. This book, by one of the leading authorities in spinal disorders, introduces the reader to the new age of modern technology and spinal abnormalities and is both educational and entertaining. I recommend the book wholeheartedly and enthusiastically. Enjoy!

» Preface to the First Edition «

The suggestion to write this book came from one of my patients. I was awoken at 2:00 am one Sunday to learn of a young woman who had just arrived in the Emergency Room, paralyzed from the waist down from a spine fracture suffered in a fall from the Santa Monica pier. I've always treated new paralysis as an absolute emergency so I gave orders to rush her to the operating room while I drove to the hospital. She needed a huge operation, opening the chest and abdomen, removing fractured bone from the spinal canal, placement of grafts, plates, and screws. As she awoke in the recovery room after her ten hour surgery, her first words were very L.A.—"Call my assistant! Cancel my appointments!" But the good news was that sensation was returning to her toes. By the following day she was starting to move her legs. When I saw that on her first post-operative day, I explained the exciting significance of the movement, the possibility she would recover and walk again. Lying there in her intensive care bed, her main question was if there was a book she could read that would explain what had happened, and what had been done to her.—It turned out she was a literary agent—that's how it goes in West L.A.

The fact is that there was no book to recommend. There are many books about back pain and about how to avoid surgery, and about how mind and body can work together to heal the spine, but no detailed accessible work for the general non-medical reader that would explain the various aspects of spine surgery. It was then some years in the making, but this book got its launch that day.

This book is intended to fill a major void by providing a comprehensive and authoritative reference source to patients facing spinal surgery. Although there is no substitute for direct communication with your own physician, I have greatly enjoyed the opportunity to gather together in one volume a thorough overview of the entire topic. I have always believed that the more a patient can understand about the entire process the better the overall outcome will be.

My own involvement with the spine goes back some 25 years. Because of an interest in evolution I started a masters degree program in Physical Anthropology at the University of Chicago in the same year that I started medical school. Although I originally intended to study brain evolution, Professor Russell Tuttle directed me to work on the evolution of the human and primate spine instead—he said that he knew too little about the brain to advise me and that no one knew very much about how the spine had evolved. With my masters completed, I took a five year break from medical school to study the spine as a PhD student at Harvard University. There, my advisors, colleagues and teachers—Irven DeVore, David Pilbeam, Terry Deacon, Farish Jenkins, Fuzz Crompton and the late lamented Stephen J. Gould provided intellectual encouragement as I raced through the unexplored details of spinal evolution, embryonic development, anatomical function and neuroscience of the spine in every creature that had one, from sharks to dinosaurs to human ancestors. In the end, I created substantial new knowledge about what the spine was and how its function could be understood, In addition, I did the fundamental work that later led to many of my inventions and technical innovations that are helping to advance this field.

As a neurosurgical resident in Seattle and registrar at Atkinson Morley's Hospital in the UK, I learned spinal surgery from Kim Burchiel, Paul Anderson, Sean Grady and Mark Mayberg and learned even more about what it meant to be a surgeon from Tony Bell, David Uttley and Richard Winn. My sub-specialty skills in spine and nerve surgery developed in fellowship training with Duncan McBride, Ulrich Batzdorf and David Kline. And from the start of my fellowship on through the day this is written I continue to learn from my teacher, friend and colleague J Patrick Johnson whose physical and intellectual energy as a surgeon continues to help drive the field forward.

I have also benefited in many ways from the shared experiences of the participants in the weekly conferences of what used to be the Comprehensive Spine Center at UCLA—Edgar Dawson, Rick Delamarter, Jeff Wang, Joshua Prager, and Asher Taban. The intellectual focus for spine surgery in Southern California has now shifted a few miles eastward where an unparalleled group of experts participate in the Institute for Spinal Disorders at Cedars Sinai Medical Center. I also benefit from the collaborative interactions with Ian Armstrong, Marshall Grode, Todd Lanman, and Serge Obukhov who I work with at Century City Hospital.

My colleagues at SynGenix LTD in Cambridge UK, Andrew Lever, Mark Bacon, and Tom Saylor as well as Franklyn Howe and John Griffiths at St. George's Medical School in London have helped me advance a new class of pain medications which I believe will help transform spinal surgery in the future.

I've been privileged to work with Jay Tsuruda and Grant Hieshima who have helped me create the new field of MR Neurography imaging and to begin to provide it on a widescale basis. I also thank Brad Jabour who has made it possible for me to develop the Open MRI guided percutaneous therapy program.

Valuable suggestions for the direction of this book came from Joan Bossert, Jodie Rhodes, and Frances Bagetta. Joe Bloch has been enormously helpful with the illustrations and Maura Roessner at Oxford University Press together with the entire editorial team have been a pleasure to work with. I owe a great debt of thanks to Marvin Cooper, my brother Matt, Jodean Haynes, Candice Canady, and Shirlee Jackson who have helped me maintain a busy surgical and imaging practice while completing this book.

Heartfelt appreciation is also due to all of my patients as I have learned something from each and every one of them.

Most of all, I thank my parents, my wife Lise and my kids Rachel and Wyatt for all their love and support.

» Preface to the Second Edition «

In the eight years that have elapsed since the publication of the first edition of this book, spinal surgery has undergone a relentless transformation that has moved it to the center of medical technology. In the 1990s, spinal surgery was at the margins of neurosurgery and orthopedics—a secondary interest for many of the physicians who took care of spine patients. By the time the first edition of this book was written, however, advanced training in spinal surgery fellowships was becoming the new standard for neurosurgeons and orthopedists who increasingly became complete specialists in a unifying field of spinal surgery.

The beginnings of widespread use of synthetic implants to help spinal surgeries took place in the 1980s, and the technical requirements of mastering the implant systems was an important driving factor behind the emergence of spinal fellowship training during the 1990s. In 2004, many surgeons who took care of spine patients were trained as surgical "carpenters" with a variable amount of training with the first advanced spinal implants and devices. In 2012, there are hundreds of technology corporations involved in a vast multi-billion dollar industry of spinal innovation. Gaining familiarity with the constantly advancing and diversifying array of devices and implants is now a critical component of spinal surgery training.

Spine specialists are riding a rapidly moving wave involving hundreds of new devices emerging annually that must be mastered, evaluated, understood, and applied. Scores of special problems in spine surgery that affect small numbers of patients have now also drawn the attention of the spine technology industry. Overall, the impact for patients has been increasingly effective with complex repairs and correction through progressively smaller and less invasive surgical approaches.

To handle the complexity of the requirements of spinal surgeons and their patients, devices and implants have become more elaborate, subtle, and intricate.

If the pedicle screw was the symbol of spinal technology in 2004, the advanced multi-material, flexible, artificial disk is more the symbol in 2012.

There have been similar advances on the biological front as well. In 2004, the first biotechnology products for manipulating bone regrowth were entering widespread use. In 2012, stem cells and a wide array of advanced biotechnologies are under development. The potential of intervening to accomplish true regeneration and regrowth of tissues is beginning to emerge.

Surgical treatments for nerve problems have also advanced dramatically. The widespread arrival of new imaging technology capable of giving doctors a detailed view of nerves is starting to come into universal use in the evaluation of nerve symptoms. New minimal access surgery, the use of real time MRI guidance during surgery, and increasingly complex electronic monitoring during surgery have increased the scope and effectiveness of treatments.

In the field of pain medication, a number of new arrivals and innovations have reduced pain and improved the success of post-operative healing. Pharmaceuticals have begun to bridge the gap between simply treating symptoms and the more appealing possibility of actually helping to repair and resolve spine and nerve problems directly, without the need for surgery.

Patients have benefited from the emergence of a large, diverse, and well-trained pool of subspecialist physicians who are experts in advanced spine and nerve treatment. In many practices and hospitals, the spine patient is now taken care of by several subspecialists—physiatrists knowledgeable about rehabilitation and exercise, neurologists, pain specialists, and even psychologists, along with an array of therapists who work with surgeons to craft individualized approaches to spine and nerve care.

There are still many difficult frontiers. Advanced biologics, microelectronics, and robotics are beginning to make a real impact in the battle to restore those with severe spinal cord and nerve injuries. The overall effectiveness of diagnosis and treatment in spine and nerve surgery is also still a critical focus of medical technology. And while new types of materials are being developed to aid in restoration, the costs of spinal surgeries need to be controlled so that the health system can afford the increasingly complex technology.

In many ways the prospect of successful treatment of disability and pain from spine and nerve disorders has advanced greatly. The emergence of a large spine technology industry has applied entrepreneurship and the energies of venture capital into a competitive drive to find new solutions to the problems of spine and nerve patients. Public confidence in the ability of spine and nerve specialists to solve their medical problems has also grown along with the capabilities.

Looking forward to the decade ahead, there will be more focus on advanced biologicals, robotics, microelectronics, and new materials. Restoration of normal function and alleviation of pain will be further refined.

Today, at the moment that a person develops a new spine or nerve problem, there are a wide array of well-trained experts to provide advice, recommendations, and treatments. Nonetheless, it is now even more important for the patient to be knowledgeable about the options and the technology. The patient is most likely to be successful if he or she understands what is taking place in this dynamic medical field.

The first edition of *Do You Really Need Back Surgery* has been very successful and has helped tens of thousands of patients navigate the medical system to find their way to the best treatments. This new edition adds information about dozens of new spinal technologies, adds coverage of herbal medications, and has been expanded to include two chapters on the symptoms and treatments of nerve disorders that overlap with spine problems. Understanding whether a given case of sciatica is due to nerve pinch from the piriformis muscle in the pelvis or due to a spinal disk bulge is obviously critical to success in treating the problem.

I thank all of the readers and patients who have made comments and suggestions, and once again thank the great team I have worked with at Cedars Sinai Medical Center in Los Angeles and in our office in Santa Monica. I wish you all the best of success at getting the optimal treatment and moving past any current spine and nerve problem to regain a full and pain-free lifestyle.

» Disclaimer «

The medical information provided in this book is intended only as a means of helping to improve the effectiveness of communication between patients and their doctors. The mention, description, or explanation of utility of any treatment, implant, or device in this book in no way implies that it is appropriate for use in the care of any individual reader or patient. Dr. Filler does not provide medical opinions or clinical advice to any patient whom he has not personally examined. Recommendation of any treatment is always based on the findings of a physician who has taken a history, done a physical examination, and reviewed the results of all appropriate tests and evaluations. The choice to proceed with a treatment rests with the individual patient. Listing of risks and complications in this book is meant to be extensive but may not be completely comprehensive. The treatments and methodologies described in this book represent the state of technology at the time of publication. Medicine is an ever-changing field. New treatments and tests are being developed. Treatments thought to be helpful at one time may later be found to be less effective than originally believed. Medical devices and implants may be used by physicians in various types of treatment with or without approval by the US Food and Drug Administration. Various countries have their own regulatory environments and device approval processes. In some cases a physician may obtain specific consent from a patient for the use of a device or implant that has not been approved or that has been approved for a different use. Illustrations of implants and devices in this book may appear because the manufacturer has granted permission for use of the illustration by Dr. Filler in this book. Such permissions should not be considered as a recommendation or advertisement for use of the device by the manufacturer or an endorsement by the author. Dr. Filler has no financial relationship with any of the device, implant, equipment, or pharmaceutical manufacturers mentioned in this book, with the exception of the biotech firm Molecular Synthetics, in which he is a substantial shareholder.

Do You
Really Need
Back Surgery?

How to Use This Book:
Two Dozen Visits to Your Doctor

Do You Really Need Back Surgery? is meant to give you the chance to learn just about everything you might want to know about every phase of trouble with your spine. There are very few people who will want to sit down and read it cover to cover. But there are many people who may eventually want to read most of it. The best way to use this book is in conjunction with a series of visits to the doctor as your spine problem progresses. The first half of the book covers every aspect of knowledge relevant to keeping your spine and nerves healthy and understanding their pains and sprains. The second half of the book explains all aspects of medical and surgical spine and nerve treatment, from injections to surgeries.

Do you need to know what is happening when you first experience a severe back spasm, such as will it go away, what does it mean, how can you make things better? This is all laid out in chapter 1. What about pain medicines? Which kind should you take? What is pain, anyhow? Should you take pain killers, or will you be masking some urgent message from your body to rush to the hospital? What are the important issues around using herbal medicines? Answers to general pain questions are in chapter 2. Are you interested in some general information that helps you prevent back problems? Chapter 3 covers work and home ergonomics and spine protective lifestyle options. Chapter 4 presents exercise programs and nonmedical therapies.

To understand what is happening and to communicate effectively with various spine care professionals, you need to know the language, so chapter 5 is devoted to a detailed overview of normal spine anatomy. This is followed up by chapter 6, which explains all the standard types of spine breakdown: herniated disks, bone spurs, and nerve pinches.

How does a doctor go about tracking down the source of a spine-related pain? That is the subject of Chapter 7: which disk will send pain to your big toe and which will make your biceps weak? Congenital problems and their implications are laid out in chapter 8. What pains could actually be from a pinched nerve and not from the spine? All the common nerve entrapments are covered in chapter 9. Tests such as X-rays, MRIs, and CTs are the subject of chapter 10—what are the differences, how do they work, are there risks, what can they reveal, how can you be sure you're getting the best quality test? Chapter 11 explains some basic facts about injury and recovery of nerves and spinal cord.

The second half of the book answers your questions about treatments and surgeries. If it turns out that you need surgery, you should get your information directly from your own doctor, but can you remember to ask all the questions you meant to ask? Do you get overwhelmed and find yourself looking for any excuse to end the appointment and run from the building? Is your doctor so excellent, famous, and successful that he or she has only five minutes to answer your two hours' worth of questions? Part II of this book can help.

Chapter 12 explains all sorts of injections and treatments carried out by needle through the skin. Chapter 13 describes the basic elements of a patient's experience during any trip to the operating room. All the basic types of routine spine surgery are explained and illustrated in chapter 14.

More unusual and delicate surgeries on the spinal cord and spinal nerves are explained in chapter 15. Chapter 16 introduces the complex subjects of spinal fusions and implanted spinal hardware (screws and plates). Details of complex spinal surgeries in the neck are presented in chapter 17 and in the mid-back (thoracic) in chapter 18. Chapter 19 describes surgeries in the low back (lumbar). Surgeries for nerve pinches in various locations around the body are explained in chapter 20.

What about new technology? Should you have your surgery now or should you suffer a little longer to hold out for the next big advance or miracle cure? There's no way to predict the future, but the future does arrive in medicine relatively slowly. A breakthrough in 1990 may reach final approval for patient use only in 2012. Chapter 21 can tell you a great deal about the pluses and minuses of what's just around the corner.

If your surgery is already scheduled or just completed, you may want to know all about the various risks (chapter 22) or about what to expect in your recovery (chapter 23). How about the costs and insurance coverages? This is a complex subject, and chapter 24 may help you understand at least how to ask the right questions.

I am an active practicing nerve and spine surgeon. I attend all the latest meetings. I'm an inventor who has created some of the important advances in the field. I work in a community of thirty or forty spine surgeons in West Los Angeles who compete to provide the best spine care in the world to a very well-educated and demanding patient population—we all talk to each other and share discoveries, problems, and challenges. I'm also a teacher who has trained spine and nerve surgeons at UCLA and Cedars Sinai, taught students at Harvard, and spends dozens of hours each week educating and learning from my own patients. I do surgeries, I do injections, and I do yoga.

What I've tried to do with this book is to empower patients to understand what is happening when there is trouble in their spines. I find that patients want their doctors to take care of them, but they are also looking for a partner with a sincere interest in their well being. I enjoy the partnership aspect, but this works best if the patient can understand as much as possible about what is taking place. In summary, then, this book should be used as a resource to help you to get the most out of your visits with your own spine care professionals. In the end, you have to rely on the judgment and advice of your doctor. This book doesn't begin to provide enough information for you to know what they know in giving you their opinions and advice. However, it should help you ask the right questions and better understand the answers.

I thank you all in advance for taking the time to read *Do You Really Need Back Surgery?* I wish you all the best for a successful recovery from your spine problem.

Part I

Spine and Nerve Health

Acute, Chronic, and Recurring: A Quick Tour of Neck and Back Pain

Perhaps the least glamorous aspect of the shared human experience is the episode of severe immobilizing back pain. Fortunately for me, I've shared in this rite of passage only twice in my life. The first and most memorable of these episodes caught me just after I'd finished the last formal medical rotation in my neurosurgery residency. My fiancée and I headed north from Seattle, across the Canadian border, for a four-day weekend in a ski lodge at Whistler Mountain. It had been eight very long years and I intended to truly celebrate and unwind. We booked a suite and got an upgrade. It was magnificent: two stories, a huge, round bed with mirrors, an oversized Jacuzzi—just exactly what I had in mind for the occasion.

It was late Friday afternoon when we arrived. I think Lise expected to spend the entire four days in the suite, but I headed straight for the slopes. It was the end of the day, the runs were icy, and the temperature was a bit warm, so the remaining snow was wet and heavy. I'd been on call seven days a week, twenty-four hours a day, for the past ten months, so I wasn't at my athletic peak. That first ski run was my last.

Halfway down the hill, l thought I had stopped atop a mogul, but I suddenly realized I was still sliding sideways. As one ski turned downhill, the other caught in the heavy snow. As I fell, my body twisted and I had the strange sensation that I was bending into a position that the human body was not meant to bend into. I pulled myself back up onto my skis and headed down the hill, noticing just a small bit of pain in my lower back. I headed for the ski lift, but my back was getting stiff and a little sorer as each minute passed. Changing plans, I headed for the lodge, then turned to release my skis. The stiffness was increasing rapidly.

Walking back to the room, I noticed more pain with each step. I tried to bend a bit to the right as I walked to relieve the gathering back spasm, but with each adjustment it seemed that I had to bend a little further, and so on, until I realized I couldn't really walk. I leaned my back against the wall of the corridor and gradually eased my way down the hall until I reached the door to our room.

When Lise opened the door, I eased myself down onto the floor, lying flat on my back. Although Lise and I both initially laughed, for the next seventy-two hours, I remained pinned to the floor. With Lise's help I made one valiant attempt to make it into the hot tub on the second day, but there was no hope. The slightest movement triggered overwhelming pain. It settled to a dull roar only when I lay perfectly flat on my back-no twists, no bends, no sitting, and certainly no standing. It was actually very entertaining because I truly believed it would end and resolve completely, as I could control the pain by lying flat and because I was at a place and time where I could accommodate the predicament.

Fortunately, by the morning of our fourth day at Whistler, the storm in my back muscles started to relent. I made it up into a stiff sitting position. Then, with one arm around Lise's shoulders, I managed to take a few steps. Next, I tried walking solo, holding myself rigid as a pole. The vibration of the car on the long ride home actually felt warm and soothing as the spasm unwound. Within two days, it was all just a fond memory.

I've had only one recurrence, six years later, after carrying my two-year-old daughter through the streets of Barcelona for four hours. Again, I spent a day flat on my back on the floor of a hotel room, and once again, the storm relented and the pain disappeared without a trace. A few years later, I carried my two-year-old son on my shoulders as we walked for hours through the San Diego Zoo, with no adverse effect. As a surgeon, I lean over patients for hours in the operating room. My life proceeds with no shadow cast by my own two experiences with back pain's agony and immobility.

Low Back Pain

Abdominal pain, headache pain, or chest pain with sudden severe onset and unrelenting persistence over many hours is almost always a reason to head for the doctor's office or emergency room. Very strangely, this is not the case with back pain. One of the truly maddening aspects of back pain is that a severe, overwhelming pain that goes on relentlessly for days can signify nothing more than a passing annoyance: no impending medical disaster, no terrible injury, and no entree to disability—nothing at all, really, except for the pain itself.

Most Back Pain Goes Away without Treatment

Amazingly, 10 or 20 million times a year in the United States, this sort of low back pain happens to someone and then, a few days later, disappears without a trace. In many cases, it either never returns or doesn't happen again for many years. You usually don't need to do anything to make it go away, except to wait. It's actually a very good thing that it goes away by itself, because modern medicine can offer virtually nothing to help with this particular problem.

Imagine your frustration when you've been pinned to the floor by low back pain for hour after hour and finally decide that somehow, you have to make it to the doctor and be seen. Getting off the floor into the car is a searing experience. Every bump and vibration along the way is a new peak of agony. Then you have to sit in a chair, which may be extraordinarily painful, unless you dispense with all social convention and just lie down on the floor in the middle of the waiting room while the secretary asks you for your insurance card, social security number, and so on. Finally, after you make it into the exam room, your trusted doctor arrives, pokes here and there, taps on your knees, prods your back, and advises you to go home, lie down, and take some Motrin.

The catch here is that not all such pain is benign. In rare circumstances, some very unusual medical disasters are first revealed by back pain. A severe stomach ulcer perforating the back wall of the stomach; a giant expansion in the blood vessel that leads to the heart, the *aorta*, which is starting to rip and bleed; an inflamed pancreas; even a bad kidney infection—all of these can initially show themselves as back pain. There are even infections and tumors that can invade the back and cause severe pain. But these conditions are very rare. If you can convince yourself that you just have a mechanical problem with the muscles and bones of your back, then you can forget about those bigger worries and accept that your situation is more akin to a sprained ankle than to the need for a heart transplant.

If you do go to the trouble of seeing a doctor, don't expect him or her to know how to relieve the back pain. The objective is to get reassurance that all you have, in fact, is back pain.

Numerous Causes and Numerous Courses

Even within the confines of low back pain alone, numerous different parts of the *lumbar spine* can be responsible. In the low back, there are five lumbar disks, ten vertebral facet joints, about fifty parts of the lumbar vertebrae, nearly 100 different ligaments, and over 200 separately identifiable muscles. Any part of any one of these can be responsible for the whole situation, and it's usually extraordinarily difficult to track down exactly which demon among these hundreds of candidates is actually causing your problem (see Fig. 1.1).

It is certainly helpful to figure out whether any movement causes pain. This is because then there's something you can do about it: Stop moving. Other pains are constant, no matter what you do. Some will relent only when you find the perfect position. This could be simply lying flat on your back. It could be lying flat with your legs up in the air against a wall. You may need a small pillow at just the right point behind your back. Some pains are relieved by curling up into a ball, others by lying on your stomach over a large pillow. Some chairs make the

Figure 1.1 Lumbar spine and ligaments. The lumbar and sacral spine include numerous bone elements, muscle attachment points, ligaments, joint surfaces, and contact points between vertebrae and nerves. Successful treatment often requires identification of a single key pain generator. Frank Netter illustration reproduced with permission from www.netterimages.com © of Elsevier Inc. All rights reserved.

pain worse; some chairs provide complete relief. In general, if there is a change in activity or change in position that can relieve the symptoms, then you are in luck. First, you have a chance of temporary relief that no doctor or medicine may be able to provide. Second, this scenario is good evidence that the problem is in your muscles, bones, and joints.

Constant, severe back pain that is not relieved by rest or position and is not calmed by anti-inflammatory medicines such as Tylenol, aspirin, or Aleve may still be *musculoskeletal*—a pulled muscle or a strained ligament—and ultimately harmless. However, this type of pain is more of a concern; here the difficult experience of going to see a doctor may be even more worthwhile for the assurance of the doctor's opinion that the pain is indeed coming from the muscles and ligaments of the low back.

Sciatica: Buttock and Leg Pain

Among the most sensitive of all nerve tissues is the spinal cord. The good news is that the spinal cord does not extend into the low back; in 99.9 percent of humans, the spinal cord ends just below the level of the ribcage. Therefore, in most of the relevant parts of the low back, there are nerves but no actual spinal cord tissue. This is important because nerves are resilient but spinal cord is most certainly not resilient (see Fig. 1.2).

Where Does Sciatica Come From?

A nerve can be crushed, squeezed, twisted, pulled, and compressed, which can cause all sorts of unpleasant consequences, but for the most part, once the trouble is relieved, the nerve will bounce back and function normally. The spinal cord, however, cannot tolerate just about anything done to it, and if it is harmed it is unlikely to recover fully. That's why it's reassuring to know there's no spinal cord in the low back. Even if you have nerve symptoms along with your low back pain, everything should be fixable.

The most common nerve symptom that goes along with low back pain is a pain that travels across the buttock, down the back of the leg, and out into at least one of your toes. This is called *sciatica*. Sometimes back pain arising in the spine's joints or disks will also cause pain to be experienced in part of the leg; this is a type of *referred pain*, which is pain perceived as occurring somewhere other than the location of injury. The most famous example of referred pain is the kind that makes your left arm hurt when you're actually having a heart attack. Sciatica differs from referred pain in the leg, however, because sciatica pain usually extends all the way past the ankles and, most commonly, to your toes.

For some people, sciatica is worse when they are sitting; others find it worse when walking. Some get relief by lying down, some by standing up. This is due to the variety of causes of this type of pain. The most common cause of sciatica is a slipped disk in the lumbar spine that is pinching a component of the *sciatic nerve*, the main nerve that runs down the back of your leg. There are other causes, such as muscle tears and sprains in the pelvis that can pinch this nerve, but these types of sciatica either extend only to the ankle and rarely have any associated back

Figure 1.2 Spinal cord and peripheral nerves. The spinal cord extends just past the lowest rib, ending at the level of first lumbar vertebra. Below this, the spinal canal is filled with the cauda equina—"horse's tail" of nerve roots. Frank Netter illustration reproduced with permission from www.netterimages.com © of Elsevier Inc. All rights reserved.

pain or involve all of the toes rather than just one or two. The "toe selectivity" of sciatica that is due to a slipped lumbar disk is a simple and convenient feature that anyone can identify; the reasons behind it are explained in Chapter 7.

Grades of Severity: Pain, Numbness, and Weakness

When a nerve pinch results in sciatica, a mild pinch causes only pain; a more severe pinch causes numbness; and an even more severe pinch causes weakness in the calf, ankle, and foot. As I've said, nerves are resilient, and if your sciatica involves pain but no numbness or weakness, you don't absolutely have to get the nerve pinch fixed. One of my colleagues (who is also a spinal neurosurgeon) dragged around with his sciatica for eight years—most of the way through his residency. Sometimes it was worse, sometimes it was better, but it never went away completely. Finally, he was brought home flat on a board after a failed helicopter skiing expedition. On arriving home, he finally had surgery for his slipped lumbar disk, was back to work three days later, and has never had trouble since.

Pain comes and goes. It can be masked and your attention can be distracted from it in many ways. Numbness is an odd sensation but usually causes little specific harm by itself. But although nerves are resilient, they are not indestructible. When you choose to leave a painful nerve pinch untreated, you take on a small risk of subsequently developing a chronic pain that will not respond to treatment. This risk is less than 1 percent, but it is not zero. If there is numbness, your risk goes up. If there is weakness, however, the situation is very different.

Actual weakness from a nerve pinch is more serious for several reasons. First, a nerve pinch causing weakness is by definition a more severe nerve pinch. Also, once you've got pain, numbness, and weakness, the body doesn't have any more warning signals, so if the pinch gets even worse, you won't be alerted by new symptoms. In this fashion, a severe and permanent injury can develop without any noticeable additional sign. Because of this, the symptom of weakness in your calf, ankle, or foot is the end of your full freedom of choice. If you want to be sure you'll be able to use your foot for normal walking in the future, you're going to have to get a full medical evaluation and possibly spine surgery as well. If the weakness comes on suddenly and is very severe, the surgery should be arranged as an emergency. Emergency surgery may also be needed if you begin to have abnormal function of your bladder or bowels with numbness in the low pelvis between your legs, or if weakness develops in both legs.

Fortunately for the typical sciatica sufferer, if none of these ominous things is happening, you don't absolutely have to consider surgery. Sciatica pain usually goes away on its own. If it's still there after three months, it may be time to see a doctor about it. Surgery can be done to relieve sciatica after just a few months or after years of pain, but as long as you're willing to put up with the pain of sciatica you may never have to have surgery for it.

Claudication Pain in the Legs and Back

Another type of leg pain with origins in the spine, called *claudication*, is very different from sciatica or referred pain. Unlike sciatica, claudication usually affects both legs, is very often worse on the front of the legs, and almost never extends to the toes. The most distinctive feature of claudication pain is its close association with walking. The pain begins a few moments after walking is begun, and then gets progressively worse until walking is impossible. When the sufferer stops walking and rests, the leg pain is usually relieved, whether or not the sufferer sits down. The back pain that goes with claudication, however, is usually more of a stiffness, and it does not come and go the way the leg pain does.

All of the usual treatments for other back pains are useless for claudication. It can sometimes be relieved with a type of injection called an *epidural*, and surgery is very effective, but virtually nothing else works. Claudication accounts for about 5 percent of the cases of chronic back and leg pain, so it is uncommon, but not rare. It occurs almost exclusively in older people in their sixties, seventies, and eighties or in younger people with congenital spine abnormalities.

Although some claudication cases are due to a spinal problem, others are actually due to problems in the blood vessels. Progressive pain in the legs with activity, particularly a burning pain that is most intense in the skin, may also be due to nerve diseases called *neuropathies*. Both claudication and neuropathies need to be evaluated by a doctor. In general, it's helpful to consider these more specialized problems in the course of reassuring yourself that you have just "garden variety" back pain that is likely to resolve without the help of a medical doctor or surgeon.

Pain in the Neck and Thoracic Outlet

You're stopped at a red light, watching for the signal to turn green. Out of the corner of your eye, you see a vehicle in your rear-view mirror racing toward you. Then, wham! Your car lurches forward, and your neck snaps backward, followed by a sharp rebound snap driving your chin down toward your chest. Immediately, your neck is throbbing, there's tingling in your fingers, you have a headache, and you feel unstable and dizzy. This is "whiplash," and it is the fastest way to get neck pain.

As its colloquial use suggests, a pain in the neck can be a major nuisance. Although neck pain generally lacks the severity and persistence of back pain, the nerves and spinal cord are more likely to be involved in a case of neck pain than in a case of back pain. Treatments such as spinal manipulation, which is quite safe in the lumbar spine, can carry far greater risks when applied to the *cervical spine* (in the neck). However, it is also worth considering that the failure rate of surgical treatment for the neck is far lower than the surgical failure rate for the lower back.

Bone Spurs and Hand Symptoms

In the neck, bone spurs from arthritis, as well as slipped disks, can cause the vertebrae to move abnormally and lead the neck to hurt when it moves. When you have back pain, it's reasonable to try to avoid moving your back, but attempting not to move your neck in the course of the day is essentially impossible. A neck collar may help, but no collar or similar device is capable of holding the neck completely still.

Neck pain is very commonly accompanied by pain in the shoulders, arms, and fingers. In fact, numbness and lack of coordination in the hands is often the most noticeable effect of a problem affecting the cervical spine. This is in part because the sensation and movement of your fingers is usually highly detailed and precise—a quality that neurologists sometimes refer to as being *eloquent*. Some numbness and clumsiness in your big toe, for example, is almost impossible to notice, but the same symptoms in your thumb and first finger can be a very obvious problem. In fact, these two digits are normally so sensitive that even the slightest numbness will be immediately evident.

The perception of numbness reflects an interference that is preventing sensations at your fingertips from reaching the brain, which often happens when one of the nerves in the cervical spine is pinched. The clumsiness comes about because your brain normally receives subconscious sensory signals from nerves in the joints and muscles of your fingers. These signals tell the brain exactly where the bones of your fingers are in space relative to each other, how far each joint is bent, and how much tension each finger is resisting in the course of its work. Without this incoming information, the brain can't accurately move and position the fingers, so you experience clumsiness and start to drop things even though your hands don't actually seem weak.

Whiplash and Neck Muscles

Whiplash can also tear the muscles that attach to the spine. Once torn, some of these muscles may heal improperly, leading to continuing neck pain. In many cases, the irritated muscles put abnormal tension on the numerous nerves of the neck, causing additional pains. One example is the set of *occipital muscles* that attach along the back of the base of the skull. These may pinch the small nerves that go to the scalp, resulting in chronic headaches. A similar problem involves the *scalene muscles*, which can pinch the nerves that emerge from the *thoracic outlet* at the base of the neck. The anterior and middle scalene muscles run from the cervical spine to the first rib and form an opening between them shaped like an upside-down V. Many of the major nerves, arteries, and veins headed to the arm and hand pass through this upside-down V or triangle, which is often termed the thoracic outlet. Compression at the thoracic outlet can lead to hand weakness, clumsiness, and numbness, most commonly affecting the little finger and ring finger.

Shoulder pain is a common problem for many reasons and is often due to problems in the shoulder itself. However, neck problems can also affect the nerves to the shoulder, and this can lead to a confusing situation. When both neck pain and shoulder pain are present, only a detailed, expert evaluation can sort it out.

Unlike low back pain, pain in the neck raises concerns about the spinal cord. Pain can result from abnormalities inside the spinal cord that do not directly involve the muscles and bones. Pain from the cervical spinal cord is usually less responsive to position and movement than pain from the muscles, bones, and nerves in the neck. Also, when the spinal cord is involved, symptoms are more likely to affect both the right and left side at the same time, and also may affect the legs, feet, balance, bowel control, and bladder. Surprisingly, injuries affecting the spinal cord in the neck may not cause any pain at all. The first symptoms may actually be problems with balance and whole-body coordination. Although these may be more subtle and less attention-grabbing than pain, the types of spinal cord problems they can signify are actually among the most serious of all spinal conditions. The cord is unforgiving and needs to be taken care of as soon as problems develop.

The Spinal Cord Can't Be Ignored

If there is pressure on the cervical spinal cord from a slipped disk, a malpositioned vertebra, or a narrowed, arthritic spinal canal, then surgery is usually the best and safest treatment, and there should never be any use of chiropractic manipulation. All good chiropractors and therapists who treat neck symptoms perform careful checks to assure the safety of the situation before they begin any neck manipulation or therapy.

Because of the higher sensitivity of the neurologic structures in the neck, as well as the effectiveness of surgery, many neck pain sufferers will turn to medical doctors, neurologists, and surgeons far more readily than sufferers of low back pain. For those seeing surgeons, back patients are more likely to see either orthopedic surgeons or neurosurgeons, while neck patients will most commonly tend to see neurosurgeons. As with back pain, if it is certain that the spinal cord and nerves are not at risk, you are presented with a wide array of options for managing neck pain. Also as in the back, there are hundreds of individual bits of anatomy in the neck that can be responsible for the pain. This is why something that works for one person may not work for someone else.

One helpful similarity between neck and back pains is that most will go away on their own whether or not you do anything. When a pain gradually resolves during the course of weeks of therapy, it's often hard to tell whether the therapy led to the improvement or if it was just "window dressing" for the passage of time. Nonetheless, the cervical spine is very responsive to various kinds of nonsurgical therapy. Although surgery plays an important role when the nerves or spinal cord are involved, surgery is rarely the first choice for treating neck pain alone.

Upper Back Pain

Pain in the upper back always requires a full medical evaluation before it is treated as simple musculoskeletal pain. The thoracic spine, between the neck and the low back, is naturally stiff and rigid and is the least likely part of the spine to develop mechanical problems. However, problems with the lungs, the heart, the great blood vessels, or the esophagus (the tube carrying food from your throat to your stomach) can all initially show up as pain in the upper back. So many serious medical conditions can first present themselves this way that a visit to the doctor is an absolutely necessary starting point.

On the flip side, a slipped disk in the upper back may cause a sharp pain that wraps around to the front of your chest and sends you rushing to the emergency room for an electrocardiogram time after time. The pain may get worse with shouting, coughing, or singing and may hurt with each breath, giving the impression of shortness of breath. If the doctor doesn't consider the spine, then the source of the pain may remain a mystery.

Because of their rarity compared with heart problems, pneumonia, tumors, blocked arteries in the lungs, and lung tissue disease, pains caused by the thoracic spine are not always considered as a possible cause of chest pain. Accurate medical diagnosis of pain in the upper back and chest is therefore extremely important in ruling out any serious internal medical condition before shifting the focus to an appropriate spine treatment. Overall, and happily, thoracic spine pain is almost always less ominous than the other medical problems for which it is often mistaken. Compared with other spinal problems, however, thoracic spinal problems are often difficult to treat either by nonsurgical or surgical approaches. Fortunately, because the thoracic spinal canal is usually large in diameter, the risk of spinal cord problems there is much lower than in the cervical spine. Compared with low back and neck pain, thoracic back pain is also relatively rare.

Approaches to Calming the Spine: A Three-Month Rule

Once all the serious medical worries are cleared away, once any threat to the nerves or spinal cord is ruled out, there is still the pain to be dealt with. Tens of millions of people each year suffer sudden severe pains in the neck and back that essentially cannot be treated by a medical doctor. There are a few general over-the-counter medicines that may help, such as anti-inflammatories (e.g., Motrin, Aleve, aspirin), and there are prescription medications to treat muscle spasm (e.g., Soma, Flexeril, Baclofen, Valium), but none of the antispasmodic medicines are highly effective, and they often have side effects of drowsiness or even addiction.

Starting with Gentle Spine Treatments

For spine pain with no severe nerve numbness or weakness, most medical spine specialists postpone any significant evaluation and treatment until the problem has been present for at least three months. The reason for the delay is that the vast majority of spine pains "burn themselves out" by that time. From a mass public health perspective, the three-month wait before starting extensive tests and examinations makes excellent sense and saves the economy tens of billions of dollars in potentially unnecessary health care costs. However, it is also important to look at this from the very different perspective of the prospective patient: you.

What we're talking about is a formal policy by which someone in immobilizing pain is intentionally left ignored and untreated for not one hour, not eight hours, a few days, or a week, but for at least three months. If you're counting while you have back pain, three months is 13 weeks, 91 days, 2184 hours, or 131,040 minutes during which the medical profession is guided by the general policy of letting you suffer without evaluation or treatment.

This lack of service creates a powerful vacuum, and many different types of spine care providers have rushed to enter it. In this vast area of health care need, traditional medicine provides little or no competition, and no single approach is standardized. Chiropractic treatment is often very effective, but anyone who has visited three or four different chiropractors knows that there may be little detectable similarity between the treatment offered by each of these practitioners.

To a degree far exceeding almost any other area of health in the United States, spine pain sufferers make choices based on the advice and experience of friends, acquaintances, co-workers, or people they run into on the street who recognize that they're having back pain. Perhaps only in the area of dieting are more books read that have been written by non-specialist authors, as few physicians have bothered to write accessible books about what to do. The array of possible schools of treatment is mind-bending: Rolfing, Pilates, yoga (seven different types), stabilization, chiropractic, acupuncture, acupressure, shiatsu, Feldenkrais, Mensendieck, osteopathy, Tai Chi, Hellerwork, reflexology, physical therapy, back school, Reiki, massage (many types), Trager, hypnosis, Alexander, and more (see chapter 4). It can be fairly said about all this that "the writing is on the wall." When there are at least twenty-eight different schools of thought on how to treat spine pain, with different practitioners using a variety of widely different approaches within each school, it's obvious that there is no single right choice and that no one really knows for certain what to do.

The Problem of Choosing

No matter how much anyone sings the praises of any given method, one can't help but believe that if any one of these were truly superior, it would dominate the field. With spine pain being so distressing and urgent, any surefire treatment would certainly push all the others aside. What seems to be the case is an interesting phenomenon. All of these methods work, and most of them work fairly well. Of course, if you don't do anything, the pain also goes away, which in turn makes it very hard to assess the benefits of any of these methods. The whole problem is further complicated by the facts that neck and back pain can be due to several hundred different specific causes and that there are very few ways to sort out which cause is most responsible in any given sufferer.

What most of the just-listed therapeutic methods have in common are the following essential aspects: (1) a reassuring practitioner who gives you reasonable hope of getting out of trouble, (2) something that you personally can do to help to resolve the situation, and (3) some sort of contact: a type of pressure, rubbing, a more-or-less gentle pounding, or pushing or pulling or massaging of the uncomfortable area. This basic approach—"laying on of hands," in essence—is as old as human civilization, and fortunately it seems to help most people most of the time.

In fact, most of these methods are so reliably effective for spine pain that failure to get relief by any of them is an excellent reason to see a medical or surgical spine specialist. Conversely, assuming that all medical and neurologic problems other than musculoskeletal pain have been ruled out already, then you really should avoid seeing a physician or surgeon for your spine pain until you've tried one of these nonmedical approaches to treatment. It is important, nonetheless, to keep a few guidelines in mind as you progress through the world of nonmedical or "alternative" therapy. If your condition is getting worse during any form of treatment, you need to take the initiative to stop that treatment. Many nonmedical practitioners base their approach to spine care on a philosophy rather than on the empirical scientific method. This kind of approach certainly has its place in the world, but you need to keep in mind that this tells you something about the bias and mindset of your therapist. If you are getting worse, the therapist's strongly held philosophy may lead him or her to persist in recommending the therapy despite all objective evidence of its failure.

Changing the Plan When There's a Change in the Pain

More important, if new symptoms develop during the course of treatment, these must be addressed. The practitioner needs to make a convincing case to you that the new symptom is well understood or is to be expected in the normal course of things. If you have any doubt about the safety or reasonableness of treating or ignoring the new symptom, then it's time for an outside opinion, possibly from another alternative practitioner or from your physician. These considerations are, in part, why chiropractors are among the most popular classes of practitioners treating spine pain. For the most part, chiropractors have some grounding or orientation in anatomy and medicine and so are more likely to recognize something that should change the treatment plan or lead them to send you to a doctor.

Many people are familiar with this problem in working with alternative practitioners in the area of childbirth. Among all the thousands of happy results, everyone has also heard occasional horror stories of a family who insisted on using an unsupervised midwife at home for childbirth and then came to catastrophe when danger signs were not recognized or were ignored. Fortunately, the stakes are not always so high in spine care as in childbirth, but the problem is similar. Passionate philosophy, fear or distaste toward standard medical approaches, frustration at past failed medical treatment, or even anger at a system that has left you to find your own way through three months of pain can all lead to bad choices. The best that you can do is seek out a practitioner you feel comfortable with who works with a philosophy, an office setting, and a physical approach that makes you feel relaxed and confident. Also, just as it may be too soon to see a spinal medical specialist before three months, longer than three months is too long to continue with an alternative therapy if you have not improved by that time.

Basics of Self-Care

What if you don't want to go to any practitioner? What are the best things to do? In general, extended bed rest is not a good idea. It may be unavoidable for a few days, but overall, the best therapy seems to be a return to most of your usual activities with a few exceptions. You need to analyze your work, home, and recreational activities to identify the things that place the greatest stress on your spine. If your work entails lifting heavy objects or leaning forward for hours, this may be a problem. Your employer may accommodate some *ergonomic* changes in your work place—alterations in the design of your workspace that help you do your work safely—and you may ultimately be able to return to a full work level. However, you will face challenges in limiting the stress to your spine during your recovery. This may mean figuring out how to hold and lift a child in a way that minimizes strain. It may mean frequent breaks from computer work that allow you to stand and to move around. The objective is to get through the acutely painful episodes so that you can resume your normal life. Some of the changes you introduce during an episode of spine pain may be things that you can continue after the episode resolves, which may help you avoid future trouble.

Walking, swimming, or keeping up a continuous level of moderate activity will help strengthen your spinal muscles and make them more resistant to abrupt failure in the future. Simple range-of-motion exercises help your joints lubricate themselves and help smooth the gliding surfaces between your ligaments and tendons. Warm baths and gentle massage are always nice and encompass some of the common features of various alternative therapies.

One of the key determinants of whether you need the guidance of a therapist or you can manage all this on your own, however, is your own personality. Some people thrive with reliance on a counselor, but others chafe at this. Some need the discipline of being forced to attend to themselves and to relax, while others tense up when given directions. Another fundamental divide is how you respond when someone talks about holistic mind-body approaches, balance in nature, and oneness with your body. For some people, such talk is extremely soothing, and others find it like fingernails on a chalkboard and want to run screaming from the room.

Spine pain is one problem for which you have to choose your own path. None of this is much fun, but you should expect to get better. Once you hit that three-month point, however, if the continuous pain has never resolved, you're going to have to rethink your situation, assemble more medical and technical understanding of your situation, and prepare to journey deeper into the spine-care world.

Mission

It should be very obvious that this book is based on a philosophy of empowerment through knowledge. I'm a subspecialist, neurosurgical spine expert who does surgery to repair the effects of unsuccessful operations by other spine surgeons. I have a PhD from Harvard University, where I spent five years studying every imaginable detail of the spine and back muscles in an effort to fill in the gaps of what has been learned by Western science and medicine up until now. I have led an advanced research group trying to discover new types of medicines that fill in the huge gaps in treatment of spine pain. My clinical practice is guided by formal outcome studies that ask hard questions about what works and what doesn't work. I've invented advanced diagnostic techniques that help to tackle the weakest point of surgical spine care, which is mistaken diagnosis.

By sharing what I personally consider to be the most important aspects of knowledge about the spine, I hope to help you with your choices. I want you to understand not only your spine, but also your spine doctor and the underlying elements of the treatments that may be recommended. This is a lot of information to cover—but there are a lot of very motivated readers. Let's get started.

2

The Nature of Pain and How It Is Treated

It may very reasonably be said that pain is nature's way of letting the mind know that the body has a problem. It is very effective. The alert comes through immediately and gives some information about the type of problem and the location. The drawback with pain, however, is something like the drawback with a very effective car alarm that helps protect the car but won't stop blaring outside your window. That is, once the message is received, there is no convenient way for you to turn off the signal—the pain—without resolving the problem that triggered your body's alert system in the first place. Because of this "little" problem, a tremendous effort is being made in medicine, pharmacology, and a variety of allied health care areas to find ways of getting the necessary information from the pain but then turning off the signal by relieving the pain. This endeavor is independent of attempts to treat the pain's underlying cause.

Paying Attention to Pain

An important issue that affects all types of pain at the highest level of the *central nervous system* (the brain and spinal cord) is the issue of attention. Pain, as I said earlier, is a kind of alarm, a way of making you pay attention to something that is going on with your body. One interesting consequence of this is that someone suffering from even a severe or chronic pain may experience a kind of relief from pain based on attention. Whether it's answering an e-mail on the computer, having a conversation, reading, or even sleeping, while the individual's attention is turned away from the pain, it ceases to be a problem. Unfortunately, pain is designed by nature to overcome your ability to ignore it. As soon as the attention is brought back to the pain, the pain becomes a problem again in full force.

Types of Pain

Pains vary in regard to the way your nerves transmit them, the quality of discomfort they cause, and the types of medications that may be able to control them. Understanding the type of pain is often very helpful to communication between patient and physician and can be the key to making the right diagnosis and choosing the right treatment.

Somatic Pain

Generally speaking, pain can be divided into a number of major categories. The first is what may be called *somatic pain*. This is pain that arises in the body tissues and is best viewed as a report from the nervous system that some sort of damage has occurred somewhere in the body. How does this signal come about? Some nerves with sensory endings in the skin are sensitive to stimuli such as temperature, pressure, or vibration, which are perceived as painful stimuli. Many of these nerve endings will generate a perception of pain when stimulated to a very high extreme; other nerve endings will precipitate a sensation of pain even with the mildest stimulus, for instance, a pinprick.

How does a nerve recognize a painful stimulus? Well, part of recognition is accomplished by what is in effect direct monitoring for sensations that might be harmful. A good example are the nerve endings that report pain when they perceive a sharp point pressing on the skin. If the skin is contacted by something that has an impact in a very small area and the neighboring skin position sensors detect that the point is starting to indent the skin, then the brain is sent processed information perceived as pain. Other nerves are sensitive to tissue damage. When any tissue is damaged, there is a common pathway of release of chemicals of injury. Similarly, the process of swelling, redness, and pain experienced in an area of irritation—called *inflammation*—also involves a release of specialized body chemicals. Some nerves are essentially chemosensory receptors that detect the chemicals released by injured tissue or inflammation and then send a signal to the brain, which perceives the signal as pain.

Neuropathic Pain

Another stimulus that can produce pain is a pinch or injury of a nerve. This type of pain is broadly called *neuropathic pain*, that is, pain arising directly from a problem with a nerve, where the nerve itself is injured or where pressure on the nerve is producing pain. An odd quality of the pain that results from nerve irritation is that at least part of the pain will be perceived as coming from the location where that nerve goes, called its *distribution*. A very common example is a herniated lumbar disk that is pinching a nerve in the spine. If the nerve pinched is the nerve that goes out to your big toe, you will feel pain in your big toe even though the actual problem is in the spine, two or three feet away from the toe. So, any pain that arises from a nerve itself poses an extra challenge in determining where the pain comes from and also in treating it. Directing treatment at your toe, when the problem actually lies in the nerve that's being pinched in your back, will not be effective, so the treatment has to be directed at relieving the pinch at the point of the nerve irritation.

In addition to causing pain in the distribution of the affected nerve, a neuropathic pain will also sometimes cause pain in the location of the nerve irritation or damage itself. This is due to the fact that nerves actually have little nerves called *nervi nervorum* (in Latin) that report irritation of the nerve tissue itself. Because these "nerves of the nerves" detect the site of the nerve tissue injury, you may feel pain where the nerve is pinched as well as at the nerve's destination.

One reason that it is important to understand whether a pain is somatic or neuropathic is that the types of medications that are effective for one type of pain are not effective for another. When an injury in the skin, for example, produces chemicals that nerves detect as pain, the pain can be treated by blocking the chemicals; however, if the pain sensation is due to a nerve being injured or pinched, then blocking those pain chemicals won't help. That's why the proper selection of pain medicine depends on understanding the source and type of the pain.

Chronic Pain

Yet another category is what may be called chronic pain, pain that has been present for a long time. At one level, chronic pain means just that: something has been irritating a nerve or irritating another body tissue, and you have not been able to get it fixed, so it keeps on hurting, and the signal keeps on coming through to your brain. However, an area of special interest in chronic pain is the question of whether the nervous system actually "learns" or memorizes the painful stimulus, so that the pain essentially becomes automatic and is perceived all the time.

The idea of the nervous system learning a particular stimulus can be understood by thinking about learning to swing a golf club. There is a transition, a period of time when someone first starts to play golf, when trying to swing the club involves thinking very carefully, putting the club in a certain position, swinging it through in a thoughtful, step-by-step way, then reflecting on it again, adjusting it until you have a better course and sequence worked out, and doing it again and again. With practice, you reach a point where you lift the club, look at a spot down the golf course, and the whole sequence of events just fires off: the club comes down, the iron strikes the ball, and the ball flies exactly where you're looking, all in an automated sequence.

The nervous system can actually remodel itself through a process caused *plasticity*, forming new connections that make certain kinds of signals or patterns into "built-in" functions, similar to the learned behavior of golfing. But with chronic or *central pain*, the idea that the central nervous system can learn about pain signals is not a beneficial thing. Instead of the spinal cord and parts of the brain learning to dodge around the signal or helping you to ignore the pain, this learning sometimes has the effect that once the painful stimulus is removed, the central nervous system continues to believe that the pain is ongoing, so that chronic pain can become difficult to treat even by removing its original cause.

Reflex Sympathetic Dystrophy, or Complex Regional Pain Syndrome

Among the different types of central or chronic pain, the one most difficult to treat is termed *reflex sympathetic dystrophy* (RSD). Other names for this are complex regional pain syndrome (CRPS) or *causalgia*. This is a category of pain that develops an abnormal quality and takes up residence, in a sense, in the central nervous system, becoming unresponsive to most medications and to most treatments for the original source of pain. In many cases, RSD or CRPS involves a part of the nervous system called the *autonomic nervous system*, which controls such involuntary bodily functions as the dilation (opening) and constriction (shrinking) of blood vessels. For this reason, people suffering from RSD or CRPS may have changes in skin color from red to blue, changes in skin temperature and sweating, and even a shininess that develops in the skin as a result of changes in tissue tension and hair pattern. The abnormalities in blood supply that contribute to these conditions can also lead to thinning of the bones. A unique quality of this type of pain is that an external observer can actually see the symptoms. Most pain is subjective, in that only the sufferer knows about it firsthand, but with RSD and CRPS it is sometimes possible actually to observe the symptoms and see what part of the body is affected by the pain.

Treatment of Pain

To make pain go away, you have to either remove its cause or somehow influence the reporting system so that although the cause may still be present, the brain is not made to pay attention to it.

Relieving Tissue Injury

The best choice is always going to be to relieve tissue injury, and this is certainly the case for somatic pain. If a patient with abdominal pain from appendicitis is treated with pain medication so the pain doesn't bother him or her anymore, this really doesn't do any good. His or her appendix is going to go ahead and rupture, and then what was a relatively treatable problem can become lethal.

Masking pain that is due to tissue injury makes sense in certain defined situations: once the details are known and a search for the cause has begun, once the cause is understood and a plan for treatment is developed, or once it is determined that the problem can't be treated. Even in some of these situations, it may be necessary to allow the pain to reemerge temporarily in order to reassess progress. In any case, relieving the primary problem is always the best choice. When that can't be done, then the reporting or perception of pain itself may need to be addressed.

Immobilization and Healing

A related issue is simply the healing of tissue injury—whether it is a wound associated with trauma or with a surgical incision—with the elapse of time. As healing progresses, the pain resolves and ceases to be a problem. An important effect of pain can be to promote healing by reducing mobility. A good example of this is a bone fracture, where what hurts is actually the *periosteum*, or the lining of the bone, which has nerve endings in it. There is normally no movement along the edge of the bone, and the periosteum perceives any such movement as pain; that's why splinting or casting a fracture will make the pain stop. Once most movement across a bone fracture is stopped, healing of the fracture will progress.

Quite often, stopping movement will also relieve other types of pain but will not aid in healing. For example, in pain that arises from nerve adhesion (a nerve abnormally bound in place onto a neighboring muscle or bone), decreasing movement will decrease pain. Movement causes traction on the nerve and produces pain. In this case, however, immobilization may actually allow the adhesion to worsen. The only solution may be to do a surgical release of the adhesion. Similarly, painful joints that are not moved may become frozen. In that situation they may have to be replaced with synthetics or, when it won't cause too much disability, be fused so that they stop moving altogether.

Distracting Stimuli

There can be situations in which there is no medical way to repair the tissue injury, the injury can't be found, or normal healing is not taking place. The body may fail, for various reasons, to heal certain injuries. There can also be pains, particularly those that develop a central or chronic aspect, that become unresponsive to medication. In such circumstances, one other way of treating the pain is to create what may be called *distracting stimuli*. This often involves placing electrodes on the tissue near the nerve in question, or even within the spinal canal. An externally controllable electronic generator attached to the electrode then can provide a sufficiently complex "buzz" so that a rapidly changing but nonpainful stimulus is supplied to the nervous system, and the original pain signal fails to claim attention over the distracting stimulus. Thus, the distraction moves the attention away from the original pain and may be a way of relieving the perception of pain even when no other part of the pain transmission cycle can be successfully interrupted.

Medication for Pain

Because of the many types of pain, the many different situations in which pain arises, and the tremendous impact that pain has on human life, an extensive range of medications exists for the treatment of pain. New and even futuristic medications with various beneficial effects are also being developed. It is important for a pain sufferer to understand what the medication options are, why certain drugs are prescribed, and why some may be more effective than others. Unfortunately, patients who are having a difficult time getting relief for their back pain problem may have a tendency to try all available medications out of desperation and frustration, without taking enough time to understand the relative benefits and risks. For all of these reasons, it is worth having a detailed understanding of the different types of pain medications and how they work. The following explanations make reference to the types and mechanisms of pain already described in this chapter.

Anti-Inflammatories and Pain Relievers

Anti-inflammatories are the most common type of medication used for pain relief. They are also called *nonsteroidal anti-inflammatories*, abbreviated as NSAIDs, to distinguish them from the steroidal anti-inflammatory medications. The prototypical anti-inflammatory, and the most ancient, is aspirin. The most widely used pain reliever that is not anti-inflammatory is Tylenol (acetaminophen). The other most common anti-inflammatories medications are Aleve, Naprosyn, or Motrin (ibuprofen; see Table 2.1).

In general terms, NSAIDs work against pain by interfering with the cycle of inflammation, which ordinarily produces chemicals to signal damage and pain in injured tissue. By blocking the production of those signaling chemicals, anti-inflammatories prevent pain-sensing nerves from learning of nearby injury. But some of the other effects of inflammation, such as swelling and increased blood flow to the injured area, are actually helpful in the body's healing response; therefore, the best NSAIDs are more effective at blocking the chemicals that lead to pain transmission than they are at blocking the chemicals that lead to tissue healing. The different NSAIDs act by slightly different pathways and have different sets of side effects.

For aspirin and many other anti-inflammatories, the most common concerns are stomach irritation or pain, easy bruising or easy bleeding, and even the risk of a bleeding ulcer. This is because some of the blocked chemicals that would be communicating painful stimuli are also involved in normal blood

Table 2.1 Non-Steroidal Anti-Inflammatory Drugs (NSAIDs) and Pain Relievers

Class	Name	Chemical Name	Risks
Over-the-Counter NSAIDs			
	Alleve	naproxen	BT, GI, KT
	Aspirin	acetyl salicylic acid	BT, GI, KT, FO
	Motrin	ibuprofen	BT, GI, KT
Pain Reliever			
	Tylenol	acetaminophen	LT, KT
Prescription NSAIDs			
	Arthrotec	Diclofenac with misoprostol	BT, FO, KT, CR
	Clinoril	sulindac	BT, GI, KT
	Daypro	oxaprazosin	BT, GI, KT
	Indocin	indomethacin	BT, GI, KT
	Orudis	ketoprofen	GI, KT, BT
	Relafen	nabumetone	BT, GI, KT
	Toradol	ketorolac intravenous	BT, GI, KT
	Voltaren XR	Diclofenac	BT, GI, KT, CR
	Flector Patches	Diclofenac topical	BT, KT
Prescription NSAID Cox-2 Inhibitors[b]			
	Bextra*	valdecoxib	GI, KT, LT, FO, CR
	Vioxx	rofecoxib	GI, KT, LT, FO, CR
	Celebrex	celcoxib	GI, KT, LT, FO, CR

Note: All pain medications listed in the text and table of this chapter have side effects. In addition to those listed as special risks for each of these medications, there are serious but unusual side effects that occur rarely such as decreased production of blood cells by the body. All medications are risky for anyone who may be pregnant or who is breast feeding and require special attention before prescribing. With the exception of over-the-counter drugs, all of these medications should only be taken · with a prescription for the patient and under the direction of a physician. Liver toxicity and kidney toxicity usually do not occur, but routine blood tests for signs of these problem are essential if they are taken on an ongoing basis. Topical preparations can deliver higher doses to a particular body location with lower general toxicity and risk.

(BT)—blood thinning; (FO)—fetal/obstetrical effects; (GI)—gastric irritation; (KT)—kidney toxicity; (LT)—liver toxicity, CR—possible cardiac effects.

[b]Cox-2 = cyclo-oxygenase 2 inhibitor—these generally cause less stomach irritation than other NSAIDS. * = discontinued in U.S.

clotting, and related chemicals play a role in stimulating the *gastrointestinal tract* (the stomach and intestines) to produce a normal lining. If the normal lining is not produced properly, irritation and *ulceration*—breakdown of the stomach lining—may start. If they are severe enough, there may be internal bleeding; and if normal blood clotting is impaired, what might otherwise have been a small hemorrhage turns into a large one. That is how chronic or excessive use of aspirin can lead to the potentially fatal complication of a bleeding ulcer.

When you are using aspirin or other anti-inflammatories, you have to be very conscious of this possibility and must take the development of stomach pain or evidence of internal bleeding quite seriously. Internal bleeding sometimes becomes apparent when a person actually vomits up some blood, but more often it takes the form of black stools (black is the color of digested blood), which may be equally ominous, though less dramatic, as many people don't associate black stools with intestinal bleeding.

History of Tylenol

Tylenol—a brand of paracetamol—is probably the most widely used medicine for treatment of fever and pain. It is not an NSAID, as it does not affect inflammation. Rather, it is thought to act in the brain and spinal cord by affecting some of the chemical communication among nerve cells that carry information about pain. Although anti-inflammatories such as aspirin have been used for thousands of years, Tylenol has a very different history. In 1866, two physicians in a hospital in Strasbourg, Germany were directed by their professor to give a patient the chemical naphthalene to try to treat an infection. The naphthalene was thought to be a useful "internal anti-septic" (the first important antibiotic—penicillin—would not be discovered until 60 years later in 1928). By accident the pharmacist gave the doctors a chemical called acetanilide, which was used for chemical synthesis work but was not supposed to be given to patients.

The doctors noticed that their patient's fever dropped, which had never been seen before with naphthalene. They investigated, found the pharmacist's error, and then introduced the use of acetanilide as a fever reducer. Within a few weeks they also discovered that it was a pain reliever. It had some potential toxicities so chemists set to work to remove a toxic component and—in 1893—produced the much safer molecule (paracetomol) that is still used as Tylenol.

Tylenol does not have any impact on blood clotting and does not usually cause stomach irritation. It does carry a risk of liver injury or even liver failure. Excessive ingestion of Tylenol can be lethal and is one of the most common reasons for liver transplants.

Advances in NSAIDs

Pharmaceutical companies are constantly trying to develop better, safer, and more specific anti-inflammatories. The ideal would be a medication that blocked only those chemicals communicating about pain and that didn't affect those contributing to blood clotting or affecting the stomach lining. In this area, significant progress has been in the development of medications called *COX-2 inhibitors* (COX stands for cyclooxygenase, which is involved in the body's production of signaling chemicals). The two most widely used COX-2 inhibitors are the widely advertised Vioxx and Celebrex. These have a relatively weak anti-inflammatory effect, but they work for many people. A new more potent COX-2 inhibitor is Bextra, and more will be developed. It is often the case that an individual can take these medications without suffering the stomach irritation that results from many other anti-inflammatories.

Some of the strongest of the anti-inflammatories, such as Diclofenac or Voltaren, are more effective than the COX-2 inhibitors but have more side effects. One of the anti-inflammatories, Toradol, is unique in that it can be administered in a very powerful intravenous form. This is an important medication for pain treatment in the hospital. It can reduce the need for narcotics and reduce the risk of unintended postoperative blood clots in the veins. However, it does increase the risk of bleeding at the site of surgery if it is administered too close to the time of surgery.

Many NSAIDS can cause problems with the kidneys if they are taken for too long. This is an occasional problem that does not affect most people, but it is worth keeping in mind. If you are using NSAID-type medications for an extended time, it is well worthwhile for your physician to check some blood tests periodically to make sure there are no developing kidney or liver complications.

Celebrex and the similar medications Vioxx and Bextra were found to present a risk of serious cardiac side effects—some potentially lethal—if used in too high a dose. In November of 2011, Merck—the manufacturer of Vioxx—was fined nearly a billion dollars because of Merck's failure to adequately investigate the cardiac risk. Celebrex proved to have a lower risk. Bextra had an even higher risk—both Vioxx and Bextra were withdrawn from use in the United States. Other NSAIDs that are not COX-2 inhibitors (such as Motrin and Alleve) present a slight cardiac risk. Voltaren (Diclofenac) was found to be more of a problem, but not sufficient to be withdrawn from use.

Diclofenac has proved extremely effective and very safe when applied in a topical patch (Flector patches) or as a gel (Voltarol). At present Flector patches are far more effective than virtually any other medication for relieving spine and nerve pain if it comes from a particular area that can guide placement of the patch. Most patients who cannot tolerate the stomach irritation from other

NSAIDs are able to use Flector patches. With an oral medication, a very large dose is delivered to the stomach, then a fair amount spreads through the entire body, and then a tiny amount actually reaches the target site where your pain is coming from. Flector patches turn this pyramid upside down by providing a very high dose just at the spot of trouble, with much less spreading through the body and very little reaching the stomach.

Steroids

Steroids are natural chemicals that can relieve pain but have their own array of side effects. One form of steroid medication that is used after surgery, called a Medrol Dosepak, has the feature of starting with a significant dose and then tapering off. This is because steroids can affect a number of body processes and, when taken, are best stopped gradually. Steroids affect the salt and water balance of the body, may cause rapid weight gain, and can even cause confusion in some people; therefore, steroid use in pain treatment is usually very limited. Because of the very high risk of stomach ulcers, it is very important that a patient taking a steroid medication also take some sort of stomach protectant such as Tagamet or Ranitidine.

Compounding and Muscle Relaxants

Certain types of pain medications are not available on a standard basis at a drug store but can be specially formulated as compounded medications. Many of these are for *topical use* (applied to the skin) and may include mixtures of locally acting anesthetics, anti-inflammatories, and even muscle relaxants.

Muscle spasm plays a role in many cases of back pain. None of the muscle relaxants are really extremely effective, but they can often reduce the tension in muscles and play an important allied role in reducing pain. The very strongest muscle relaxants are medications such as Valium, which have their own pitfalls of potential dependency, drowsiness, mood effects, and abuse. However, some of the milder muscle relaxants, such as Soma, Flexeril, Zanaflex, Skelaxin, or Robaxin, have relatively few side effects and may be an important additional measure when muscle spasm plays a role in a pain problem (see Table 2.2). One sleeping medication that can be helpful with muscle spasm is Ambien (Zolpidem)—so this may be a good medication for people who mostly have a problem with pain interfering with sleep.

Anesthetics

Yet another type of medication for pain treatment, most widely known to most people from its use in the dentist's office, is based on shutting down the nerves that carry a pain stimulus. The term for a medication that simply blocks a nerve's pain transmission is an analgesic, whereas a medication that completely blocks all of the

Table 2.2 Various Locally Acting Medications for Pain

Class	Name	Chemical Name	Risks
Steroids			
	Medrol Dosepak	methylprednisolone	GI
Muscle relaxants			
	Flexeril	cyclobenzaprene	DI, DR, CE
	Soma	carisoprodol	DI, DR, A1
	Robaxin	methocarbamol	DI, DR
	Skelaxin	metaxalone	DR, LT
	Baclofen	lioresal	DI, DR, WI
	Parafon Forte	chlorzoxazone	LT, A1
	Valium	diazepam	A1, MC, DI, DR, RD
Local anaesthetics			
	Lidoderm	lidocaine patch	CE
	Mexilitene	lidocaine derivative—oral	CE
Anti-hypertensive for relief of nerve pain			
	Catapes TTS	clonidine patch	LB

See also the notes for table 2.1; (A1)—some addiction potential; (CE)—cardiac effects; (DI)—dizziness; (DR)—drowsiness; (GI)—gastric irritation; (LB)—low blood pressure; (LT)—liver toxicity; (MC)—mental clouding; (RD)—respiratory depression; (WI)—withdrawal risk

nerve function in the area is an anesthetic, that is, it temporarily eliminates all the sensation and movement that would normally be carried out by that nerve.

Local anesthetics can be injected at the site of tissue injury, or near an area where a nerve is being pinched, to block that pain. Local anesthetics can also be helpful in the course of diagnosing a pain problem, because most of them act for only a relatively short period before being washed away in the bloodstream. Local anesthetics don't usually cause any problems with blood thinning or with the liver or kidneys, but an excess amount of local anesthetic getting in the bloodstream does have some significant risk of complications, such as making the heart race, affecting breathing, or causing other neurologic symptoms.

In addition to the widely known injectable anesthetics such as novacaine, lidocaine, or Marcaine, local anesthetics can be administered in other ways. One method is a topical patch called Lidoderm, which is applied to the area that's involved in pain and provides the anesthetic lidocaine through the skin. This is a very important alternative for patients who can't or don't want to take narcotics and who have trouble taking anti-inflammatories. An oral form of lidocaine is

Mexilitene, which is used more commonly as a heart medicine. Patients who are having abnormal heart rhythms are sometimes given intravenous lidocaine. For those people who have a very high sensitivity to local anesthetics and who do not experience side effects, an oral anesthetic such as this provides yet another means to attack pain.

Narcotics

Aside from NSAIDs and steroids, *narcotics* are another type of medication commonly used to treat pain. Some of the narcotic medications are natural, some are created by chemically altering natural compounds, some are purely synthetic, and some are even made of substances that are entirely different from natural narcotics but have the same effect in the body (see Table 2.3).

Table 2.3 Narcotic Pain Medications

Class	Name	Chemical Name	Risks
DEA Schedule III narcotic compounded medications—standard prescription			
	Tylenol #3	codeine, Tylenol	A1, LT
	Empirin	codeine, aspirin	A1, GI
	Vicodin, Lorcet, Norco	hydrocodone, Tylenol	A1, KT
	Vicoprofen	hydrocodone, ibuprofen	A1, KT, GI
	Darvocet*	propoxyphene, Tylenol	A1, LT, CE
	Darvon*	propoxyphene	A1, GI, CE
DEA Schedule II narcotic compounded medications—security prescription			
	Percocet	oxycodone, Tylenol	A2, LT, WI
	Percodan	oxycodone, aspirin	AS, GI, WI
DEA Schedule II narcotic medications—security prescription			
	Dilaudid	hydromorphone	A3, MC, RD, WI
	Duragesic	Fentanyl patch	A3, MC, RD. WI
	Actiq	fentanyl oral swab	A3, MC, RD, WI
	Oxycontin	oxycodone slow release tablet	A2, MC, RD, WI
	Oxy-IR	oxycodone fast release tablet	A2, MC, RD, WI
	Demerol	meperidine injection or tablet	A3, MC, RD, WI
	Kadian	morphine slow release	A2, MC, RD, WI
	MS Contin	morphine slow release	A2, MC, RD, WI

See also the notes for table 2.1; (A1)—some addiction potential; (A2)—significant addiction potential; (A3)—high addiction potential; (CE)—cardiac effects; (GI)—gastric irritation; (KT)—kidney toxicity; (LT) – liver toxicity; (MC)—mental clouding; (RD)—respiratory depression; (WI)—withdrawal risk; (*)—discontinued in U.S.

Pros and Cons

Narcotic medications operate through a mechanism completely different from that of the anti-inflammatories, affecting the way that the central nervous system processes the pain signals it receives rather than blocking the nerves' initial response to them. Narcotics not only affect the perception of pain but also play an important role in the area of attention and attitude toward pain. The pain may still be present, but it doesn't bother the patient as much, it doesn't seem as important as it did, and the patient doesn't attend to it. This is an important quality of narcotic medications.

Narcotics also affect the way the gastrointestinal tract works. Imodium, which is a treatment for diarrhea, actually has a narcotic in it, because narcotic medications decrease the mobility of the intestines and can actually cause quite a bit of constipation. That is why patients who are taking narcotic medications for pain after surgery very often require stool softeners at the same time. But narcotic medications don't cause kidney trouble, liver trouble, bleeding, or stomach breakdown; rather, the side effects are unwanted effects on the central nervous system, including *euphoria*—what is colloquially described as "being high," drowsiness, and decreased breathing.

The government tightly controls the prescription of narcotic medications because of the potential for abuse. Narcotics are abused for their tendency to produce euphoria. It is well known that some people, when given the opportunity, will take narcotic medications to achieve more and more euphoria, sometimes even leading to death. A narcotic is also a particularly "personal" medication in that it produces *tolerance*: That is, an individual may require greater and greater amounts to achieve the same amount of pain relief that was previously achieved with a lower dose. Not only does the body become dependent, needing higher and higher amounts for the drug to be effective, but a psychological dependence can develop as well.

For these reasons, many people are hesitant to take narcotic medications out of fear that addiction will develop. When pain is present and its course of treatment with a narcotic medication is expected to be relatively short, addiction is usually not an issue. When chronic pain is treated with a narcotic, many people are able to stop taking the medication once the pain is relieved, but tolerance and addiction are nevertheless major concerns.

Combination Medications

Narcotic medications can be divided very roughly into two different levels of effectiveness and availability. In the United States, narcotics are monitored by the government's Drug Enforcement Agency (DEA), which maintains a classification system that affects both patients and doctors. Milder narcotic medications, those with the lowest abuse and addiction potentials, can be prescribed by your doctor just as a standard prescribed medication would be. When your medication runs out, the pharmacy can call the doctor on the phone for a refill authorization. These milder medications universally include a mixture of a narcotic with an anti-inflammatory. The most common of these combinations is Vicodin, which contains Tylenol and a narcotic called hydrocodone. This combination comes in various strengths (usually 325 or 650 milligrams of Tylenol with 5, 7.5, or 10 milligrams of hydrocodone) and has a number of different brand names, but they all share a relatively low abuse potential and are relatively well tolerated by many people. Similar narcotic medications containing Tylenol include Tylenol no. 3, which is Tylenol with codeine, and Darvocet, which is Tylenol with Darvon or propoxyphene. Narcotic medications may also be compounded with aspirin, and there are others, such as Vicoprofen, that combine Motrin or ibuprofen with hydrocodone.

There are also now some purely synthetic molecules that act on the opiate receptor sited in the brain and spinal cord (causing pain relief similar to opiates) but without some other effects—fewer mood effects and fewer addiction risks. These include tramadol (Ultram or Ultracet when compounded with Tylenol) and Nucynta.

In fact, the Tylenol is actually included in part to serve as a kind of poison in these narcotic combination medications. It does help improve the effectiveness of the medication by adding the anti-inflammatory effect, but at the same time it places a limit on the amount a patient can take. If these medications are taken in excess, the Tylenol dose can become lethal long before the mild narcotic can produce a "high." The doctor warns the patient about this and both the physician and the DEA can feel that these medications will not play a significant role in narcotic abuse.

Triplicates, Patches, and Swabs

There is a range of stronger narcotic medications, either with or without Tylenol, that are available with a *security (triplicate) prescription*. This refers to the fact that the prescription had to be written on a special form issued by the federal government that generated three copies. In many states, a simpler security prescription system has replaced the triplicates, but the monitoring of prescribing is still maintained.

The prescriptions are numbered in sequence so they can be closely tracked. For triplicates, one copy stays in the physician's office, one copy goes to the pharmacy, and one copy makes its way back to the DEA. They expire two weeks after they are written. The prescription includes your birthdate and address for identification purposes. There are no refills on a triplicate prescription; they can't be phoned in, faxed, or sent by e-mail. Many doctor's offices will issue them only directly to your pharmacist, and they are often mailed by secure trackable services such as Federal Express. All the paperwork reflects their higher abuse or misuse potential. They can be easily tracked if they are stolen or sold.

Although many of the triplicate medications are very important for pain control for patients with severe spinal conditions or chronic pain—there is great concern about abuse of the system. The simpler security prescriptions actually rely on electronic transmission of the information as opposed to delivery of paper components in the older triplicate system and definitely do not represent a relaxation of the monitoring system. Here, the delivery of information is rapid and tightly monitored. A patient who presents a falsified, duplicated, or otherwise inappropriate prescription can suddenly trigger a complete personal lockout nationwide. They will be surprised to discover that essentially every pharmacy in the United States will immediately refuse any narcotic prescription with their name on it. Once this happens—it is immediate "cold turkey" and it is very difficult to get the shutdown reversed—a full DEA investigation may be required.

Among the most commonly used of the stronger narcotic pain medications in the past were morphine or its slow-release form, MS contin, demerol, and hydromorphone (Dilaudid). At present, the most widely used triplicate narcotic pain medications are based on oxycodone. This is compounded with Tylenol and called Percocet, or with aspirin and called Percodan. It is also prescribed without a combination NSAID in a long-acting form called Oxycontin, and a short-acting form called oxycodone or oxycodone IR. This is a very useful method of prescribing narcotics. A continuing background dose is maintained with a long-acting or slow-release version of the medication, while occasional severe pain episodes are covered with a quick acting form. In this way, the patient is less likely to seek a very high dose to cover all potential pain episodes all the time.

Some of the synthetic opiates can be taken in forms other than a pill. Two such widely used medications are Duragesic, which is Fentanyl delivered through patches of various strengths that are applied to the skin and can be worn for three days at a time, and Actiq, which is Fentanyl delivered through an oral swab that effectively starts and stops immediately as the swab is placed in the mouth or taken out.

The use of a long-acting and a short-acting narcotic medication achieves separate, but sometimes complementary, effects. If you have a chronic pain with occasional worsening, providing a constant, continuous level of pain treatment through a medication taken once a day or every twelve hours (or a patch replaced every three days) removes an important aspect of your pain, which is the anxiety component. It is helpful not to be worrying all the time about when your next pain pill is coming. If you take a medication every four hours, it may begin to wear off once you reach the third hour or so, and then you begin to look at your watch and think increasingly about how severe your pain is as you wait for a few more minutes to go by until you can take your next pain pill—and that effect is not what's intended. Therefore, providing a more continuous level of medication often makes it easier to keep your attention away from the pain. However, when the pain occasionally worsens, you need to be able to take a short-acting extra amount of medication for rapid-onset pain relief. That's what the short-acting oxycodone or the Actiq oral swabs are for; as soon as the swab is removed from the mouth, the extra medication dose is removed.

This may all sound good, but remember that these medications have very significant abuse potentials. Many people can't tolerate one or another of the narcotics because they experience nausea, drowsiness, or even an allergic reaction (itching, swelling, difficulty breathing), and a pain specialist may have to prescribe different types of narcotic medications to find the one that will be most suitable for the patient.

Dealing with Pain Medicine Addiction

Addiction is a combination of physical abnormalities and psychological problems. When a patient uses narcotic medication for an extended period of time, the body develops tolerance for the medication. This means that the body requires more and more of the medication to achieve the same pain relieving effect. At the same time a sort of psychological tolerance can develop. In effect, instead of feeling a high when narcotics are taken, the patient notices a lack of a high when the medication is taken away.

Even if a patient is still in pain, the patient or the physician may feel that it is necessary to go through some sort of detoxification to reduce the amount of narcotic medication required for pain relief.

An even more troubling situation can arise when a patient has had successful treatment of their pain, such as with an effective surgery. When the pain is gone, the addiction can still remain. Fortunately, the vast majority of patients can take narcotic medication for pain and then stop using the medication rapidly when the pain is gone. Some people, however, have great difficulty with this. There are social and psychological aspects. A patient may try to deny the addiction out of sheer embarrassment, by insisting that the pain still remains and that the medication is still needed for pain control. It is often the task of an experienced psychologist to tease out the actual state of affairs.

Addiction is often treated by addiction specialists (addictionists). Withdrawing from narcotic addition can be fairly straightforward once the will is there on the part of the patient. It is not necessarily very pleasant, but there are several medications (clonidine, Xanax) that can greatly ease the process when given under the close supervision of a pain specialist physician.

The fear of addiction should never be a reason for a patient to suffer in pain without treatment with appropriate narcotic medication. However, when addiction develops and becomes a problem in and of itself, it needs to be recognized and treated as part of the successful management of the original pain problem.

Anti-seizure Medications for Pain

Although narcotic medications are effective for many types of pain, they work best for somatic pain, and somewhat well for some types of central pain, but are relatively ineffective for many types of neuropathic pain. Unfortunately, the anti-inflammatory medications generally don't work for neuropathic pain, either. This problem leads us to another category of pain medication, which is actually anti-seizure medications that are used for patients with difficult neuropathic-type pain problems (see Table 2.4).

Table 2.4 Various Centrally Acting Pain Medications

Class	Name	Chemical Name	Risks
Compounded Over-the-counter			
	Fioricet	tylenol, caffeine, butalbital	DI, A1
Anti-seizure medications for pain relief for nerve irritation			
	Neurontin	gabapentin	DR
	Lyrica	pregabalin	DR, SI
	Tegretol	carbamazepine	DR, LT
	Dilantin	phenytoin	DR, DI, CE
	Topamax	topiramate	MC, DI, SI
	Lamotrigine	Lamictal	DR, SA, SI
	Keppra	levitiracetam	DI, DP, SI, WI
Anti-depressants for pain relief			
	Elavil	amitripyline	DI, MC, SI, WI
	Cymbalta	duloxetine	DP, SI, WI
Centrally acting analgesic			
	Ultram	tramadol	A1, MC, SZ, SI, WI

See also the notes for table 2.1; (A1)—some addiction potential; (CE)—cardiac effects; (DI)—dizziness; (DP)—depression, (DR)—drowsiness; (LT)—liver toxicity; (MC)—mental clouding; (SA)—severe allergic reactions; (SI)—suicidal ideation, (SZ)—seizures, (WI)—withdrawal risk

This surprising use of anti-seizure medications (or *anticonvulsants*) is based on the idea that a pain syndrome can be like a seizure, or an excess of activity, in the pain-sensing portions of the spinal cord. In a seizure, nerves are firing abnormally; in the brains of patients who have seizures, anti-seizure medications work by raising the *threshold*—that is, the severity of stimulus required for the activation of the nerves—thus making it harder for the nerves to be triggered and fired, and this may be all that's needed to stop the event. Similarly, in patients who have excessive transmission of pain stimuli, anti-seizure medications make it harder for that pain stimulus to trigger a response.

The most widely used of these medications is Neurontin, or gabapentin. In many patients, anti-seizure medications have very few side effects, but some people find they can't take Neurontin because of resulting drowsiness and dizziness or weight gain. Lyrica is a new chemical form called pre-gabalin and it greatly reduces the side effects of the gabapentin enabling many more patients to take advantage of this. Other related anticonvulsant medications are sometimes used for pain treatment until one can be identified that is effective for the individual and doesn't cause the side effects. Another helpful recent addition to this area of treatment is Cymbalta. It has some anti-depressant capabilities as well. Unlike gabapentin, Cymbalta tends to be stimulating and to make it a bit more difficult to settle down to sleep.

Blood Pressure Medicines and RSD Pain

One of the most feared types of pain is the intense burning that is experienced by patients with nerve pain (neuropathic pain) that arises in the autonomic or sympathetic nerves. Often this type of pain is completely unresponsive to NSAIDs, opiates, and even to the anti-convulsants. Because the pain involves the chemical transmitters that also control blood pressure—one treatment option for the burning is the use of clonidine patches. The clonidine can lower the blood pressure (not a problem if you have high blood pressure—but a definite issue if you have low blood pressure). Treatment for this kind of pain has been extremely difficult so clonidine should be considered. This is an "off label" type of use so it is something that an individual pain specialist has to decide to prescribe. It does not work for all sufferers of burning pain but is a reasonably safe and helpful option for the pain specialist trying to treat patients for whom all other medications have failed.

The Food and Drug Administration (FDA) reviews studies on new drugs and implants to determine whether they have been proven safe and effective. However, the FDA controls labels on containers and information used in marketing but it does not actually control how physicians practice. This is why it can be said that some drugs are "off label." A given manufacturer will spend hundreds of millions of dollars doing a trial of a new drug for a specific use. If the data is good, the FDA will approve the drug for that use and only for that use. The company may choose to ignore medical conditions that affect fewer people because the expected income from drug sales will not be large enough to pay for the costs of the research and the FDA application process. This is why physicians may choose to use a drug or implant "off label," which means they are using a drug that is known to be safe but for which there is no full-scale, very large study paid for by the manufacturer showing the clinical result. The physicians' choice could be based on hundreds of academic scientific papers or on personal experience. This is entirely legal and very common. The drug company, however, is not allowed to mention, promote, or support any type of "off label" use. Many insurance companies choose not to pay for any medication or implant that is being used "off label."

Biotechnology and Pain Medication

For the future, an area of interest is the use of gene therapy in neurons that are affected by a chronic, untreatable pain problem. This is a means of changing the way those neurons function so that they no longer transmit the pain signals. But meanwhile, a tremendous amount of research is taking place to develop new, more effective, and more specific types of pain medicines.

The *opiates* (derivatives of opium) presently used as medications are based on a type of chemical called *alkaloids* that are produced in plants such as the opium poppy. Current research is investigating the design of proteins that can mimic the actions of the opiate medications. The human body's own source of opiate function comes from short proteins, or *peptides*, called the *endorphins*. Redesign of the endorphins by bioengineers may lead to more accurate and effective advanced medications to take over for the narcotic medications used today.

A type of neurotoxin derived from snails (ziconotide—Prialt) has been investigated, but it has many serious side effects, so an improved derivative of this molecule is more likely to be sought and may prove useful in the future. The only moderately safe way to apply it so far involves direct administration into the spinal fluid—which is neither routine nor currently useful.

Many of the new high-tech approaches to pain treatment rely on new methods of drug delivery, that is, new ways of getting medication into the targeted cells. One such approach that I've helped to develop is the use of a natural process called *axonal transport*. This allows medication to be introduced into skin or muscle and then to be carried only to those nerves that are specifically involved in the pain. This type of approach may be used, for instance, to provide analgesia by targeting the pain nerves only, without the broader blocking effect of

Figure 2.1 Advanced medications from biotechnology. Biotechnology promises to develop new medications for the treatment of pain, muscle spasms and nerve injury. These drug-delivery vehicles include a targeting element and a chemical backbone that carry multiple drug molecules. They are injected into muscle near an area of injury and then travel via an "intraneural" route- inside the nerve-using a natural property of nerves called axonal transport. Image reproduced with permission of Molecular Synthetics Ltd.

anesthetic on the general sensory nerves. Axonal transport may also prove to be the key to getting several days of postoperative pain relief from a single injection (see Fig. 2.1).

Research into a wide variety of new drug-delivery techniques—through the skin, nasal sprays, oral sprays, and oral swabs—may provide more benefit, quicker or longer times of action, or fewer side effects. These are all ways in which there are potential new avenues for expanding the range of possible treatments for the very complex array of pain problems faced by patients and their doctors.

Enbrel—Antibodies for Neuritis

The most important advance in pain medication may be coming from the very high-tech world of antibody synthesis. Some patients who have inexplicably high levels of nerve pain despite apparently successful surgery to remove entrapments and compressions have proven to have an auto-immune neuritis. This is similar to arthritis that affects joints, asthma that affects the lung, or colitis that affects the colon. Enbrel, Remicade, and Humarin are some of the important medications of this type. Enbrel has proven to be the most effective for pain treatment in a variety of formal studies.

These medications are immune suppressants so there is an increased risk of infection while they are being used. In addition, they work by attacking a protein called tumor necrosis factor (TNF), so they may reduce the body's natural resistance to cancer. Essentially, the body maintains internal surveillance for abnormal cells. If such cells are detected, TNF is sent to trigger a destructive attack on the abnormal cells. This suppresses tumor formation. However, sometimes TNF apparently gets misdirected at nerves that have been irritated by compression—rubbed raw essentially. Then the TNF starts to direct a painful continuing attack on the nerves. A good blood test for this is still lacking, so patients may be given a trial of Enbrel (etanercept) treatment in which they self-administer a subcutaneous (under the skin) injection once a week for four weeks. If there is some response—such as a flu-like syndrome—then it is likely that the person does have excess TNF and a second four-week course is given. The pain relief progresses slowly over weeks and months. Some physicians administer the Enbrel directly into the area of pain.

This is new, off-label, and carries a variety of risks. However, it is proving to be the fact that if a patient's unusual pain is due to an autoimmune neuritis, nothing else will work. If TNF is not the cause, Enbrel will have absolutely no beneficial effect but instead will provide only risks. These types of medications are in widespread use for patients who have a type of arthritis linked to psoriasis and in patients with inflammatory bowel syndromes that don't respond to steroids.

Herbal Medicines and Back Pain

Herbal medicines are important in dealing with spine and nerve pain for two reasons. First, they are widely used by people seeking ways to get relief. Second, the side effects of herbal medicines can greatly increase various risks during any surgery for spine or nerve problems.

The term *herbal medicines* refers to medications that are made from plant sources on an essentially informal basis. There are many formal medications—FDA approved, prescription protected, and commercially prepared—that come from plant sources. Among the most famous examples are the heart medicine digoxin that is made from the flowering plant fox glove (*Digitalis purpurea*) and aspirin, which was based on the salicylates originally derived from the bark of the willow tree (*Salix alba*). Both of these medications have been in use for thousands of years and most likely had been used as herbal medicines for thousands of years before recorded history.

A herbal medicine will actually be made from a plant substance. Aspirin and digitalis are examples of molecules that are synthesized chemically by modern pharmaceutical companies even though the active molecules were originally purified from plants. A herbal medicine may be made from seeds, roots, barks, berries, flowers, or juices. Plants may be dried and ground up or leaves may be prepared in a tea-like infusion or soup.

Unlike formal medicines, herbal medicines are unregulated and untested. This has two important implications for the patient. First, just because someone says a particular herbal agent has a particular effect or function doesn't mean that it actually does anything at all. There is no testing requirement (think "they say it is good for the joints," spoken in conspiratorial voice by a dark gypsy sorceress). If it is on the label of the herbal medicine bottle at the drug store—it still doesn't mean anything certain. This is because the FDA assures that nutritional claims and therapeutic claims on foods and medicines are accurate, but it has no involvement or responsibility for herbal medicines. You are on your own.

One of the problems with herbal medicines is that there is no standardization from one preparation to the next. This fact has several causes and meanings. First, one strain of a plant could have a higher concentration of an active ingredient than another strain. A given strain might even vary from year to year on a given farm, based on weather and soil conditions. Because the active ingredient is not extracted and purified, there is no way to differentiate between a very little or an excessively high dose. In addition, a plant may have many active ingredients—some of which could be responsible for undesirable side effects. The amount of the undesirable compounds also varies without any monitoring or regulation.

Fox glove and digitalis offer another point. Digitalis was often used as a lethal poison. An overdose of digitalis causes sudden death. That it is made from a plant and is natural does not mean that it is not also highly toxic. This applies to any herbal medicine.

So what is the appeal? Many people believe that because a medication is natural, it is somehow fundamentally more healthy. This belief reflects the anxiety and distrust regarding corporations and factories, corruption and industrial accidents, chemicals and solvents—even a generalized fear of modernity. For other people, it is just more fun to use plant substances. Still others are affected by cultural norms and traditions. It may simply be that you enjoy working with a particular practitioner who is recommending one herbal medicine or another. This is a frequent situation with herbalists, chiropractors, naturopathic medicine practitioners, and traditional folk practitioners such as Chinese or Indian practitioners that have strong traditions of herbal medicine use.

Many people reasonably feel that if a herbal medicine seems to make them feel better and has no obvious side effects—why not use it?" After all, they are usually relatively inexpensive.

Table 2.5 Herbal Medicines Relevant to Spine and Nerve Pain

Name	Biological Name	Actions	Risks
Black cohosh	Actea racemos	IF, MS	BT, BP
Black haw	Viburnum prunifolium	MS	
Boswelia	Boswelia serrate	IF	BT
Bromelain	Ananus sativus	IF, MS	BT
Burdock root	Arctium lappa	P, IF	BT
Cat's claw	Uncaria tomentosa	IF, IB	BT, BP
Cayenne pepper	Capsicum frutescens	P	
Celery seed	Apium graveolens	IF, MS	BT
Chamomile	Matricaria recutita	IF, MS	BT, AG
Coriander	Coriandrum sativum	P	
Cramp bark	Viburnum opulus	IF, MS	BT
Curcumin	Curcuma domestica	IF	BT
Devil's claw	Harpagophytum procumbens	P, IF	BT
Echinacea	Echinacea purpurea	IB	SE
Ephedra	Ephedra sinica	EB	CS, BP
Evening primrose	Oenothera biennis	IF	BT, CS
Feverfew	Tanacetum parthenium	IF, P	BT
Garlic	Allium sativum	BP	BT
Ginger	Zingiber officinale	IF, P	BT
Ginkgo	Ginkgo biloba	MM	BT, CS
Ginseng	Panax quinquefolius	IF, P	BT
Ginseng, Siberian	Eleurtherococcus senticosus	EB	BT
Goldenseal	Hydrastis canadensis	IF	BT
Grape seed	Vitis vinifera	IF	BT
Horsetail	Equisetum arvense	IF	BT, LK
Kava kava	Piper methysticum	DP, P	LT, SE
Lavender	Lavandula angustifolia	IF, MS, SL	BT, SE
Licorice	Glycyrrhiza glabra	IF	BT, LK, BP, IW
Meadowsweet	Filipendula ulmaria	IF	BT
Milk thistle	Silybum marianum	GH	LBS
Mint	Mentha spicata	P	
Mustard seed, black	Brassica nigra	IF, P	BT
Mustard see, white	Sinapis alba	IF, P	BT
Primrose	Oenothera biennis	IF	BT
Rosemary	Rosmarinus officinalis	IF, MS	BT, BP
St. John's wort	Hypericum perforatum	IF, P, DP	BT, IW
Saw palmetto	Serenoa repens	IF	BT
Turmeric	Curcuma aromatica	IF	BT
Valerian root	Valeriana officinalis	SL, MS	SE
White willow bark	Salix alba	IF, P	BT
Yarrow juice	Achilllea millefolium	MS	AG

(continued)

Table 2.5 (Continued)

Possible beneficial effects

Anti-spasm/muscle relaxant =	MS
Anti-inflammatory =	IF
Pain relief—	PR
Immunity boost—	IB
Mental function/memory—	MM
Anti-depressant—	DP
Sleeplessness—	SL
Energy boost	EB
General health	GH

Side effects relevant to surgery

Blood thinner	BT
Blood pressure	BP
Sedation	SE
Allergy	AG
Liver toxicity	LT
Interferes with Warfarin	IW
Causes seizures	CS
Lowers potassium	LK
Lowers blood sugar	LBS

Table 2.5 offers a list of herbal medicines common in general use and herbal medicines especially thought to be useful for back pain or nerve pain. Table 2.5 also addresses the downside of interactions with other medicines and special risks for surgery.

Three special risks arise when a patient uses herbal medicines. The first and most important of these is that any medicine that has an anti-inflammatory effect can also be a "blood thinner"—that is, it may increase the risk of bleeding during and after surgery. In general the surgeon or the surgeon's staff will warn you not to use Alleve or Motrin or aspirin, but they won't even ask about herbal medicines. Many anti-inflammatory medications have a "platelet poisoning" effect that can inhibit and prevent blood clotting for as long as two weeks after the medication is discontinued.

Although Table 2.5 mentions known "blood thinner" effects for more than a dozen herbal medicines, you should probably stop *all* herbal medicines at least two weeks before any surgery. Some may have blood thinning effects that have never been properly tested or reported. A mistake on this issue could result in abnormal bleeding during and after surgery that ruins the surgery, requires a reoperation, or even can be life threatening.

The second risk involves herbal medicines that increase blood pressure. Others simply interfere with medications that the anesthesiologist needs to use during surgery, thus causing unpredictable interactions and side effects that make blood pressure difficult to control during surgery. This poses a risk of heart attack or stroke during an operation.

The third special risk includes sedative effects that can cause unexpected depth of drowsiness—even to the point of trouble breathing—when the doctors think they are using normal and appropriate doses of medicine and anesthetic agents. Even if you disclose your herbal medicines, your doctor may not know which ones are sedating, and other caregivers in the hospital—such as nurses and the anesthesiologist or any covering physicians taking care of you—may not be familiar with herbal medicines. Even if they are familiar, unpredictable variations of doses due to the lack of standardization of herbal medicine could cause a very dangerous effect even when the listed herbal medicine is usually very safe.

The bottom line here is that prior to any surgery or even prior to any deep injection such as an epidural, you should fully disclose all of your herbal medicines to your doctor and you should probably stop all herbal medicines at least two weeks prior to any procedure. Some herbal medicines have to be stopped gradually, so give yourself plenty of time if that's the case. What should you do if you suddenly realize on the morning of surgery that you forgot to mention your natural herbal medicines to your doctor and that you are still taking them? You should probably cancel the surgery. Even if your mother-in-law flew across the country to take care of the kids after the surgery and you have arranged two weeks off work—you should probably cancel and chalk it up to a life experience not to be repeated in the future.

3

Keeping the Spine Healthy: Ergonomics for Life

Back pain, herniated disks, and problems with the joints and ligaments of the spine seem possible in just about anyone and at just about any time during adult life. It is worth pointing out that even if you are absolutely careful and take every precautionary measure, back problems may develop because of your natural anatomy and normal activities.

The fundamental wear and tear on the spine from life really can't be prevented. In fact, the bones and ligaments of the spine require activity to maintain them. Bones and joints lubricate themselves as they move and come under pressure, and the muscles become strengthened as well. Bones actually gain strength as they are stressed, so the complete avoidance of activity and stress would only tend to produce more spine abnormalities. In fact, one reason for the high incidence of spine problems today may be reduced activity.

One of the research studies that I carried out as a graduate student involved studying ape vertebrae that had been collected during the nineteenth century from a large population of gorillas and chimpanzees, our close relatives. A significant incidence and frequency of pathologies occurred in these other primates just as in humans: bone spurs, stenosis, narrowing of the spinal canal foramina foramen and the back joints. It appears that back problems may really be a part of our nature and can't be blamed entirely on the ills of modern life. However, significant solid evidence shows that there are things we can do to reduce our chances of back and neck problems—at the very least, to reduce their severity and how much trouble we have in recovering and returning to our usual activities. A variety of measures have been well supported by scientific studies demonstrating their usefulness. Many of these measures are common sense, and others have come from the science of *ergonomics*. Ergonomics refers to the design of everyday activities, workplaces, and living spaces in such a way that we reduce stresses on the body. In this chapter, I try to provide an overview of a variety of ways in which people expose themselves to accelerated wear and tear on the spine in the course of normal life. People commonly focus on work-related ergonomics; however, ergonomics play a role in many aspects of life, including home, travel, and leisure activities as well.

Workplace Ergonomics

A great many work-related neck and back problems are the result of unexpected trauma, such as falls and other impacts. There are certain basic, commonsense measures that can be taken to reduce these accidents in the workplace, but as accidents, by definition, they really can't be reduced to zero. It is certainly important for any employee who notices something about a workplace that makes accidents more likely to happen to report the problem and try to get the situation corrected.

There is also the issue of psychological stress, which can lead to muscle tension and anxiety, which in many people can lead to physical pains. Trying to achieve a low-stress workplace is an often-cited objective; some individuals, however, thrive on stress, and a low-stress workplace only puts them to sleep or makes them bored and ineffectual. It is probably better to recommend that employees strive to find a type of work where the level of stress, whether high or low, feels appropriate to them and to consider changes in employment or in associates, if possible, when the level of workplace stress seems to be associated with back and neck pain or other symptoms.

Desk Work

One of the easiest things to get right is to have an ergonomically appropriate desk chair, with good lumbar support, that is comfortable and places you at a good working level. Anyone who uses a computer also needs to be sure that the keyboard is low enough and the screen is also situated at an appropriate height. There are many guidelines and manuals on what's appropriate for deskwork positions, and ergonomic design of office work stations and computer equipment is now supported by policy in most companies.

For telephone use, the advent of comfortable, convenient headsets should help to eliminate the habit of holding the telephone receiver between the ear and shoulder. Although there is no solid evidence that this crunching habit is particularly bad for you, it seems clear enough that when you wear the headset, your neck movements are going to be more normal during the course of a telephone conversation.

Lifting and Carrying

Another widespread area of exposure to spinal wear and tear in the workplace is the vast array of jobs that include lifting, carrying, pulling, and pushing. For all of these, it has proven helpful for employees to have training in advance as to the best postures, to use the whole body for lifting "with the trunk," avoid bending or twisting, and avoid taking on sudden, unexpectedly heavy weights. All of these strategies can reduce the development of disk herniations and back muscle strains. Companies that rely on employees to do a significant amount of lifting and carrying should have guidelines in place for maximum amounts and for the use of supplementary carrying devices such as dollies and trolleys.

Spine Protectors

In workplaces where lifting and bending is an important part of the job, corsets and braces can be very useful in lending additional support to the spine so that it is less prone to injury when sudden or unexpected weights are applied. Another important consideration is minimizing extremes of vibration. For example, a forklift operator may need a padded seat that reduces the transmission of the forklift's vibration and impacts into the spine. Repetitive strain can affect the spine just as it affects the nerves in the arm or hand, so abnormal vibration should be controlled as a way of extending the ability of the spine to tolerate wear and tear in the workplace.

Home Ergonomics

You don't need to go through your entire home and exchange all the furniture for expensive ergonomic furniture, but you should give some thought to the feel of your furniture and not just the look, particularly when choosing furniture that you will be spending many, many hours on (for instance, while sleeping or watching television).

Beds and Chairs

One of the most important measures you can take in the home to improve the health of your spine is to have an appropriate mattress. It is very clear that soft mattresses that allow the spine to shift into abnormal positions during the night or that cause gradual shifting of the posture can lead many people to experience back pain that can then be resolved when they switch to a more firm or supporting mattress. This is often true for individuals who are beginning to experience back pain and are trying to minimize its progression. Similar principles also apply to favorite chairs. A chair that reduces the weight on the spine and provides some lumbar support may impart just enough relaxation that it cancels out the tensions applied to the spine during other aspects of normal activity.

House Cleaning

The field of ergonomics also applies to equipment such as brooms and vacuums, which should be usable from a comfortable standing position. House cleaning can act in many ways like exercise, providing a range of activities that build and strengthen the spine. But if there is some part of your normal housecleaning that you know requires twisting, straining, and reaching off balance, it may be worth your while to think carefully about what could be done, either to change the layout of your home in that area or to change your equipment to reduce your risk.

Carrying a Child

Picking up and carrying a child is one of the joys and necessities of life, and it is well worth looking at parenting books and talking to your pediatrician about ergonomic ways to do this. Your kids may not want to cooperate, but particularly if you are beginning to have trouble, it is very important to figure out ergonomic lifting and carrying methods that work for you and your children so that you don't become unable to carry them at all.

The issue of spine problems that develop during late pregnancy is a real one and is addressed well in a number of parenting books. These problems have to do with the altered distribution of weight in the pregnant woman's body and also with some relaxation of ligaments that is brought about hormonally late in pregnancy as a prelude to delivery. When warning signs of back pain start to appear, it is important for the expectant mother to pay attention, because severe back pain may be very distressing both in finishing up the pregnancy and in trying to care for a small child after birth. You can certainly consult your obstetrician. Walking, an exercise program, stretching, strengthening, relaxation, and attention to optimizing your posture are important. In the last month or two of pregnancy, it is particularly important to consider carefully how the change in your center of gravity affects some of your normal work or home activities.

Travel Ergonomics

There is tremendous variation in car seats, with very high-end cars typically offering a large number of controls that adjust the position of the lumbar supports, the angle of the back, and the tendency of the car seat to resist the individual's sliding from side to side. All of these adjustments can help to avoid the development of back pain during routine driving. In cities such as Los Angeles, where many people drive as long as an hour or an hour and a half to work and back as part of their daily commute, the design of the car seat is especially important. You may consider a car-seat insert or even pay extra attention to the types of seats and seat controls available when choosing a new car.

Driving style can also affect the wear and tear on your back: Acceleration and deceleration are part of the fun and necessity of driving but can place undue strain and stresses on the spine if your car seat is not optimally designed.

Making Car Accidents Minor

One of the evils of modern life, and a frequent cause of back and neck pain, is the motor vehicle accident. Clearly, the thoughtful design and engineering of cars and of the driving environment has had a large effect on the level of injury suffered in motor vehicle accidents. The addition of roll bars, seat belts, and air bags has dramatically decreased the rate of death and serious spinal injuries from accidents, independently of any change or decrease in the frequency or number of motor vehicle accidents per year. But there is no way to repeal the laws of physics, even in the best-designed vehicles. In many more minor accidents, there is still a tremendous range in the amount of injury suffered by the cars' occupants, depending on how the design modifications of the car environment apply to different types of impacts.

Rear-End Impacts

The rear-end motor vehicle accident may be rare in some cities, but again, in places like Los Angeles where there are always hundreds of thousands of vehicles stopped intermittently on freeways, rear-end impacts are very frequent. Most important among the design factors to compensate for this type of impact has been the advent of good headrests, so that in the case of an impact where the car is propelled forward and the body is thrust back, the neck doesn't snap back over the top of the seat (which, as logic dictates, isn't very good for the spine or for the muscles of the neck). Overall, the best design for a car seat is one in which the sudden application of a tremendous force, such as a rear-end impact, applies uniform pressure to the entire spine without suddenly bending or twisting it. This can be achieved by a seat that fits well against the curves of the back and neck.

Imagine that in your car seat the natural curvature of your spine is not met by a lumbar support, and so your shoulders and perhaps your hips are resting against the seat: in an accident, the mid-portion of your back would snap unnaturally straight between the upper and low back. A sudden acceleration like this can strain ligaments and cause disks to herniate. With a lumbar support properly in place, however, the impact would produce a movement of the entire spine with the rest of the body and without the individual spine regions moving relative to each other. Modern headrests prevent extremes of hyperextension of the neck during rear-end motor vehicle accidents, but because there is no curved support behind the neck itself, the normal neck curvature can flatten abruptly.

This is one reason that an accident can cause multiple cervical disk herniations and tearing of neck ligaments—even with the best of current seat designs.

Another important aspect of vehicle design to counteract rear-end collisions has to do with the bumpers. A bumper that absorbs force changes the rate of acceleration of the car seat against the back of the driver or passenger. Think of a large spring with a heavy object moving toward it at a high rate of speed: When the object hits one end of the spring, the spring starts to bend, and although the front of the spring may still move forward, it's going to move forward more slowly than if that heavy object had struck a solid piece of metal. That's how bumpers that deform or bend with impact, rather than strictly transmitting all of the force directly through the car's metal frame, can reduce the rate of the seat's acceleration against the spine.

I have personally experienced the benefits of a bending bumper. I had just bought a new car, a Mercedes, and it needed to have some parts added, so the dealership gave me a loaner. The loaner was a very high-end, late-model Mercedes, which had every aspect of advanced seat and bumper design—fortunately for me. Driving from the dealership on the freeway, I came to a full stop behind a line of vehicles and was hit from behind at about forty-five miles per hour by a car full of sixteen-year-olds who hadn't noticed what was in front of them. Their vehicle was severely damaged, with the front end telescoped in; fortunately, no one was badly hurt. My loaner Mercedes came out without a scratch because the bumpers apparently deformed and bounced back. Thanks to the design of the seat, I suffered no strain or impact whatsoever, and spent the next day carrying my three-year-old around Disneyland on my shoulders.

Unfortunately, it is not possible to prescribe a top-of-the-line Mercedes for everyone with potential back problems. But the point is that the safety-conscious design of bumpers and seats can have a tremendous impact in any car, and if you have a choice this should be a factor to consider along with a vehicle's styling and financing. It is certainly worth making sure that when you're shopping for a new car, it has the feel of fitting to your back or has an adjustable seat that helps. Information is also available through Consumer Reports, which reports on car safety and can shed light on the ability of different makes and models to get you through the minor bumps and crashes that are an inevitable part of our motor vehicle-based life.

Front-End Impacts

It is difficult to implement a restraint system that holds a person flat without bending in the case of a head-on car accident. When a front-end impact is at all severe, the seat belts and air bags come into play, but the neck may snap forward over the seat belt and the body may bend forward sharply as well, which will greatly compress spinal disks and vertebrae. Air bags can reduce severity of injury in a front-impact accident, but air-bag technology is tricky and involves an explosive expansion of the bag to limit the driver's or passenger's movement very quickly. This, of course, carries its own risks, particularly for children and small adults. There are obviously lots of reasons beyond avoiding neck and back strain to choose a vehicle with air bags.

Side Impacts

Lessening the severity of side impacts also relies on the seat-belt system, but the shoulder belt and lap belt do allow the body to bend to the side. The worst of all side impacts are those that cause a powerful twisting that can apply harmful *torques* (rotating forces) to the spine. Here, a seat design that is more of a bucket seat than a bench may limit your sliding, and if the seat is soft enough that you are driven back into it at all, it may provide support against a side impact. Side-impact air bags can also help in these situations. It is difficult to recommend any particular type of posture to take during a motor vehicle accident, as there is usually not enough warning to do anything; and even if there is any warning, it is hard to think in that frightening moment of what posture might be best.

Overall, design modifications enabling cars to absorb impacts in an elastic fashion can slow the rate of acceleration of the spine and reduce the severity of any injuries. After a motor vehicle accident, it is common for neck and back strain to develop progressively over the following days. It is important in this case to maintain usual activity, take anti-inflammatory medications, and, if there is any significant or severe pain, visit the doctor and perhaps have X-rays or other imaging tests. Although it should be possible to get through a minor motor vehicle accident without suffering long-term strains, the stress of the event, particularly if litigation follows, may make it difficult to avoid the development of a pain problem. Therefore, the early resolution of stress and any dispute are also very helpful.

Strengthening the Spine

If any single piece of advice is widely relevant in helping to reduce the impact of normal life on the development of back and neck pain, it is the finding that general exercise to strengthen the body is beneficial.

Exercise and Sports

Although a number of studies have examined particular types of exercise, it is difficult to recommend any individual method across the board. There are specific strengthening and stretching exercises for the back, and then there is simply the overall toning of body and spine that comes from regular physical activity, be it walking, running, or participating in other sports.

There is some evidence that strong abdominal musculature can help relieve strain that would otherwise have to be carried by the spine. However, as with the arms, legs, shoulders, and hips, the key is always to avoid sudden and excessive strains. You certainly can't predict every surprise when a load shifts, a box gives way, you lose your balance, or you just pick something up that turns out to be a good deal heavier than you thought it was. What you can do is to maintain an awareness of the potential consequences of failing to listen to your body. If a load or stress feels like a severe strain or overload, try to stop and back off. There is a sports mentality some of us learn in high school—"no pain, no gain"—this implies that you have to keep on pushing even when it hurts or you'll never amount to anything on your team. This sort of advice may play a role in high school football, but if you're over eighteen, it may be time to start unlearning it.

Another important issue where sports and exercise can affect your dose of spinal strain concerns excess body weight. It sometimes seems mandatory for every medical voice in the world to weigh in against being overweight. In fact, a moderate amount of excess weight is unlikely to affect the spine; however, individuals who are significantly overweight have greater mechanical stress on all of their spinal elements. If an injury does occur, then recovery, with or without surgery, is rendered that much more difficult.

Stretching and Toning the Spinal Musculature

The key elements of a self-directed spine maintenance program are as follows: (1) Fully ranging the spine through the various natural directions—forward bends and toe touches for flexion, arching backward for extension, lateral bending to each side, and rotation of the trunk clockwise and counterclockwise over a fixed pelvis. These movements should be done without weights and they should be developed progressively—that is, when you first start doing them, they should be slow, gentle, and limited. Gradually, with time, the range through which you can move comfortably will increase. (2) Loading and working the spinal muscles. This type of exercise is safest when it is done as an isometric activity; that is, you place your body or arms against a wall or other fixed structure and you try to build up force to move through each of the directions listed above for range of motion but don't actually move. This will help avoid the risk that comes with using your muscles to overload the spine when it is turned or bent into a compromised position.

By doing these exercises on a regular basis, you may make the spine better prepared to resist any excesses of movement or pressure that are demanded suddenly by surprise, such as turning to catch a heavy falling suitcase or losing your balance while reaching. There are many types of formal back exercises, but you should approach all of them with initial caution. You need to make sure that you are in condition to do the conditioning without harming yourself.

Posture

Beyond exercise, good posture when sitting, standing, and walking seems to have a general positive influence on spine health. However, although there are strong advocates for the critical role of posture, this area does not readily lend itself to exact quantification and application of scientific methods to prove what's the best way to stand, to work, or to go about life. The body is flexible and has a great range of adaptability. It is therefore hard to provide broad guidelines other than what's just been said about maintaining generally good physical shape with exercise.

Common Sense

The preventive and ergonomic recommendations given here have to do with individual scenarios or activities. It is often within particular circumstances that it is most feasible to identify a problem and design an appropriate correction. Although applying general solutions to various aspects of life may be satisfying from some points of view, it is not a very useful approach to proving or learning what's really effective. Nonetheless, common sense and careful attention to some of the points outlined in this chapter may help you, whether in the specific situations described or in similar situations. Reflection about your own activities, workplace, or living space can lead to adaptations that contribute to preserving your spine's health.

4

Renewal Without Surgery: Schools of Therapy

Surgery is only very rarely the solution to the problem of spine pain. This is because problems in the spine that cause neck pain, back pain, or radiating pain into the legs or arms are only rarely due to a structural abnormality that can be fixed with surgery or even with injections. The majority of people, for the majority of episodes of back and neck pain, can resolve their problems without any interventions and most likely even without any medications.

The "natural history" of back pain bears mentioning. This simply means that most back pains will resolve no matter what you do, but that not all will resolve. Because most episodes go away on their own eventually, it is sometimes difficult to understand the importance of the wide variety of nonsurgical treatments and how they affect recovery. If you are likely to recover without some sort of special massage, but you do have that massage, and you do get better, can you say that you got better because of the massage, or were you going to get better anyway? This is a very difficult question to answer.

Attempts have been made to carry out large-scale, randomized trials to compare the rate of recovery from back pain with no special measures taken versus the rate of recovery with any one of a variety of nonsurgical approaches. A few treatments seem clearly to have an effect; for others, the jury remains out. Even when objective tests have shown a given treatment method to be ineffective, the method may still have many strong advocates whose belief systems suggest that it should work or who suspect that any test results that go against it are somehow biased or wrong. Because of these issues, it is difficult to strongly recommend any one of the various nonsurgical techniques discussed in this chapter. Nonetheless, they all seem to play a role in accelerating recovery from back pain. The decision to use any of these treatments, and the selection of which type or which individual version to use, is in many ways a personal choice that should depend on the treatment's expense, its availability, and its fit with your own expectations. Some types of surgeries and injections have the dramatic effect of rapidly relieving pain on a lasting basis, whereas others have outcomes like the nonsurgical treatments; that is, their outcomes are uncertain, and their impact on rate of recovery remains undetermined.

Bed Rest versus Activity and Exercise

One important issue in nonsurgical treatment is that research has clearly demonstrated that the old medical recommendation of bed rest for the onset of severe back pain was wrong. *Patients do better, recover more quickly, and have more lasting benefit if they try to resume and to maintain normal activity—and actually get worse with bed rest.* Directed activity, such as stretching and strengthening exercises, also may be helpful if you are able to do these things; but in general, trying to commence a program of exercise during an episode of back pain is difficult. Nonetheless, the clearest difference in outcome is between normal activity versus bed rest.

Rehabilitation for the Joints of the Spine

For some types of spinal pain, it is possible to carry out specific externally applied medical interventions that can repair and soothe the relevant areas creating pain—the *pain generators*. The choice to use one of these therapies, as well as the likelihood of success, generally requires a very precise medical diagnosis before proceeding. The diagnostic process leading to this choice may include X-rays, MRI scans, consultations with medical or surgical specialists, and even image-guided injections. The outcome of the evaluation may be the identification of a specific type of problem that can be repaired with very specialized, directed external treatments.

Loading and Lubrication

From the field of orthopedics, we know that when most joints with healthy cartilage are placed under pressure or stress ("loaded"), they actually produce more joint fluid. This has made it possible to design very specifically controlled exercises, often involving complex, computer-driven equipment, that are capable of loading and lubricating the joints of the body.

Traction

A much simpler type of mechanical measure is traction, which benefits many patients with disk or joint problems in the cervical spine. The basic setup often involves wearing a neck harness attached to a pulley, which can be strung up over a door and is attached to a weight. Another version involves an inflatable collar that expands to push your head away from your shoulders. Traction applied to the cervical spine may help a disk that has been bulging to slip back into place and it may unload the muscles and ligaments that are straining to return to their

Figure 4.1 Home cervical traction. These Pronex devices help to apply a stretching force to the neck. In many cases, when used properly under the supervision of a physician or physical therapist, they can allow a herniated disk to recede into a normal position. Figure reproduced with permission of RS Medical Direct.

normal balance. It is usually easy to carry out with a variety of equipment types now available that have proven to be safe and effective (see Fig. 4.1). With some types of traction equipment, you can even sit in a chair reading a book while you have cervical traction at home.

Lumbar traction, however, is more difficult to accomplish and is only sometimes helpful. The biggest problem is that it is hard to apply traction in an effective way to the lumbar region of the spine. Also, the devices and equipment for lumbar traction may be large and complex and are often limited to a specialized practitioner's office.

Physical Therapy

Physical therapy involves trained practitioners using a variety of modalities, or types of treatment, such as ultrasound, heat, massage, and electrical stimulation, as well as strengthening and range-of-motion exercises, which are helpful in various conditions. Physical therapy is generally offered only with a doctor's prescription, after an examination.

Individualized Programs

Because the techniques that are helpful in the case of a strained muscle may be very harmful in the case of a pinched nerve, physical therapy regimens must be individualized to ensure that the techniques employed do not have any chance of being harmful. Specific modalities and exercises used in physical therapy can help some patients recover from an episode of back pain, but it is important that both the practitioner and the patient remain aware that any modality or exercise may be helpful for some individuals but harmful for others. A general physical therapy practice may not specialize in the spine or may have a one-size-fits-all treatment.

If no improvement is seen with physical therapy, even on a short-term basis, it may be that the particular modality or even the physical therapy in general should be abandoned. Sometimes there is the misguided impression that because physical therapy includes the word "therapy" it must be good for you, but unfortunately that is not always the case.

Back School

One type of physical therapy that is often recommended for back pain is back school. This involves training in posture for the workplace and for home, in strengthening and stretching, and in the psychology of living with back pain. Back schools are more popular in some countries than others. Despite the commonsense appeal, this is an area in which it is difficult to prove any benefits that lead to recovery.

Braces and Corsets

Another aspect of physical therapy is the application and proper use of braces and corsets. These supports have both beneficial and harmful effects. A brace or corset can take the pressure off the spine and can allow muscles to relax and "take a breather" from straining to do their usual work. Long-term use of braces and corsets, however, can weaken the muscles; when weak muscles are forced to go back to work, there is a much higher risk of developing new muscle tears, sprains, and spasms.

Multidisciplinary Pain Management

One nonsurgical treatment area in which the medical profession has gotten heavily involved is the *multidisciplinary pain management* group. These are made up of a battery of professionals, such as physical therapists, anesthesiologists, and psychologists, who address the patient's response to pain and apply various modalities and medications on multiple fronts to try to hasten the end of the back-pain episode. This approach has the disadvantages of being extremely costly and time-intensive, and unfortunately it is again difficult to prove whether it is beneficial relative to other types of nonsurgical treatment.

Multidisciplinary pain management probably has its greatest benefit in people with severe, chronic pain who have not been able to achieve a positive result with any other treatment, including patients who have already had back surgery and have failed to improve or have gotten worse. Among the common causes of failure to improve after back surgery is simply the possibility that the surgery itself was inadequate and needs to be redone; once that has been ruled out, and a pain problem still remains, then a multidisciplinary pain management group may be an appropriate choice of treatment.

State of Mind

Aside from all the physical causes of back pain and tension, it is very clear that many individuals suffer from these symptoms simply as a reflection of their psychological state. This doesn't mean that the pain is imaginary—rather, mental or emotional stress contributes to mild muscle tension, which then produces a cascade effect of causing pain. Another theory holds that stress and tension cause excess activity of the autonomic nervous system (a set of nerves that control the "fight or flight" response with effects on sweating, body temperature, and heart rate), so that *pain fibers* are activated and blood flow is abnormal in the muscles. This leads to suggestions that one's mental state can affect inflammation in the muscles and joints. There is very little reliable evidence on the specific mind-body mechanisms involved, but it is clear that a significant number of individuals with back pain can get better through one or more of a wide variety of treatments directed at their state of mind, including those discussed in the following sections.

Introspective Methods

Meditation is a simple and ancient method that allows the individual to use relaxed reflection to achieve a calming effect throughout the body. Although meditation may take place under supervision and with guidance, it is ultimately an internal, personal process. In general, the meditation is not directed at the pain itself but at the overall mental state of the individual.

Another essentially introspective technique is based on helping the individual to accept fully an idea with relevant psychological impact on the pain. One of these ideas is to instill the conviction and convince oneself that there is really nothing physically wrong with the body. Obviously, the practitioner encouraging this should be sure of this fact before this sort of "awareness" therapy begins. The message, essentially, is that there is no mechanical cause for the pain, that there is no damage taking place in the body, and that the individual's own psychological state is the driving force behind the pain. Pain sufferers for whom this is true constantly need to remind themselves of these facts. This is not carried out at the level of hypnosis but is instead a matter of convincing the rational aware mind that there is no physical problem.

When it becomes clear that a psychological state is driving the pain, it is sometimes recommended that all physical treatments—that is, all of those which do not have their basis primarily in psychology—be stopped in order to help the person accept that there is no mechanical problem and that no mechanical treatment is required to relieve it. Therapy is limited to dealing with psychological issues such as tension, stress, depression, and feelings of helplessness.

Interactive Therapies

One of the most effective methods of psychological treatment for back pain is spa therapy, which involves a variety of calming and relaxing baths, lotions, and other soothing activities. There is no common formula for spa therapy; it seems to be more the sense of well-being and state of relaxation that drive the benefit rather than the specific type of body wrap or oils used.

A more aggressive psychological treatment is psychotherapy based on the assumption that some people with repressed anger and anxiety experience their suppressed emotions as physical pain. When meditation, awareness, cessation of physical treatments, and even spa therapy don't work for back pain, there may be a place for counseling and psychological therapy in helping to resolve the conflicts possibly underlying the sufferer's physical problem.

One rapid way for a person to connect his or her psychological and physical state is through *biofeedback*. This usually involves some monitoring equipment that allows the person to observe readily some of his or her own autonomic responses such as heart rate. This provides a rapid feedback to the individual as he or she tries to vary his or her mental state and get information back about how this affects muscle tension in the body.

Placebo Effects

Simply stated, the *placebo effect* means that the very fact that a person is undergoing some kind of treatment, or at least thinks a treatment is being given, can help to improve that person's psychological and physical state. The placebo effect clearly exists in many health care situations. This often makes it difficult to prove whether many nonsurgical interventions are helpful, because some patients will improve through a placebo effect no matter what is done. Although the effect is real, it doesn't apply to everyone in all situations; instead, it reflects the response of a proportion of individuals in some situations and should not be seen as a reason to dismiss the differences among the various nonsurgical treatments for back pain.

Other Schools of Therapy

The numerous specialized schools of treatment often reflect the individual philosophy of the founding practitioner. Some of these treatments are recent phenomena that have been available for only a few years; others, such as some of the yoga techniques, have extremely long histories. They fall into certain categories, and like the other nonsurgical measures, they work for some people and not others. In general, any one (or more) of these therapies should be selected based on availability, cost, and what feels right for you.

Point-Based Treatments: Acupuncture, Acupressure, and Shiatsu

The first category, called *point-based treatments*, doesn't necessarily address the precise locations of damage in the body but is rooted in the idea that locations or points at or near the body surface can be affected in such a way as to relieve pain in surrounding or related regions.

The oldest of the point-based treatments is *acupuncture*, which involves placing a series of needles into the skin according to an ancient pattern. Modern interpretations suggest that the distracting stimulus of the needle redirects the attention of the sensory and motor nervous systems. Any actual basis in fact for the traditional beliefs about the nature of acupuncture remain to be clarified. Nonetheless, acupuncture and electrical acupuncture, which further accentuates the impact of the needle, are among the most widely used nonsurgical treatments for pain. There is also abundant medical data to show that acupuncture may help in a variety of situations. So despite any controversy over the mechanics of how acupuncture achieves results, there is agreement that it is beneficial for a variety of individuals in a variety of situations.

There are many research studies that have failed to confirm fully the beneficial effect of acupuncture. Typically, matched groups of patients with back pain are randomly assigned to acupuncture, medication, massage, or chiropractic treatment, and outcomes are assessed afterward. In some of these studies acupuncture appears to be effective for back pain. In other studies it proves ineffective. Sometimes back pain sufferers combine medication, massage, and acupuncture. In my practice, I feel confident recommending that patients with moderate back pain should try acupuncture as an additional treatment. Some patients will then report it provided huge benefits; others will return quite irritated that I've wasted their time. The published studies don't provide a definitive answer. My recommendation to the reader is the same as for my patients: I do think it is worth trying, but be prepared for the possibility that it will not help.

Acupressure is based on the same idea but relies on applying pressure rather than introducing needles. *Shiatsu* massage is another step along the intensity or severity continuum, involving more vigorous pressure at triggering locations. This point-based treatment bears some relationship to injection therapies with trigger-point injections, which are also founded on the premise that certain locations on the body surface can control pain in other regions.

Exercise-Based Treatments: Yoga, Pilates, and Aquatherapy

Another very extensive group of therapeutic techniques is the category of *exercise-based treatments*, involving specialized types of controlled movement.

Yoga is the oldest example of these exercise-based treatments and also among the most varied. Yoga utilizes a combination of mental state and physical exercises to achieve all of the desired goals of relaxation, stretching, and strengthening. Although it can be very helpful, yoga can also be carried to extremes. It is not uncommon for the physician to see patients with herniated disks, nerve pinches, and other mechanical problems that arose in the course of yoga practice, especially during the performance of difficult positions that didn't go as intended. This is one reason why it is important for a back pain sufferer to be very careful in selecting a yoga instructor to find an individual who is motivated by the pursuit of relaxation rather than the pursuit of more and more extreme distortions of the body.

There is not really any completely standard or uniform approach to back pain treatment through yoga. One theme is to emphasize stretching of the hamstring muscles. The idea is that the pelvis may be tilted backward around the hip joint by stiff hamstring muscles in the legs. The tilted pelvis places strain on the lumbar spine. Strengthening and stretching of the hamstrings corrects the pelvis orientation and thereby returns the back muscles to their correct length and tension.

Another aspect of yoga is the use of poses held for extended periods. The poses used in yoga have been developed over a great length of time over many generations and are therefore generally well tested. They can help soothe muscle spasm in some people. The introspection and focus on breathing during yoga also helps the mental state of the back pain sufferer. In general, yoga carried out on a regular basis can help protect against muscle strain because yoga provides general exercise, improved flexibility and improved strength.

Pilates is a kind of Western-methodized version of yoga concepts, using specialized equipment for stretching, strengthening, and isometric exercises in which muscles develop tension without allowing them to cause actual movement.

Pilates also combines a psychological component with the exercises and is very effective for some people. This isn't an option for everyone, because you can't really participate effectively unless you are in fairly good condition to begin with—good strength, good flexibility, no severe strains or sprains at the outset. As with any physical method involving exertion, a good instructor is a must and you can't avoid some risk of suffering a new injury or worsening an existing one as a consequence of your chosen form of therapy.

Aquatherapy, or pool therapy, usually amounts to walking and exercising in a pool of water. This has the benefits of both supporting the weight of the body and slowing the movements of the back pain sufferer. With proper instruction, pool therapy can provide a psychological as well as a physical method of relaxation and strengthening.

Posture and Process

An ancient prototype for this type of therapy, *tai chi*, involves both a psychological component and the assumption of certain postures and movements according to a formal method. Other approaches, such as the *Alexander* and *Feldenkrais* techniques, emphasize posture and positioning both in routine aspects of daily life and in the work environment.

Manipulation: Chiropractic and Rolfing

The field of *chiropractic* is based on the idea that many types of back pain are due to misalignments in the spine. Although X-rays often can't show the misalignment, it is still assumed to exist, and repositioning by directed pressure along the spine is very often extremely effective. The reasons that chiropractic is effective are still not completely understood; the manipulations may briefly shock the joints, muscles, and nerves of the spine into settling their chronic pain response.

The down side of chiropractic treatment is that it usually is effective only for a very short time, and therefore can be very expensive because it may require many, many sessions. If the pain does not improve with repeated sessions of chiropractic, it's important for both the practitioner and the patient to consider seeking further diagnosis and possibly a medical visit.

The chiropractor also plays a role in obtaining X-rays and looking for structural problems that may make spinal manipulation risky. Chiropractic is one of the few types of nonsurgical therapy that actually does carry a risk of severe injury when it is misapplied or is given to the wrong patient. That is why the chiropractor must be aware of these potential risks and attentive to the possible need for X-rays or other tests, or even referral to a doctor, before proceeding or continuing with chiropractic procedures. Partly for these reasons, chiropractors receive extensive formal training analogous to the basic course work for medical training. A chiropractor doctor should be licensed to carry out chiropractic treatment in your state and should have national board certification.

Rolfing is somewhat similar to chiropractic, involving vigorous hands-on manipulation, but is directed more at the muscles and ligaments of the spine or other parts of the body. Like chiropractic, Rolfing carries a significant risk of injury and should be performed only by an experienced practitioner who is aware of the potential for injury. Training for Rolfing is less formal than chiropractic treatment and typically involves two to three months of practical and course work training. Similarly, the certification process for Rolfing is far less formally organized than for chiropractic treatment.

Choosing Your Own Path

With so many alternatives and so little hard evidence to rely on, how can an individual decide on a way forward? Is it best to just sit home in a bath of Epsom salts and write off the whole outside world of therapy? One reason that it is difficult to make uniform recommendations is that there are so many different individual situations. An excellent treatment approach for one person can be a disaster for another. However, there are some principles and guidelines that may help you make the best choices.

A useful way to approach the question is to work out your own individual set of risks, needs, and objectives. The relevant types of risks concern age, exercise tolerance (how's your heart?), existing or preexisting injuries, time, availability, and mind set. Time and availability may play a very large role. Can you get away for an hour every day to attend to the needs of your body? What are the therapies and options available nearby that you can take advantage of? How great is the range of choices and the quality of competition among the various practitioners in your area? If you live in Manhattan and there are five nearby Pilates studios competing for you, then there may be a lot of personal attention and individual programming at your disposal. If your town has one overworked physical therapist doing everything for everybody, you may not be able to get any useful help.

Assuming, however, that you have the time, the will, and the options, your choices can be guided by a few underlying principles. First, it is clear that you can minimize the occurrence and the severity of injuries if your body is in good condition. This means that you are not overweight, you have built up your exercise tolerance (how long you can be active for), your joints are limber, and your muscles are strong. This is a valuable state to attain and there are many, many medical studies showing the lifetime value of this. Aside from improving your life expectancy and reducing your injury risk, being in good shape just tends to feel good. For most people, it makes life seem better.

To get in good shape, the first recourse is to natural body activities such as walking and running. These don't work for everybody because walking enough to get in shape is very time-consuming and because running is an impact activity that demands a good exercise tolerance. Nonimpact activity such as swimming or exercise machines and isometrics such as yoga and Pilates are attractive alternatives. Unlike running, they require gear, such as pools, studios, instructors, machines, memberships, or classes. What all of these activities do have in common, however, is that they fit into a lifelong fabric of activity and health. For most people, returning to their usual preferred exercise activity can prove to be therapeutic for back and neck strain while helping to reduce the risk of future injury.

However, if you are suffering from a new pain that seems to get worse with your preferred activity, you can give it a few tries, but eventually you need to back off and consider switching to a class of activity that is more specifically configured as a means of treatment for an injury. Treatments that don't require a visit to a doctor include point-based approaches such as acupuncture. Before moving on to more vigorous approaches such as shiatsu or chiropractic treatment, it may be time to have a medical evaluation in order to gain some assurance that there is no major injury, such as a herniated disk, that can be worsened by physical treatments. Once your doctor says you're in the clear, a massage or chiropractic type of treatment becomes a reasonable next step for that pain that just won't go away.

These treatments can be expensive and time-consuming even if they do make you feel better for short times. You can't emphasize enough to the practitioner the fact that you have an injury and you need him or her to go easy. It will be up to you to be vigilant against any supposed therapy that may actually risk making you worse. A good rule of thumb is to limit any treatment of this type to three months. If the problem isn't getting better by then, you may be barking up the wrong tree. If the doctor still finds no physical problem, then you need to reflect seriously on whether a round of psychological therapy may be in order.

Your next step, if the problem persists, is to consider whether you may be seeing the wrong doctor. At this point, six to nine months will have passed. It is rare for any problem that does not have a medically treatable physical basis to persist for this length of time. If you have been seeing your internist or family practice doctor, request a referral to a spine specialist. At the very least, you may get a prescription for some expert physical therapy.

In the end, you may find that you have improved significantly but that despite a carefully verified clean bill of health from your doctor, you just can't get back to your pre-injury condition. This is also a reasonable outcome. Not all spine problems are repairable, you may only get back to 85 percent of your previous vim and vigor. Before you accept any diminished health, you want to be sure that there is no medical problem and that all reasonable therapies have been tested. Often, time will have a way of righting some wrongs inflicted by the wear and tear of life. You may need to change your usual form of exercise—abandon running in favor of swimming, change to a less aggressive yoga instructor, join a less wired health club. However, you should try to find an alternative that helps you to maintain your fitness. This is the surest way to help ease your aches and pains into oblivion and to head off the development of new ones.

5

Anatomy 101: From Bones, Disks, and Joints to Mind, Muscles, and Nerves

Trying to navigate your way through the details of understanding the break-downs of the spine and how it is repaired is challenging in many ways. One of the very basic aspects, however, is simply the problem of learning about the basic anatomy and organization of the bones, muscles, nerves, and ligaments of the spine and learning the technical names for all the anatomical parts. This chapter describes the various parts and how they fit together and provides a basis for understanding both the failures of the spine and the plans for repair.

Using the precise directional terms of anatomy is also helpful in describing the parts of the vertebrae. *Anterior* means toward the front of the body, *posterior* or *dorsal* means toward the back. And of course *lateral* is to the side, whether right or left, while *medial* is toward the middle of the body. The technical word for upward, toward the head, is *cranial*, and for downward, *caudal*; but we can also use *superior* and *inferior* for up and down or top and bottom, which may be more convenient terms for thinking about the different surfaces and parts of the vertebrae and disks. The term *superficial* indicates something closer to the skin, while *deep* means being farther away from the skin.

The Vertebrae

Although the bones of the vertebrae have a similar design throughout the spine, they are organized somewhat differently and have unique features in each of the major spinal regions: the cervical, thoracic, lumbar, and sacral regions. Between each of these regions, and also between the cervical vertebrae and the *cranium* (the skull), there are transitions where the vertebrae have intermediate features. Nonetheless, certain characteristics, with very few exceptions, are common to all vertebrae.

Essentially, each vertebra has a *vertebral body*, which is the cylindrical portion that carries most of the weight borne by the spine. The vertebral body is like a round box, with walls of hard *cortex* and an inside filled with soft *marrow* (a thick liquid soup of blood cells and of tissues that actually make new blood cells) as well as *cancellous bone*, which is made up of a fine mesh of tiny bone *spicules*, or hard spike-like strands. Because of this organization, most of the strength of the vertebral body is in its outer wall. The top and the bottom of the cylinder are called the *end plates*, and these face the disks above and below the vertebra.

Immediately posterior to-that is, behind-the vertebral body is the *spinal canal* where the spinal cord and-in the lumbar region-a "horse's tail" of nerves, the *cauda equina*, are found. The floor of the spinal canal is formed by the vertebral bodies, and the roof is formed by the *lamina*, which are flat segments of bone (laminar or lamina means "flat"). The side walls of the spinal canal have windows, essentially, which are the nerve canals, or *foramina*, and that's how nerves pass from inside the main spinal canal to outside the spine. The hard part of the side walls between these windows are the *pedicles*, which are very strong, roughly cylindrical, supporting columns. For each vertebra, the pedicles attach the lamina at the back of the spinal canal to the vertebral body at the front of the canal (see Fig. 5.1).

Spinous Processes, Transverse Processes, and Ribs

On each lamina, there are two to three different types of bony extensions, called *processes*. The most striking extension is the *spinous process*, pointing straight back toward the skin behind the spine. It is a long, tapering structure, usually with a small bulbous portion on its posterior tip, which flows smoothly down the sides of the spinous process and onto the lamina. This laminar surface and spinous process is where many of the back muscles attach to the spinal column.

The set of laminar extensions pointing out to the sides are generally called *transverse processes*. The transverse processes take very different shape and form in different portions of the spine. In the lumbar region, these processes are short and strong and have many muscle attachments on them. In the thoracic region, they point back toward the posterior surface and play an important role in the attachment of the ribs to the thoracic vertebral bodies. In the neck, the transverse processes are small and complex; they extend from a part of the cervical vertebra called the *lateral mass* because its base is very thick, and they carry openings for a major blood vessel, the *vertebral artery* (see Fig. 5.2).

Articular Processes, Joints, and Facets

The third type of process on the lamina at the back of the vertebrae is involved in the joints of the spine. These extensions are technically called *articular processes* because they form *articulations*, or joints. The articular processes attach the vertebrae to the joint surfaces, or *facets*. These processes and facets also take very different forms in different portions of the spinal column.

Most of the vertebrae have four of these facet surfaces—right and left superior, and right and left inferior. At the very top of the vertebral column, the first, or C1, vertebra supports the skull at a special facet called the occipital *condyle*, or joint. About 50 percent of the head nodding movement occurs at the occipital condyle.

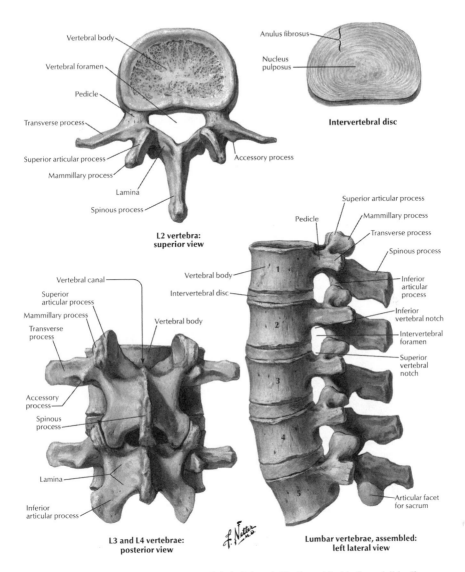

Figure 5.1 Lumbar spine detail. The main weight of the body is carried by the vertebral bodies and disks. The lamina, facets, and spinous process are major parts of the posterior elements that help to guide the movement of the vertebrae and to protect the spinal cord. Frank Netter illustration reproduced with permission from www.netterimages.com © of Elsevier Inc. All rights reserved.

In the cervical and thoracic region the facets are small and flat, but in the lumbar region the upper facets on each vertebra are at the end of long, stout, supporting arms (articular processes). In the sacrum, the first, or S1, vertebra has superior facets only, but there are no other facets in the sacrum since the posterior parts of the sacral vertebrae are naturally fused together in virtually all humans.

Figure 5.2 Cervical spine detail. The vertebral bodies are relatively small in the cervical spine because there is less weight to carry when compared with the work of the spine in lower parts of the body. The joint surfaces are extensive, however, because the cervical spine has such an extensive range of movement compared with other parts of the spine. Frank Netter illustration reproduced with permission from www.netterimages.com © of Elsevier Inc. All rights reserved.

Vertebral Numbers and Special Shapes

The cranial or top-most end of the spinal column is complex, because the first and second cervical vertebrae, C1 and C2, have unique shapes based on their functions and their roles in head movements. Movement in the spinal column—turning, twisting, and bending—is generally evenly distributed among the vertebrae, but C1 and C2 have special roles. As noted previously, about 50 percent of

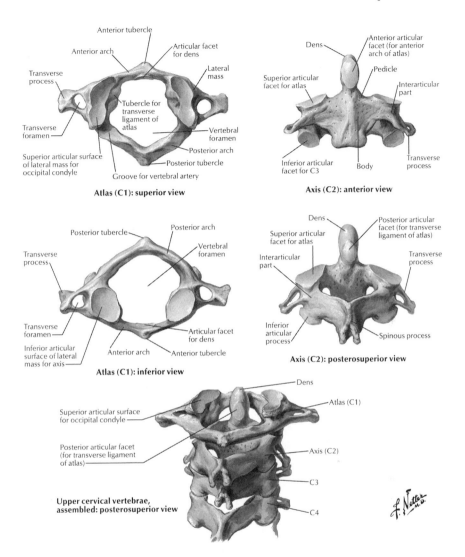

Figure 5.3 High cervical spine: C1-C2. The highest two vertebrae in the cervical spine have very specialized shapes and functions. The joint between the C1 vertebra, or "Atlas," and the skull is responsible for 50 percent of the flexion and extension in the neck, such as nodding the head. The joint between the C1 vertebra and the C2 vertebra, or "Axis," provides 50 percent of the side to side turning in the neck, such as shaking the head to indicate "no." Frank Netter illustration reproduced with permission from www.netterimages.com © of Elsevier Inc. All rights reserved.

your head's nodding movement, or going forward and back, takes place between the skull and C1, and about 50 percent of your head's turning from right to left takes place between C1 and C2 (see Fig. 5.3).

The first vertebra, C1, is also called the *Atlas vertebra* because it has the job of holding up the skull. The entire C1 vertebra is a round, bony ring with essentially no vertebral body. The ring bears two very large, flat surfaces that face upward to receive the *occipital condyles*, which are the knobs on the joint at the base of the skull where it attaches to the spine. The C2 vertebra, also called the *axis vertebra*, is also uniquely shaped, because its vertebral body is actually a fusion or combination with what is, in effect, the missing body of C1. This part of C2 forms a kind of finger that points upward toward the base of the skull and serves as a pin around which the ring of C1 rotates. Another name for the upward-pointing finger of the axis is the *dens*, or "tooth."

The number of vertebrae in each part of the human spinal column is fairly standard, although not completely fixed. For the most part, everybody has seven cervical vertebrae, twelve thoracic vertebrae, and five lumbar vertebrae. There are another four or five vertebrae that make up the sacrum, and then finally there are vertebrae in the *coccyx*, or "tailbone," which extends inferiorly below the sacrum toward the underside of the pelvis, or *perineum* (see Fig. 5.4).

The number of cervical vertebrae is very well fixed at seven, with extremely few exceptions. Occasionally, the caudal or bottommost cervical vertebra, called C7, has some characteristics of a thoracic vertebra, in that it develops very long transverse (lateral) processes; in a small number of people, there may even be a cervical rib on this vertebra.

The thoracic vertebrae all have ribs attached. In general, the thoracic part of the vertebral column is stiff and unbending. This stiffness helps allow the ribs to move together in unison during breathing by keeping all twelve *costovertebral* joints—the three-part joints between the ribs and the vertebrae—strictly in line with each other (see Fig. 5.5). The relatively limited amount of movement in the thoracic region also accounts for the relative rarity of herniated disks in this part of the spine.

The Disks

Aside from the bony vertebrae and their extensions, the spine contains soft tissue: the disks and, of course, the nerves. Disks have two main components.

Annulus: An O-Ring

The outside of each disk is a retaining structure like an O-ring, called the *annulus fibrosus* or simply the *annulus*. The annulus is made of a complex mesh of heavy ligament fibers that reach from the vertebra above the disk to the vertebra below the disk. It has many layers, much like the design of a radial tire.

Nucleus Pulposus: An Elastic Core

Inside the ring is a spongy material called the *nucleus pulposus*. There isn't any blood supply into the nucleus pulposus, but it is a moist, elastic material that can dry out with age. If a disk degenerates or loses its moisture and becomes less elastic, it does an increasingly less effective job at maintaining the normal

Figure 5.4 The complete spine. There are usually seven cervical, twelve thoracic, five lumbar, and five sacral vertebrae. The vertebrae from each region have similar parts, but the shapes of vertebrae vary considerably from region to region in the spine. Frank Netter illustration reproduced with permission from www.netterimages.com © of Elsevier Inc. All rights reserved.

tension of the annular ligaments and the relative positions of the vertebrae above and below it. This then puts increasingly more stress on the vertebral joints to do the work of handling the motion between vertebrae. That's why degeneration or loss of moisture in disks may go hand in hand with the development of arthritis and bone spurs in the joints of the vertebrae (see Fig. 5.6).

The nucleus pulposus has a relationship with a very ancient, evolutionary relic called the *notochord*, which is present in the tiny fish-like animals that

Figure 5.5 Thoracic spine detail. The thoracic vertebrae are the rib bearing vertebrae. To simplify the mechanics of expanding the chest to breathe, the thoracic spine is designed to remain stiff and straight, no matter what the body is doing. Frank Netter illustration reproduced with permission from www.netterimages.com © of Elsevier Inc. All rights reserved.

are ancestors of all the vertebrate animals. Those primitive ancestors don't have any vertebrae, and in fact they don't even have any bones in their bodies, just the elastic strip of notochord for a skeleton. Nucleus pulposus is a unique material and is very important in the diseases and degenerative problems of the spine.

Figure 5.6 Details of the lumbar disk. The vertebral disk has a complex design with two major components. There is an outer retaining ring called the annulus fibrosus, which is made up of alternating layers of strong sheets of ligaments. This part of the disk helps hold the vertebrae together, limits their range of movement, and contains the inner, elastic core of the disk. The inner part is the nucleus pulposus. This is a spongy, elastic material that provides a "shock absorber" function between each pair of vertebrae. Image published with permission of Joe Bloch.

The Spinal Cord and Nerves

The vertebrae and disks provide support and protection to the crucial inner tissue of the spine, the neural tissue that carries the signals to manage the operations of movement and sensation throughout the body. This central portion of the spine is the *spinal cord* itself, which in turn gives rise to the *spinal nerves*.

Long Tracts of White Matter, Connections in Gray Matter

The spinal cord has two major types of nerve tissue in it. The first is essentially made up only out of wires of conduction, which are called the *long tracts*. Some of these actually run from the surface of the brain all the way down to the upper lumbar region of the spine without any connections or breaks. This allows the brain to speak directly to a nerve in the lumbar spinal cord. This long-tract portion of the spinal cord is also called the *white matter*.

The white matter includes those very long fibers from the brain, and it also carries other long fibers that connect one part of the spinal cord to another. This arrangement is what enables integration between your arms swinging and your legs walking: some of the signals traveling in these tracts take short hops, some take very long hops, and some go up to intermediate parts of the brain but not all the way up to the cortex. These are essentially control pathways, and that is why an injury to the spinal cord in the neck can stop motion and sensation all the way down the spine and through the legs.

The other part of the spinal cord is the *gray matter*. This type of tissue acts a little bit more like the brain in that it contains hundreds of thousands of connections between the individual nerve cells, or *neurons*, right where they are sitting

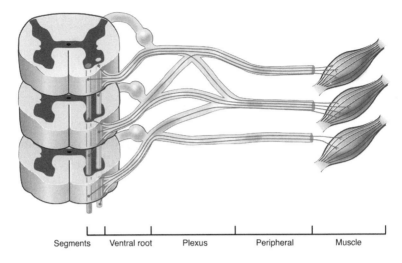

Segments   Ventral root   Plexus   Peripheral   Muscle

Figure 5.7 Neural routing in the spinal cord. The ventral (anterior) gray matter of the spinal cord contains nerve cells that send axon fibers out, through the nerves, to their end points on the muscles that they activate. Sensory information from the body and arriving instructions from the brain all cause movement by giving instructions to these "motor neurons" in the spinal cord gray matter. Image published with permission of Joe Bloch.

in the spinal cord. For example, the bit of the cervical spinal cord that sends nerves out to your index finger to operate its muscles (see Fig. 5.7) also receives sensory signals from nerves that return back from the hand. Connections there in the gray portion of the spinal cord help to provide local detailed feedback for control of movement.

At that level of the spine in the neck, for example, directions come in from the brain's long tracts that stop there while sensory information comes back in from the hand. Some signals return to the hand and others head upward to reach various parts of the brain that help to control smooth, targeted movements. The gray portion of the spinal cord processes these signals and is very, very sensitive. Any mechanical injury or disruption of the gray matter will break hundreds of thousands of fine, detailed connections between neurons, which are very hard for the spinal cord to reestablish correctly.

From this point of view, you can see that every level of the spinal cord plays both a local role, in controlling nerves that emerge from the cord right at that site, and also a long-distance role, in hosting a portion of the long tracts that are passing through it from the brain down to the lower spinal cord.

Floating and Flowing in the Spinal Canal

The spinal cord itself usually does not completely fill the spinal canal. It floats in *cerebrospinal fluid* (CSF), which is generated inside the brain in the *ventricle system*, a series of connected cavities filled with CSF. This crystal-clear spinal fluid has a few cells floating in it but looks essentially like water, although it has salts, sugars, and other nutrients in it that help to feed the nerves. In general, the CSF provides a fluid medium for the spinal cord so that with various bumps and traumas, the spinal cord can float within this space and not be impacted directly.

The CSF has a natural flow. It is produced in the brain, flows down the spinal canal inside the dura membranes, and is reabsorbed back into the bloodstream through little filters along the walls of the spinal dura. Disruptions of this normal process can negatively affect the spinal cord. Running straight down the center of the spinal cord is a *central canal*, a tiny little tube that has a tiny amount of CSF in it. If the normal flow of fluid between the outside of the cord and the surrounding spinal dura is severely disrupted, some CSF may get forced down the middle through the central canal. This can cause the spinal canal to expand from the inside out, thereby opening up a hole or cyst inside it, which is a problematic condition called *syringomyelia* (discussed in chapter 8).

From Nerve Roots to Ganglia to Spinal Nerves

At each level of the spinal cord, small motor nerve filaments, or *rootlets*, emerge from the spinal cord to form the major spinal nerves. There are also small sensory nerve rootlets that return and come into the spinal cord. The sensory nerve rootlets are located more toward the back of the spinal cord, and the motor nerve rootlets are located more toward the front. These rootlets emerge from the spinal cord and group together into the "nerve roots" as they enter the vertebral foramina, gather their coating layers that form the nerve conduit, and begin to get organized into actual nerves (see Fig. 5.8).

Just before the sensory nerve roots pass out of their foraminal canals into the body, they have a connection in a *ganglion*, which is the technical term for a clump of connecting nerve cells. Each of these ganglia, called the *dorsal root ganglia*, carries a complete set of sensory connections before its motor and sensory nerve roots join together to form a mixed motor and sensory nerve that heads out of the spinal cord and into the body. Thus, the nerve roots form a major spinal nerve at each level of the spinal column.

The spinal nerves are numbered for reference similarly to the vertebrae, although there is a trick to the numbering scheme that makes it a little different for the cervical region than for the thoracic and lumbar regions. In the neck, each spinal nerve is given the same number as the vertebra below it. The C6 spinal nerve comes out between the C5 and C6 vertebral bodies, and the C7 nerve comes out between vertebrae C6 and C7. But between vertebrae C7 and T1, the reference system changes, and the nerve is called C8 even though there is no eighth cervical vertebra. Subsequently, in the thoracic and lumbar regions, each spinal

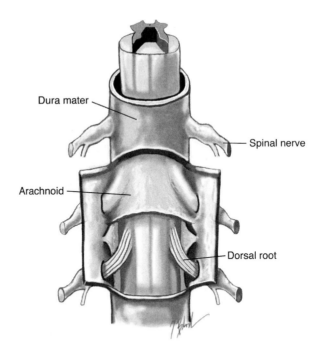

Figure 5.8 Dura and rootlets (posterior view). The nerve rootlets gather together into nerve bundles as they pass out of the arachnoid and dura mater membranes that protect the spinal cord. The exiting spinal nerves then acquire a coating of epineurium. Image published with permission of Joe Bloch.

nerve is given the same number as the vertebra above it: The nerve that comes out between vertebrae T1 and T2 is called the T1 spinal nerve, the L4 nerve comes out between L4 and L5, and so on. Why are the spinal nerves numbered differently in the different regions like this, and why doesn't anybody fix it? Well, that's a good question. The nerve numbering scheme has a history going back many centuries, and for unclear reasons, it has never been corrected. Incidentally, there is no C1 spinal nerve at all (from between the occiput and C1).

Brachial Plexus and Lumbosacral Plexus

After the spinal nerves emerge from the spine, they travel into the body and *extremities* (arms and legs). Some go through the lower cervical region and into the shoulder toward the upper arm, and some go through the lumbar region and head out into the pelvis toward the legs. In the thoracic region, the course taken by the nerves after they leave the spine is pretty simple: they run out in straight lines and lie along the undersides of the ribs as *intercostal* nerves.

The situation in the arms and the legs, however, is much more complex. In both cases, after leaving the spine, these cervical and lumbar spinal nerves start combining into a smaller number of nerves, and then they start dividing, recombining,

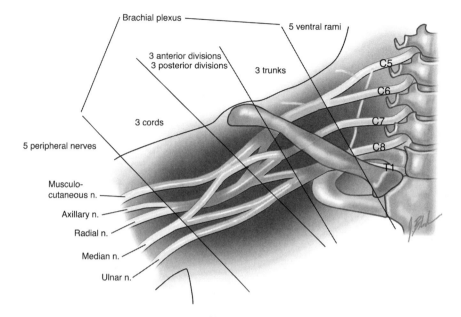

Brachial plexus

5 ventral rami

3 anterior divisions
3 posterior divisions

3 trunks

C5

C6

C7

C8

T1

3 cords

5 peripheral nerves

Musculo-
cutaneous n.

Axillary n.

Radial n.

Median n.

Ulnar n.

Figure 5.9 The nerves of the brachial plexus. The ventral rami of the spinal nerves from C5 to C8, together with the T1 thoracic spinal nerve, join together to form the brachial plexus. The nerve elements combine, divide, and combine again to mix together the various components that lead into the major nerves of the shoulder, arm, and hand (musculocutaneous, axillary, radial, median, and ulnar nerves). Image published with permission of Joe Bloch.

and redividing. Following any nerve along its course from the spinal nerve out into an arm or a leg is very complex indeed (see Fig. 5.9). The area of the nerves where this combination and division takes place in the low neck and shoulder is called the *brachial plexus*; the similar area in the lumbar and sacral region is the *lumbosacral plexus*. Once the nerves leave these convoluted clusters and enter the arms or legs, they organize into their major final groupings: in the arm, the *radial, ulnar, median,* and *musculocutaneous* nerves; in the leg, the *sciatic, femoral,* and *obturator* nerves, and a few other smaller ones (see Fig. 5.10).

Autonomic Nervous System

In addition to the major, or *somatic,* nerves, as they are technically called, there is a parallel system of *autonomic* nerves, which in turn contains both *sympathetic* nerves and *parasympathetic* nerves. The autonomic nervous system controls the expansion and constriction of blood vessels. This affects blood pressure when the size of the major blood vessels is varied. Adjustment of blood flow to the skin affects the temperature and color of your skin. Other autonomic effects control sweating, the size of the black pupil in the center of the eye, and other types of activities that are not really voluntary in the sense that one doesn't have direct, conscious control of these nerves (see Fig. 5.11).

Figure 5.10 The nerves of the lumbosacral plexus. Spinal nerves ranging from L1 and on down to S4 play a part in contributing the complex components of the lumbosacral plexus. The major nerves that emerge from this plexus include the sciatic nerve and the femoral nerve, as well as a variety of others. Frank Netter illustration reproduced with permission from www.netterimages.com © of Elsevier Inc. All rights reserved.

One of the other terms for the sympathetic nerves is "fight or flight nerves," because in a situation of extreme emotion, such as fear or anger, they activate a pattern of changes, such as sweating or operating the tiny muscles that make the hairs on your skin stand up. Overall, they provide the literal "burst of adrenalin" that prepares the body for action. By contrast, the parasympathetic system tends to be activated for activities such as eating and digestion.

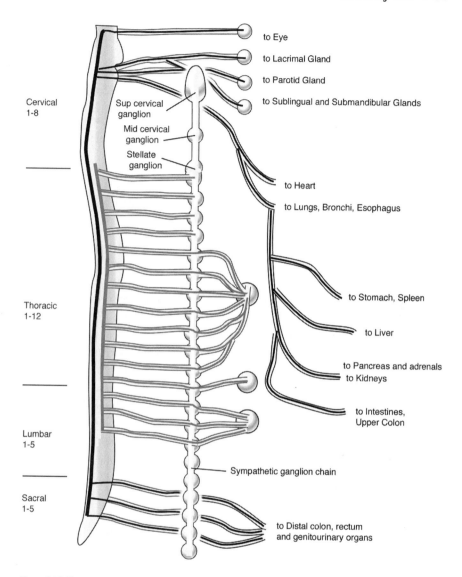

to Eye

to Lacrimal Gland

to Parotid Gland

to Sublingual and Submandibular Glands

Cervical
1-8

Sup cervical
ganglion

Mid cervical
ganglion

Stellate
ganglion

to Heart

to Lungs, Bronchi, Esophagus

Thoracic
1-12

to Stomach, Spleen

to Liver

to Pancreas and adrenals
to Kidneys

to Intestines,
Upper Colon

Lumbar
1-5

Sympathetic ganglion chain

Sacral
1-5

to Distal colon, rectum
and genitourinary organs

Figure 5.11 The components of the autonomic nervous system. The autonomic nerves emerge from the spinal cord and brain and form their own nervous system. In general, these nerves control unconscious body functions such as sweating and digestive activity. Nerves with dark line are in the "parasympathetic nervous system" and travel to glands and internal organs. Nerves with lighter lines are in the "sympathetic nervous system" and travel to reach skin, glands, muscles, and blood vessels throughout the body. Image published with permission of Joe Bloch.

Some pain syndromes involve abnormal activity of the sympathetic nerves. These nerves travel out from the spinal cord with the spinal nerve roots, but as they start to leave the foramina, they separate from the main nerves and turn back to the outside of the vertebral bodies, where they form their own chain of *autonomic* or *sympathetic ganglia*. These ganglia are sometimes the focus of treatment in complex pain syndromes.

Neural Control of Motion: How the Body Is Operated

Given all these parts and pieces, how can we put it all together to describe how the body is operated? This is a very complex process, but it is worthwhile to summarize it briefly for purposes of understanding the pains and problems described in the rest of this book.

Intention in the Cortex, Tone in the Basal Ganglia, and Sequence in the Cerebellum

Intention or thought arises on the surface of the brain in what's called the *cerebral cortex*. Most of the nerve cells in the cortex connect in complex ways with other neighboring nerve cells. However, the brain has some direct "output" connections, reaching all the way down into the gray matter of the spinal cord, to the nerve cells that operate the muscles. The cortex also has outputs that reach down into different functional centers of the brain, which carry out additional processing and preparation that control our activities (see Fig. 5.12).

One such level in the brain is called the *basal ganglia*, which controls some of the natural muscle tone in the body. You can see malfunctions of the basal ganglia in people who have problems, such as Parkinson's disease, that cause tremors. For example, when a pair of muscles for flexion and extension of the elbow can't properly balance each other, the arm is seen to shake continuously, as the control of balance and timing that is needed to leave the limb motionless is impaired. Although it seems like a natural thing to do, when you really consider it, there is a lot of control involved in moving your finger, hand, or elbow to a particular position in space and leaving it motionless. It all seems to be accomplished with a feeling of fluidity, which is how we usually perceive our limbs. The fluidity masks the involvement of thousands of nerve cells in multiple brain regions.

An even more basic level of movement processing takes place in the *cerebellum*. The cerebellum encodes complex movement patterns, such as all the different tiny steps it takes to swing a golf club and hit a ball, or to carry out the writing of a word by means of the hundreds of tightly sequenced adjustments of dozens of muscles that make your hand produce that word on paper. When you consider all of the muscles from your shoulder, elbow, wrist, and inside your fingers that have to fire in a particular sequence to generate a word as you write it, you can see that you certainly are not conscious of every little step. You sort of conceive of the motion and it gets carried out. The cerebellum has the task of carrying these patterns or codes that can be played out rapidly or adjusted in subtle ways, such as accommodating the stroke of a thick lead pencil versus a microfine gel roller pen.

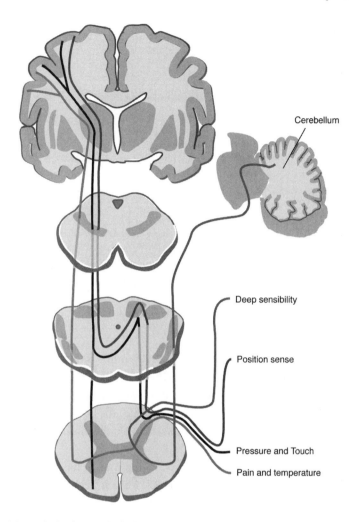

Figure 5.12 Motor circuitry, brain and body. The sensory inputs from the skin, joints, and muscles are carried up the spinal cord to reach various processing centers in the brain. This system helps the mind to understand, to track, and to change the position and movement pattern of the body. Image published with permission of Joe Bloch.

Interaction of Brain and Spine

All of the major centers of the brain—the cortex, the basal ganglia, the cerebellum, and a few others—have their own long tracts. They all run down the spinal cord and into the gray matter at each level of the cord to control movement and sensation, and in parallel, sensory inputs come back up from the cord to the brain. At each level of the spine, these different components interact, and the spinal gray matter controls the final output to the body. Signals to control movement are sent out by what are called the *motor neurons*, which are based in the spinal cord and reach all the way to the surface of the muscles. Meanwhile,

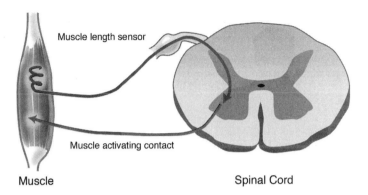

Figure 5.13 Sensors in muscle. Various types of sensors built into our muscles measure the length, tension, and stiffness of our muscles. This information can help the body to produce perfect, smooth movements. Disorders of this system can result in muscle spasm. Images published with permission of Joe Bloch.

sensory neurons come back into the spinal cord and communicate with the motor neurons that drive the muscles.

Muscles and Sensors

Everyone understands that the way we actually move is a complex process of activating muscles to contract and relax. The fine detail is even more complex. Each muscle is made up of many thousands of *motor units*, or muscle cells, that can contract or shorten and thereby generate force. The body operates the motor units by making use of a vast array of sensors within the muscles and their associated tissues.

There are sensors that determine how much a muscle has shortened. There are sensors in the tendons that tell how much force is being applied. There are sensors in and around the joints that allow the brain to understand the position of a joint in space, so that an intention to reach for something, which begins in the brain's cortex, gets converted into a series of movements of the shoulder, elbow, wrist, and fingers.

Bringing the right fingertip to the right place on your desktop to pick up your pen involves posture, position, tension, and speed, all of this continually monitored, and much of this information is processed at an unconscious level. If all that had to be done at a conscious level, you would be overwhelmed with mechanical detail (see Fig. 5.13).

When you think of the complexity of the nervous system and of the role of your spine in control, adjustment, tension, velocity, and the communication of sensation, you can see how any pinch or nerve compression that starts to impair the conduction of all or some of the signals involved becomes a problem that requires your attention. The body lets you know about the malfunction in a language of pain, weakness, numbness, and disability.

6

Disks, Spurs, Stenosis, Slippage, and Osteoporosis

One key thing to keep in mind about all the spinal disorders is that the body tends to break down in certain standard ways. In general, this occurs because those parts suffer particularly strong forces and have designs that are certainly in need of further perfection. In the human body, the spinal disks are one such weak point. Perhaps this is due to our upright posture compared with other animals, or perhaps it is due to our lifestyles. It's clear from veterinary medicine and biology that some other animals can also suffer disk problems. However, many mammal species actually don't have disks but rather have direct cartilage joints between their vertebrae. There are certainly times when the average human may wish to have been built without disks as well.

In any case, for better or worse, humans have disks, and along with a few other parts of the spinal anatomy, these have a high failure rate. The popular term "slipped disk" is actually a general term that covers several different types of spinal problems. Sometimes the term is used just to refer to any back problem. When the problem actually does arise in the disk, however, *prognosis* (what is likely to happen eventually with the problem) and treatment both depend on identifying the exact details of the breakdown.

Bulging Disks

The disks, located between each vertebra in the spinal column, act as shock absorbers. However, they can cause a tremendous range of pain and disability when they cease to function normally. To understand the different types of disk failure, it is helpful to review how the vertebrae and disks are built. The bone itself, or vertebral body, is like a cylindrical box with a hard shell or cortex outside, a softer inside, and an end plate on both the top and bottom of the cylinder. Between the bottom end plate of a vertebra and the top end plate of the vertebra below it is a disk. The disk has a kind of an O-ring structure, which is the annulus, and inside the annulus is a soft, spongy material called the nucleus pulposus, which loses some of its elasticity with age. Either part of the disk can fail—the outer ring or the nucleus itself—or they can fail together as the breakdown of one part affects the functional environment of the other.

Disk Pain: A Tear in the Annulus?

The annular ring is somewhat like a radial tire, having multiple, different fibers that are oriented in different directions, providing strength and durability. Nonetheless, with the proper amount of twisting, bending, and misapplied force, a tear can develop in the annulus. Unfortunately, this can be extremely painful. The back pain from an annular tear is usually noticeable with movement and with twisting in particular. Because of normal activity and stress on the spine, annular tears heal very slowly, and they are difficult to correct surgically, but there are a number of possible treatments for pain from the annulus (see chapters 11 and 18).

Discogenic pain is any spinal pain that comes from a disk itself. The nerve endings in a torn annulus usually report the tear, as happens in any torn ligament. It is possible, however, for a tear that doesn't actually cause any pain to show up on an imaging test, and we know that back pain can have many different causes. So, when you have back pain and imaging shows an annular tear, the next step is to prove that the annular tear is really the source of the pain. The most reliable way is with an *intradiscal injection* into the suspect disk.

A term for this kind of injection along with an imaging test is *discography*. Two major types of discography are performed. For a *provocative discogram*, fluid is injected into the disk to stress the tear and is supposed to be painful; if the pain you experience from the provocative injection is the same pain that you've been having (*concordant*), then the test is considered positive. However, many people who have a lot of back pain will experience pain from the injection but can't remember exactly which of their back pains it is, or they may be so sore that they also require sedation for the procedure and then can't really be sure what hurts.

For an *anesthetic discogram*, a long-acting anesthetic is injected into the disk, which should block any nerves that are reporting pain from the torn annulus. If the intradiscal injection of anesthetic completely relieves your back pain, then it's fair to accept the diagnosis that the observed annular tear is indeed the cause of it.

Along with the provocative fluid or the anesthetic, a dye or other imaging agent is usually used in discography. If the discogram is done with *magnetic resonance imaging* (MRI), then only the fluid or anesthetic is needed, but if it's done with X-rays, an iodine dye is also injected to show the shape and structure of the tear, which can help in planning its possible treatment. Now and then, it turns out that inflammation contributes significantly to the pain from an annular tear and it will be greatly relieved by the injection of a steroid medication. However, for the most part, discography and intradiscal injections are only diagnostic. They help to prove that the torn annulus is the source of the pain, but they don't cure it.

More information about discography appears in chapter 10, and information about other types of treatments for annular tears appears in chapter 12 and in the chapters about spine fusion (chapters 16–19).

Does a Bulge Always Matter?

Short of an annular tear, the annular ligament can simply become overly stretched and the soft material inside the disk can bulge. Sometimes bulging disk material with a stretched ligament causes discogenic pain, just as a tear can. Very often, however, simply having a bulging disk has no real significance. If it doesn't pinch a nerve, doesn't hurt, and just shows up on your imaging test, that bulging disk by itself doesn't really matter, except to alert you that a little bit of degenerative disease is present in your spine.

Herniation and Extrusion

The next step beyond a disk that is simply bulging is a disk in which the soft inner material actually begins to push through the outer ring (see Fig. 6.1). This is called a *herniation* of the disk. An *extrusion* usually means that the herniated fragment of nucleus pulposus has poked all the way through the annulus and broken off, so it's afloat, or at least disconnected, inside the spinal canal (between the bony canal walls and the fluid-filled central tube containing the spinal cord and nerves).

One big risk with a herniation or extrusion is that the extra material will actually pinch one of the major spinal nerves. This can cause a type of pain that extends in a strip from the spine out to the fingers or toes called a *radiculopathy*. When this takes place in the cervical region of the spine, it can cause arm pain; in the thoracic region, chest pain; and in the lumbar region, leg pain and sciatica. The vast majority of disk herniations and extrusions that produce symptoms pinch a single nerve. Most commonly, the culprit in the lumbar region is the L4-L5 disk between the fourth and fifth lumbar vertebrae, or the L5-S1 disk between the fifth lumbar and first sacral vertebrae. The most common cervical disks to herniate are the C5–6, the C6–7, and the C4–5. Beyond these five disks, all other disk herniations are essentially unusual or rare.

In the lumbar region, most herniations or extrusions that go toward the center of the spinal canal don't cause much trouble; however, if the disk protrusion or fragment is very large, it can compress the entire contents of the spinal canal and lead to very significant problems, including weakness and pain in both legs or even bowel and bladder dysfunction. This sort of situation is an emergency requiring immediate treatment.

Figure 6.1 Types of herniated disks. The nucleus pulposus, which is usually contained inside the annulus fibrosus, may bulge or herniate outward. Tearing through the annulus may produce back pain. If the herniation presses on one of the nerves in the spinal cord or in the foramen, symptoms may "radiate" down the leg as far as the toes. A bulging disk may later recede back into place, but an extruded fragment will remain outside the annulus. Images published with permission of Joe Bloch.

A disk that herniates or extrudes centrally in the cervical region (or occasionally in the thoracic region) can actually compress the spinal cord itself. When this happens, although the problem is in the neck, the patient may experience balance problems and jumpy reflexes. Generalized numbness in both feet and legs may then follow. This sort of problem is called *myelopathy* (literally, spinal cord dysfunction), and early surgical treatment should be considered.

Bone Spurs or Osteophytes

Aside from disk problems, the most common type of spinal abnormality affecting the nerves or spinal cord is a *bone spur*, or technically, an *osteophyte*. An

Healthy Cervical Spine   Central Stenosis

Foraminal Stenosis   Herniated Disk

Figure 6.2 Types of cervical spine problems. Degeneration of the cervical vertebra may lead to overgrowth of bone into the neural foramen-foraminal stenosis-that sends symptoms radiating out to the shoulder, arm, or hand. A herniated disk that bulges into the neural foramen may cause the same types of symptoms. In central stenosis, bone or disk compresses the spinal cord and can cause symptoms in the legs or affect bowel and bladder function. Image published with permission of Joe Bloch.

osteophyte is an abnormal bump or spike that grows on the edge of a bone. Osteophytes on vertebrae grow steadily and slowly, and, unlike a bulging or herniated disk, a bone spur that has begun to pinch into a nerve is very unlikely to recede on its own (see Fig. 6.2). The reason that spurs form in the first place is that joints don't always function in a completely normal fashion.

How Did They Get There?

Essentially, bones have predetermined shapes, and as they grow into them they ultimately reach a resting state in which they are coated with a lining called *periosteum*. Periosteum helps to nourish and protect the bone; however, if the periosteum is disrupted in any way, or sometimes if it is just inflamed, the bone will begin to grow underneath it. Bones most commonly form abnormal growths in an attempt to distribute evenly a physical stress or pressure.

The surfaces of a normally shaped and normally functioning joint are exposed to a fairly standard range of pressures. If the joint begins to fail, the cartilage becomes worn down, the natural ligaments that guide the movement of the joint become stretched or deformed, the bone begins to come into contact in abnormal ways, and areas of the bone may experience much greater pressures than they would otherwise encounter. The bone responds to this by growing, forming an expanded surface so that the force will spread over a larger area instead of being focused on a small spot or two. So in the spine, if two vertebrae come into contact in an abnormal way, the bone edges of the spinal joints will start to grow, forming osteophytes, or spurs.

Crunched Nerves and Pain

It is actually fairly common to have seen, either in ourselves or in a friend or relative, the knuckles of the hand enlarge due to arthritis. The same process, essentially, can take place in the spine. The problem is that in the spine there is really no safe place for any extra bone to grow. Each nerve canal, or *foramen*, is generally just large enough to allow the spinal nerve to pass from the spinal cord out toward the arms and legs. One of the spinal canal's walls is composed of the spine's joint surfaces, or facets, so if those facets start to expand in response to abnormal joint function, the resulting bone spur tends to grow straight down into the canal and pinch the nerve.

At the same time that spinal joints are growing abnormally and pinching the nerves, pain can also arise in the periosteum and joint surface as well. Just as arthritis in the knee or shoulder can cause joint pain, so can any abnormal spinal facets or any abnormal contact between vertebrae. Joint and bone pain felt during movement is therefore a common result of osteophyte formation, and it often accompanies the other symptoms that come from a bone spur's pinching of a nerve.

In general, the best way to check for bone spurs is with an X-ray or CT scan. This is because MRI scans tend to miss the osteophytes. MRI mostly sees the water in tissues, but bone spurs are made of dense calcium crystals in tissues with very low water content. Once an osteophyte is identified and proven to be the cause of a pain problem, a surgery can be planned in which the spur is easily drilled away. Any such removal, however, has to be accompanied by a plan to prevent the spur from reoccurring; in many cases, this involves fusion surgery.

Stenosis: Feeling the Pinch from a Narrow Canal

You can see that the problems due to osteophyte formation on vertebrae in many ways parallel the problems due to disk bulges, herniations, and extrusions. What they have in common is an abnormal shape of the vertebrae and joints, where

Severe Spinal Canal Stenosis

Ligamentum Flavum

Figure 6.3 Lumbar stenosis. Narrowing of the lumbar spinal canal can be due to either a bulging disk or to infolding of the thick elastic ligament called the ligamentum flavum or to both problems occurring at same site in the spine. Image published with permission of Joe Bloch.

a natural opening or canal is impinged on or narrowed by an abnormal tissue development. But the impinging material from a bulging disk is soft, and symptom onset is essentially sudden or rapid and may be dominated by nerve-pinch symptoms as well as pain from the torn annulus; whereas hard, vertebral bone spurs produce more of a chronic, arthritic pain with movement, which gradually develops into neurologic symptoms as well (see Fig. 6.3).

The general process of narrowing is medically known as *stenosis*. When bulges or osteophytes cause stenosis of the foramina, they can put pressure on the spinal nerves. However, if herniations or spurs form inside the main spinal canal, particularly in the neck, they can eventually press on the spinal cord itself. Symptoms of spinal cord compression are always of more concern than a pinched nerve is, simply because spinal cord tissue doesn't recover as well from pressure as other nerve tissue does.

Radiculopathy versus Myelopathy: What Exactly Is Being Squeezed?

When a disk bulges into a neural foramen, it pinches a nerve, and this causes arm, back, or leg pain. In fact, depending on exactly where the pain is felt, you can tell which disk is bulging, and the surgeon often relies on the location of the pain in determining that the problem really is a herniated disk.

For instance, if the pain goes just to the little toe, it is very commonly from the S1 spinal nerve and is almost always caused by herniation of the L5-S1 disk between vertebrae L5 and S1. If the pain goes to the big toe, it is usually caused by compression of the L5 nerve root due to herniation of the disk between vertebrae L4 and L5.

Most common in the cervical region are a C5-C6 disk herniation, which affects the thumb and index finger; a C6-C7 disk herniation, which affects the middle finger; and a C4-C5 disk herniation, which affects the shoulder. All the

Schematic demarcation of dermatomes shown as distinct segments. There is actually considerable overlap between any two adjacent dermatomes

Levels of principal dermatomes

C5	Clavicles
C5, 6, 7	Lateral parts of upper limbs
C8, T1	Medial sides of upper limbs
C6	Thumb
C6, 7, 8	Hand
C8	Ring and little fingers
T4	Level of nipples
T10	Level of umbilicus
T12	Inguinal or groin regions
L1, 2, 3, 4	Anterior and inner surfaces of lower limbs
L4, 5, S1	Foot
L4	Medial side of great toe
S1, 2, L5	Posterior and outer surfaces of lower limbs
S1	Lateral margin of foot and little toe
S2, 3, 4	Perineum

Figure 6.4 Dermatome map of the body. Each of the spinal nerves provides sensation to a predictable area of skin or dermatome. Pain radiating down the leg to the small toe in the general pattern of the S1 dermatome suggests that a herniated disk may be pinching the S1 nerve root in the spine. Frank Netter illustration reproduced with permission from www.netterimages.com © of Elsevier Inc. All rights reserved.

types of disk herniation or bone spur formation that affect or pinch a single exiting nerve or nerve root cause a condition called *radiculopathy* (see Fig. 6.4).

However, in the neck or chest, a central disk herniation or extrusion can have more significant consequences than causing radiculopathy. In the cervical and thoracic regions of the spine, the spinal canal is filled significantly with the spinal cord, and there is often very little room for anything else; whereas in the lumbar region, the spinal canal is simply filled with fluid and floating nerve roots. There is a very important difference between the consequences of a pinched nerve (radiculopathy) and the consequences of a spinal cord compression or irritation, which is called myelopathy. Myelopathy is more significant than radiculopathy for two reasons. First, myelopathy will affect everything in the body at and below the spinal level at which it occurs, not just a single arm or leg, or a portion of a single arm or leg. Second, nerves do much better than the spinal cord at recovering from pressure, so if any weakness, numbness, or other problems in neurologic function develop from spinal cord compression, the cord may not recover once the pressure is removed.

Instability and Slippage

When spinal joints begin to function abnormally and allow excess motion, most commonly the result is pain, abnormal growth of the joints, and nerve impingement. However, sometimes an abnormality of the ligaments and the joints is sufficiently severe that two or more vertebrae begin to slip out of their normal alignment in the spinal column. The existence of a slippage can be seen in a routine X-ray or MRI, but is seen in a CT scan only when specialized computer image reconstructions are performed. To prove that a static malalignment is actually a dynamically sliding vertebral pair, you need to have at least two X-rays, one with the spine flexed forward and one with the spine flexed back. Smaller amounts of slippage and instability that are difficult to see on X-ray but can still cause pain may be detected during surgery using specialized meters that detect and quantify intervertebral movement and stiffness.

Spondylolisthesis, Subluxation, and Scoliosis: A Mouthful of Trouble

A technical word for the misalignment of two vertebrae is based on the Latin root for vertebra, which is *spondylo*, and for slippage, which is *listhesis*. Thus *spondylolisthesis* is the term for slippage between two vertebrae, most commonly used with the lumbar spine (see Fig. 6.5).

Although it may sound very worrisome to have two vertebrae slip out of place, it actually can happen in the lumbar spine without causing a great deal of trouble. The amount of slippage between two vertebrae is described by a grading system, 1 through 4. Grade 1 is a slippage by as much as 25 percent out of alignment, and the slippage can go even farther, most typically between L5 and S 1 or between L4

Figure 6.5 Spondylolisthesis. The L4 vertebral body has slipped forward relative to the L5 vertebral body. This movement has reduced the space available for the exiting nerve root in the L4-L5 neural foramen. Image published with permission of Joe Bloch.

and L5, to a degree where one vertebra may be as much as halfway slipped off the one below it. Most commonly, spondylolisthesis causes back pain, but with some reflection it is readily apparent that this can also stretch and pull on the nerves; therefore, a slipped vertebra, just like a slipped or herniated disk, can be a cause of low back pain and also of pain and numbness extending into the legs.

A different term is used for slippage in the cervical spine. This is most commonly described as *subluxation*, and the level of concern about slippage of a vertebra of the neck is actually much greater. A small amount of subluxation of a few millimeters is actually fairly common when the ligaments become lax due to wear and tear or trauma. This really only causes potentially some neck pain and extra stress on the joints. However, as the subluxation becomes more pronounced, the small amount of excess space in the spinal canal may be taken up and spinal cord compression may begin, with effects as mild as a little bit of imbalance or very severe symptoms such as difficulty walking (see Fig. 6.6).

Stretching and Stabilizing

In general, once a spondylolisthesis or a subluxation has taken place and begins to cause pain and neurologic symptoms, the problem has to be corrected. Sometimes it is sufficient to correct it simply by stopping the slipped elements in place so that no further slippage occurs, and then opening up the space around

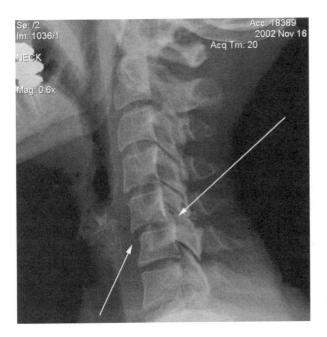

Figure 6.6 Subluxation. The C5 vertebral body has slipped forward relative to the C6 vertebra. In the neck, a slippage, or subluxation, is often dynamic. It disappears or reduces when the neck is extended backward.

the nerve canals so that any pressure on the nerves is relieved. However, often it is necessary to correct the subluxation by pulling the vertebrae back into normal alignment. In the neck, this is fairly straightforward to accomplish during surgery. This can even be done with external traction devices that pull the neck back into alignment, but usually, once the traction is relieved, the spine will slip out of alignment again; therefore, surgery is often required to correct and repair slippage in the cervical spine. This is discussed in chapter 17.

As for the lumbar spine, correction is sometimes necessary, but because the lumbar spine has a lot of weight and pressure on it and usually slips very slowly, it sometimes is difficult to correct. Fusion in place, with decompression of the nerve roots, is often the best choice. Correction of a slipped vertebra has a fair amount of risk in the lumbar spine because the nerves adapt to their altered position; when a correction is done, if it is not done with the greatest care, the correction itself poses risk to the nerves. Special devices have only recently been developed that allow the surgeon to pull the lumbar vertebrae back into alignment while fully preserving the opening of the nerve canals to protect the nerves (see chapter 19).

The term *scoliosis* (whether congenital or acquired) reflects abnormal side-to-side positioning of vertebrae. This can take place to a considerable degree without symptoms, but sometimes the slip causes local pain and nerve compression, and then similar considerations apply as with spondylolisthesis and subluxation.

Correction of scoliosis can occasionally be achieved with traction, but often surgery is needed and sometimes requires screws and rods to hold the vertebrae in alignment until they heal in a corrected position (see chapters 18 and 19).

Torn Spinal Ligaments: Spine Injuries with No Broken Bones

The types of slippage in spondylolisthesis and subluxation generally reflect chronic or degenerative changes in the spinal column. Slips of vertebrae can also occur, however, during a trauma, such as when a disk is abruptly ruptured or a spinal ligament is severely torn. In this situation, because of the sudden and relatively unconstrained movement of vertebrae, the resulting neurologic injury may be much more severe. Sometimes torn spinal ligaments and vertebral slippage can result from a trauma without any damage to the nerves, but when ligaments are torn and no longer hold the vertebrae in their normal fashion, the risk of neurologic injury is greatly increased (see Fig. 6.7).

In the course of traumatic injury, a spinal misalignment from torn ligaments can take place without any bones being fractured. So it is always important, even

Torn ligaments

Figure 6.7 Torn ligaments. Severe trauma involving the neck can pose serious risks to the spinal cord even when there is no fracture. If the ligaments and disk attachments are disrupted, the stability of the spine is compromised. A hard cervical collar will protect the spinal cord. However, if the individual is not placed in a collar and does bend his or her neck forward in this situation, a subluxation may occur, resulting in pressure on the spinal cord. This condition is detected with MRI scanning or carefully controlled flexion and extension spine X-rays monitored by a physician. Image published with permission of Joe Bloch.

if the X-rays don't show any fracture, that the natural movement of the spine be evaluated after a traumatic injury to be sure that no excess or abnormal slippage of vertebrae is affecting their alignment. This requires flexion and extension X-rays that show all seven cervical vertebrae.

Osteoporosis and Fragile Bone: Take Your Calcium

Loss of normal bone calcium is called *osteoporosis*. The presence of osteoporosis can be tested most accurately with a type of test called *dual energy X-ray absorpsiometry*, or a DEXA scan (an image in which the physics of X-rays is used to support a calculation of the density of the bone), which provides a precise measurement of the degree to which bones have lost their calcium.

In general, bone calcium can be maintained with oral intake of an adequate amount of daily calcium, usually about 1500 milligrams. Aside from food sources, the mineral can be gotten from Tums® or a wide variety of calcium supplements, and a vitamin D supplement of at least 400 international units per day may also be advisable. Certain medications can also help with osteoporosis; one is called alendronate (Fosamax), and another is Miacalcin, a nasal spray including a natural hormone, calcitonin, that promotes movement of calcium from the bloodstream back into the bones. Forteo is another medication made by genetic engineering that is given as an injection: it increases the effects of another natural body hormone—parathyroid hormone—which affects calcium processing by the body.

Both Fosamax and Forteo have been associated with significant side effects—so be sure to ask you doctor to explain the relative risks and benefits to you before you start on either. The risks seem to be low in that they occur only in a small number of the people receiving the medication, but the effects are significant. For Fosamax, it is a risk of a severe form of bone weakening called osteonecrosis. For Forteo there seems to be a small risk related to a type of cancer.

Osteoporosis occurs in a variety of situations, the most common of which is as a routine development in women after menopause. This situation arises, as far as anyone can tell, because the hormonal changes associated with menopause have an unintended and coincidental negative impact on the body's ability to balance its calcium stores. If a DEXA scan confirms the presence of osteoporosis, then a daily intake of at least 1500 milligrams of calcium is essential, and one of the promoters of bone strength (Fosamax, Forteo, Miacalcin, or other similar medications) may be prescribed to help assure that the calcium reaches the bones.

Spontaneous Spine Fractures: Why They Happen

The spine gets in trouble when its mechanical strength is reduced by the loss of calcium from the vertebrae. This is a common problem for women in their fifties and older, although it can affect women who are younger and certainly

Body of vertebra

Intervertebral disc

Collapsed
vertebra

Figure 6.8 Osteoporotic fractures. As bones lose calcium, they become softer. A common complication of osteoporosis is the collapse of one of the thoracic vertebral bodies. Image published with permission of Joe Bloch.

can affect men as well. When the calcium level in your bones gets too low, your vertebrae can become subject to sudden fractures even in the course of your normal activities. The most common of these fractures is a "wedge collapse," when a vertebra suddenly loses its normal height and becomes shortened and wedge-shaped. This can happen in a number of vertebrae in the thoracic region, thereby causing a forward curvature of the upper spine. A variety of other types of fractures can also occur, although usually only in the most severe cases of osteoporosis (see Fig. 6.8).

Soft Bones Don't Hold Screws: Fixing Things Later Can Be Tricky

If a spine surgery is needed for some reason and will entail the placement or implantation of any "hardware" into the body, both the patient and the surgeon need to consider the possible presence of even mild osteoporosis. Repairs of the spine involving wires, hooks, rods, or screws all require that the bone be strong enough to hold them in place. Osteoporosis essentially produces softened bone that doesn't hold things very well, so even a properly done spine surgery with well-placed devices may subsequently collapse as the metal parts pull through the osteoporotic bone.

A spine surgery patient who has osteoporosis may therefore need extra amounts of instrumentation and external bracing. Preferably, if there is time before a planned fusion and instrumentation surgery, a very thorough preoperative course of calcium, vitamin D, and a medication such as Miacalcin will help to strengthen and harden the bones in preparation.

7

Spinal Symptoms: Where Does That Pain Come From?

When you have a pain in your foot, your first instinct is to look and see what's wrong with your foot. However, when pinched nerves are involved, locating the source of your problem may not be so simple. Although nerves can correctly report the location of another tissue's injury—in that when something is wrong in your foot, your brain tells you that your foot hurts—they can give an incorrect location report when a nerve itself is pinched. That's why a herniated disk in your lumbar spine that's pinching the nerve headed out to your big toe leads to a message that your big toe hurts, even though the problem is actually in your back, three feet away from the toe.

The concepts of *referred pain* and how pain travels down the leg or arm from herniated disks in the back or neck are very well understood by most physicians and are familiar also to most of the general public. But oversimplification can lead to an incorrect conclusion, because there are a lot of places other than in the spine where a nerve can be pinched. When a pain develops, the process of *localization*, or finding its origin, is very important to understanding what the patient's prognosis is and what is most likely to be an effective treatment.

Is Your Leg Pain or Arm Pain from Your Spine?

Despite the tremendous number of nerves in the body and the many levels and parts of the spinal column, the problem of localizing a pain that originates in the spine is simplified in the vast majority of cases because the body tends to fail in certain standard or predictable ways.

With a car, tires go flat, transmissions fail after 50,000 to 60,000 miles, and brake shoes need to be changed after every 5000 to 10,000 miles. Not every part of a car tends to fall apart, but certain parts do go, and they tend to go after a relatively predictable amount of wear and tear. To an extent, this is also true of the body: For instance, there are particular, known details of nerve compressions and pain syndromes that enable us to predict many spine-driven pain problems.

On the one hand, this chapter lays out the most common or predictable patterns of spine or nerve failure, so that you can understand when such a problem is occurring exactly according to the textbook pattern. On the other hand, it also identifies some of the ways that a pattern of symptoms can be a little different from the standard and how the most seemingly obvious diagnosis may actually be the wrong one.

Matching Abnormalities to Symptoms

A big problem in spinal diagnosis is that many of the abnormalities that are seen on a magnetic resonance image (MRI; see chapter 10) of the spine have no actual significance. Technically, this problem can be described as a high rate of "false positive" or "true but irrelevant" findings. If a lumbar MRI is performed on 100 people who are age sixty or older and have never had much back or leg pain, as many as 60 percent of them will show bulging disks, bone spurs, or narrowed canals on the MRI but will lack any significant symptoms or need for treatment. So if you develop a pain in your leg and get a lumbar MRI scan, there is a better-than-even chance that abnormalities will be found in your spine, but it may still be necessary to prove that what's seen in the image is actually responsible for your symptoms.

The match between your symptoms and the findings on an imaging test is accomplished by a doctor who investigates very particular aspects of the symptoms that you are experiencing and connects them to the exact features of any abnormality seen in your spine. Even then, there may be ambiguities; that's why spinal injections are often required as part of the exam, essentially to test ideas and to determine which of the observed abnormalities is causing the pain.

Aspects of Sciatica: Herniated Disk versus Piriformis Pinch

The details of sciatica are a good example of the localization process. Sciatica refers to a pain in the leg that follows a particular pattern related to the course of the sciatic nerve: pain starting in the low back, running down behind the buttock and leg, then down the side of the leg and reaching around the ankle into the foot.

One of the most common causes of sciatica is a herniated lumbar disk at either the L4-L5 or L5-S1 level. These two herniations occur with about equal frequency. When the L4-L5 disk ruptures, it tends to rupture in a particular location on the posterior and lateral corner of the disk (toward the back and to the side), on either the right or the left. This disk extrusion doesn't actually pinch the L4 nerve in the foramen, or nerve canal, at the L4-L5 level; instead, it usually pinches a nerve in the main spinal canal, the L5 nerve, that's headed out through the foramen below at the L5-S1 level. That pinch almost invariably causes sciatica that runs all the way down the leg into the big toe. Similarly, an L5-S1 disk herniation usually pinches the S1 nerve and the resulting sciatica also runs down the leg, but it goes out to the little toe (see Fig. 7.1).

Figure 7.1 Sciatica pain distribution. When sciatica is due to a herniated disk, it often affects a single strip of skin, or dermatome. A far lateral herniation affects the exiting nerve root: In this picture, the L4 root is compressed by an L4-L5 lateral disk herniation. More commonly, however, the disk bulge is close to the body's midline. The illustration shows an L5-S1 disk herniation affecting the transiting S1 root but leaving the L5 root undisturbed. The patient's detailed distribution of symptoms must match exactly with the MRI findings in the spine before a surgery can be recommended. Image published with permission of Joe Bloch.

A pinch of the L4 nerve is far less common and is more complex to diagnose. It can be caused either by an L3-L4 disk herniation, which is relatively rare, or by an L4-L5 disk herniation that happens to point out laterally into the nerve canal. When the L4 nerve is pinched, the pain runs down the leg and may reach the ankle but not necessarily the toes. The other trick to an L4 nerve pinch is that the resulting pain can have a more prominent presence in the knee and on the anterior thigh. That's because the L4 nerve doesn't run into the leg entirely with the sciatic nerve; instead, part of it runs along the front surface of the thigh with the femoral nerve.

What about when both the big toe and the little toe are having sciatica pain? It could be that both your L4-L5 and your L5-S1 disk herniated at the same time; however, the chance of two disk failures happening exactly the same way and at the same time is very small. This symptom pattern tends to lead to the question of whether the whole sciatic nerve is being pinched somewhere along its course from the sacrum to the knee rather than one of the spinal nerves that leads into it.

One place where the entire sciatic nerve is pinched most commonly is in the pelvis, where the nerve exits from the inside to the outside of the pelvis through the *sciatic notch* and passes under a muscle called the *piriformis* muscle. Tension and spasm or increased muscle tone in the piriformis can cause a sciatica that affects the buttock and the leg and reaches down to the level of the ankle but does not go to any one of the toes in particular. A doctor can use physical exam maneuvers or tests to distinguish between the lumbar and pelvic forms of sciatica. The two also have some different features: piriformis sciatica tends to be worse with

Figure 7.2 Sciatica: disk versus piriformis. Physicians use physical examination maneuvers to seek out the cause of sciatica. When a straight leg raise (A) reproduces the pain, a herniated disk is often the cause. If the leg raise has no effect, the crossed leg test (B) shown below can be used to stretch the piriformis muscle to test for a pelvic location of the sciatic nerve entrapment. Image published with permission of Joe Bloch.

sitting but relieved by standing or walking, whereas the sciatica from lumbar disk herniation can often be relieved by sitting in certain positions (see Fig. 7.2).

Aside from sciatic nerve problems, entrapments of the tibial nerve at the ankle or *tarsal tunnel syndrome,* or entrapment of the peroneal nerve near the knee at the head of the fibula bone are common. Each of these will cause a specific pattern of pain numbness and weakness in the foot that can be mistaken for nerve root impingement by a spinal disk. If the physician considers these problems, they may be sorted by physical exam, electrical nerve testing, or specialized imaging such as MR neurography (see chapter 10).

Arm, Shoulder, and Neck Pain: Canals and Other Tunnels

When dealing with pains in the neck, arm, and shoulders, there is a similar set of considerations, but the patterns are obviously somewhat different. The most common cervical disk herniation is at the C5-C6 level, which tends to pinch the C6 spinal nerve, causing some tingling and numbness out to the thumb and first (index) finger. The second most common is at C6-C7, which produces symptoms out to the second (middle) finger, and the third most common is at C4-C5, which causes pain in the shoulder. Shoulder pain is complex to diagnose because plenty of mechanical problems arise in the shoulder itself, such as rotator cuff tears or *impingement syndromes* (rubbing between the two parts of the shoulder

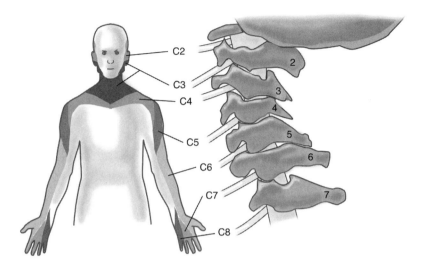

Figure 7.3 Cervical radiculopathy. Herniated disks and nerve canal stenosis in the neck most commonly affect the C5 root, causing shoulder pain; the C6 root, causing thumb and second digit pain; or the C7 root, causing pain into the middle finger. Other cervical dermatomes are only rarely affected by degenerative disease in the neck. Image published with permission of Joe Bloch.

joint complex) that lead to shoulder pain and other symptoms; nonetheless, some shoulder pains are due to disk herniation or to bone spurs in the cervical spine (see Fig. 7.3).

Although the first and second fingers can experience numbness from a C5-C6 herniated disk, a common nerve pinch that occurs in the wrist rather than the spine is *carpal tunnel syndrome*. Carpal tunnel syndrome pinches the median nerve (a nerve that powers the muscles of finger flexion near the elbow and that powers the base of the thumb and provides sensation to part of the hand as it travels past the wrist), resulting in numbness that affects the first, second, and third fingers.

Thoracic Outlet Syndrome Is Also a Player

I haven't mentioned the fourth (ring) finger or the fifth (little) finger yet. These can be affected by a problem with the C7-T1 disk, but a herniation or bone spur at the C7-T1 level is extremely rare, so when the fourth and fifth fingers are involved in the symptom pattern, two other sites of possible nerve pinch should be considered first. One of the most common is a pinched ulnar nerve at the elbow in the *cubital tunnel*, or "funny bone" area. The other is a condition called *thoracic outlet syndrome*, where a part of the *brachial plexus* (a group of combining and dividing spinal nerves near the arm) is pinched, affecting the C8 and T1 nerves about two or three inches after they leave the spinal canal. A thoracic outlet pinch often results from muscle tension in the *anterior scalene* muscle (running from the cervical spine to the first rib as it crosses over major nerves

Middle scalene muscle

Anterior scalene muscle

Brachial Plexus Entrapment

Brachial plexus

Figure 7.4 Anatomy of thoracic outlet syndrome. The nerves of the brachial plexus pass between the anterior and middle scalene muscles as they travel toward the shoulder and arm. A stretch, tear, or chronic spasm in a scalene muscle can occur in a whiplash injury or in a variety of other situations. This can cause pain and weakness in the arm and hand as the nerves are squeezed by the injured muscle. Image published with permission of Joe Bloch.

and arteries). As with the piriformis muscle in the pelvis pinching a nerve and causing sciatica, the whole pattern and quality of pain from a thoracic outlet pinch is different from that caused by a bone spur or a herniated disk and may vary much more with positioning (see Fig. 7.4).

Back Pain and Neck Pain

What about back or neck pain itself? This is among the most common of ailments, and almost everyone experiences back or neck pain sometimes. The vast majority of these pains aren't actually due to problems in the vertebrae or nerves; the most common causes are strained muscles and strained ligaments, which can be quite severe but usually resolve with some anti-inflammatory medication and a little bit of time. Nonetheless, some back and neck pains are due to failures in the spine.

Imaging and Injections

When a pain persists over months and doesn't respond to routine medications, it becomes time to do imaging tests such as X-rays, MRIs, and computed tomography (CT) scans to try to see where the problem is. When spinal abnormalities are seen on an imaging test, it is necessary to carefully analyze them to see whether they can explain the symptoms. Back or neck pain is also matched up to observed spine abnormalities by figuring out what kinds of movement and activity aggravate it; diagnostic injections may be required to help to confirm the role of the abnormality in causing the pain.

The most classic and clear of these matchings of a spine pain, an image, and an injection is in the case of a torn annulus (the retaining ring around a disk). When an annulus is torn in the lumbar region, the individual may experience excruciating back pain with any movement or with sitting. Once an MRI identifies a disk with a suspected annular tear, a test can be done by injecting a tiny amount of anesthetic into the ring. If the individual then experiences complete relief of the pain, the test has proven that the whole back pain is coming from that spot. Other spinal locations that can cause back pain are the facets (joint surfaces) between the vertebrae. Whereas joint problems often have the feature of causing significant pain when the back is extended (leaning backward), an annular tear tends to be most affected by twisting.

Can Surgery Fix Back or Neck Pain?

For back pain that is due to a problem in the spine, you are faced with a question: Can back surgery cure back pain? In the medical community, this question is longstanding and controversial. Successful surgical treatment for neck pain has been possible for many years and is widely accepted as a valid expectation of surgery. However, surgery for back pain as opposed to surgery for decompression of pinched nerves has been perfected only more recently. For this reason, many physicians were trained in an era when the received teaching was that surgery can't cure back pain. This is no longer the case.

Increasingly during the 1990s, and now as the years pass in the 2010s, the success rate and accuracy in treating severe, persistent back pain with spinal surgery is getting higher and higher. So the answer to the question is definitely yes, some kinds of back pain can be effectively and reliably cured by spinal surgery. Keep in mind, however, that this is true for only a small fraction of all back pain patients who are accurately diagnosed. These patients are often the ones with the most severe, most unresponsive pains that follow certain patterns.

This situation has to be framed with the understanding that although surgery can cure some back pain, it is not a 100 percent reliable fix because of possible uncertainty in diagnosis and the difficulty of carrying out the very complex procedures involved. Nonetheless, if the best application of the best modern technology correctly diagnoses a particular failure in your spine as being the cause of your back pain, it is fair to expect something in the range of an 80 percent success rate from a properly designed spinal surgery to cure that pain.

Other Things That Hurt the Back

A physician seeing a patient for back or neck pain always has to keep in mind the possibility that the pain is caused by something more medically ominous and life-threatening than degeneration or arthritis. A stomach ulcer about to perforate and dump infected stomach contents into the abdomen may be perceived as back pain. A giant expansion, or aneurysm, in the aorta, the main artery output from the heart, may cause an intense tearing pain in the back just before the aorta ruptures with catastrophic results. A kidney stone or urinary infection can also cause back pain. An impending heart attack is well known to cause chest pain extending down the right arm. Cancers, infections, medical metabolic disorders, nerve diseases, multiple sclerosis—all of these can seem to show up as routine musculoskeletal back pain (see Fig. 7.5).

For these reasons, the onset of a new spinal pain is a good reason to see your internist for a routine medical checkup. A spinal surgeon should be able to spot medical conditions. Nonetheless, it is best to go to a generalist or internist at the outset of a problem so that you can feel assured that nonspinal causes for the back pain have been adequately considered.

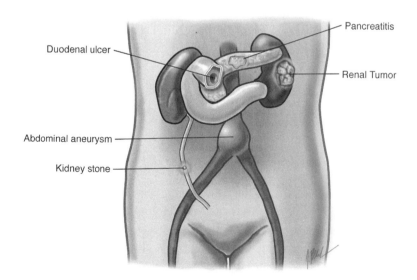

Figure 7.5 Various medical causes of back pain. The onset of back pain doesn't always mean that your spine is hurting. A variety of serious medical conditions affecting various internal organs can also cause back pain. Image published with permission of Joe Bloch.

Myelopathy: What If Your Spinal Cord Is Under Pressure?

Most people clearly understand that a pinched nerve causes pain, but what happens when the spinal cord itself is pinched? Interestingly enough, there often isn't any pain. This is partly because the spinal cord doesn't have any sensory nerve endings inside it or on its surface. The spinal cord shows symptoms of its compression by the effects on its function and not by pain. The general term for abnormal function of the spinal cord due to any pressure or injury is myelopathy, and this is a more severe concern than the symptoms arising from a pinched nerve, or radiculopathy.

Symptoms and Signs of Spinal Cord Compression

The first symptoms of spinal cord compression are usually abnormalities in the unconscious reflex patterns of the body, which can be simply tested by a doctor with a reflex hammer. When the spinal cord is compressed and keeping the normal signals from the brain from reaching the spinal cord in a normal way, the reflexes become increased or more "brisk." This is the opposite of what happens with radiculopathy: When a nerve pinch shuts those signals down, the reflexes are actually decreased, so increased reflexes may reflect myelopathy (see Fig. 7.6).

One of the other very early signs of myelopathy is balance failure. The tests for this are a little bit like what a police officer uses to test a driver for intoxication, such as walking heel-to-toe along a straight line, or standing with feet together, arms in front, and eyes closed, which can lead to unsteadiness.

When those symptoms occur and there are various motor and sensory abnormalities along every spinal nerve distribution below some point in the neck or chest, there is reason for concern. If an imaging test then shows compression of the spinal cord beginning at that level, a diagnosis of myelopathy can reasonably be proposed, and getting the pressure off the spinal cord becomes an important consideration.

Time Is of the Essence

The ability of the spinal cord to recover from myelopathy varies, as does the amount of time it can tolerate compression; but with myelopathy, time is always an important consideration and the time frame is always limited, which is a very different scenario from the compression of a nerve. The main reason is that pinched nerves will recover when the pressure is removed, even after a year or two or more of pressure, whereas the spinal cord very often makes little recovery after the relief of pressure. Surgeries are often carried out primarily to stop spinal cord symptoms from getting worse, rather than to make them better. The spinal cord does sometimes recover from a deficit arising from a compression,

Figure 7.6 Symptoms of spinal cord compression. The earliest signs of spinal cord compression, or myelopathy, can be detected by abnormalities in the physical examination performed by an experienced physician. Some of these signs include very brisk reflexes when tapping the correct spot below the knee cap, a bouncing reflex when the ankle is stretched, called clonus, and unsteadiness when standing with the eyes closed, a positive Romberg sign. Image published with permission of Joe Bloch.

particularly in younger individuals, but it recovers very slowly, often taking a year or two, and that is why any spinal cord compression warrants great concern.

That is also why, if a spinal cord compression that is not yet producing symptoms is discovered through an imaging test (see chapter 10), it may be worthwhile to relieve the compression before any symptoms develop. This is not true for a pinched nerve. If an imaging test shows a nerve canal that might eventually pinch a nerve, there is usually no reason to operate on it immediately because the pinch might never happen, and if it ever does, the surgery can be done effectively at that future time. An observed spinal cord compression, however, is reasonable to decompress even before myelopathy develops because of the difficulty of reversing myelopathy once it occurs.

8

Accidents of the Embryo: Spina Bifida and Variations at Birth

The formation of the spine during embryological development is a highly complex and elaborate process. One of the unique features of the spine, which really doesn't apply to most of the rest of the body, is its *segmentation*. In the vertebrae, along the spinal column, and even in the spinal cord itself, there are repeating elements, similar structures that appear again and again at numerous levels as you proceed down the spine. The process of segmentation, the repetition of specialized but similar units, is a very ancient part of the developmental program of embryos, in that the genes controlling this process are shared by the common ancestors of the insects and the most primitive vertebrate animals (you can read *The Upright Ape: A New Origin of the Species,* by Aaron Filler, 2007, to learn about the evolution of the spine). This process has been specialized, optimized, adjusted, and augmented throughout evolutionary history in leading to the detailed body formation plan that produces the human spine and spinal nerves.

This elaborate script from the earliest days of embryo formation plays out precisely and correctly millions of times each year in human prenatal development. However, the process is subject to minor variations or mistakes that can lead to abnormalities affecting the spine after birth. These missteps have a variety of causes. Some of them are in the environment, some are inherited, some happen only once. Some problems are simply extreme aspects of normal variation that lead to anatomy that doesn't function optimally in a child or that eventually breaks down in the adult. There are even subtle anatomical differences that leave one person's spine working perfectly without serious problems throughout a very long life whereas another begins to show minor breakdowns and degenerative changes at a relatively young age. This chapter is directed toward the more significant congenital abnormalities that lead to noticeable differences in spinal form, differences that can cause problems that are treatable by surgery.

Figure 8.1 Scoliosis. Curvature in the spine has a variety of causes. Even very pronounced curvatures may not cause any symptoms. However, pain, weakness, or postural or appearance problems resulting from scoliosis may require straightening of the spine. Image published with permission of Joe Bloch.

Scoliosis

Among the most common and widely known of these problems is an abnormal curvature of the spine called scoliosis. Scoliosis is generally a developmental abnormality, which means that some critical congenital abnormality sets the stage for it, but it develops and progresses gradually over years. In some cases the triggering factor is some mechanical, traumatic, or degenerative problem that has no congenital component to it, but many patients suffer from this because of a genetic variance in the spinal construction plan (see Fig. 8.1).

Curve Characteristics and Causes

Scoliosis can be a lateral curvature, curving like an S-curve to the left or to the right, but more often it gives the spine a concave or bowed shape, with the middle of the bow pointing to one side or the other. Problems from scoliosis can develop at various ages and have various severities. You can even have a very remarkable amount of scoliosis with a lateral curvature and twisting of the spine but with essentially no symptoms. In my own practice, I once saw a patient with a very dramatic scoliosis who was an internationally successful ballerina seeing me for an unrelated nerve problem. Nonetheless, scoliosis often results in an undesirable appearance, pain and disability, and interference with athletic activity in children, and can be a precipitator of more rapid spine degeneration in older adults.

Scoliosis apparently develops either because of subtle malformations in the vertebrae or, more commonly, because of imbalances in the spinal muscles or the nervous system components that drive them. The muscles on one side seem to apply more force to the spine than the muscles on the other side, leading to progressive curvature.

Correction of the Curved Spine

Fortunately, it is often possible to treat scoliosis by bringing the spine into proper alignment. This typically requires the use of metal instrumentation in extensive surgeries, in which screws are placed into many vertebrae, the screws are attached to rods, and the rod-and-screw construct is used to pull the spine into a normal position and lock it there (see chapter 16). It is then often necessary to fuse elements of the spine to keep it in the corrected alignment.

Correction of scoliosis was one of the first types of instrumented spine surgery to be done. This type of operation is now performed with increasing sophistication and increasingly less-invasive types of metal implants and is usually very effective. Spine specialists who focus on the treatment of scoliosis in children have made it a very successful area of spinal surgery that can open up new worlds of activity for children who might otherwise suffer progressive disability from their scoliosis.

Spina Bifida

Another very common area of congenital spinal abnormality is called spina bifida. This reflects an abnormality in the closure of the spine. In normal embryo development, the vertebrae start as a series of solid structures with the nerves of the spinal cord forming behind them; then the flat, bony lamina reach around the cord from both sides and close into a roof over the spinal canal. Sometimes, however, the closure of the roof is not complete.

Closed versus Open

In the most minor form of spina bifida, the two laminar arches reach up and stop just short of meeting each other, creating an abnormality in the bone that can be observed only with X-rays or other diagnostic imaging. Behind the abnormal bone are the back muscles and the skin, which often appear quite normal: dimples, hairs, or other subtle abnormalities at the low end of the spine may indicate the presence of spina bifida, or there may be no sign at all. Spina bifida with minimal external signs is called *spina bifida occulta*, which means "hidden spina bifida."

The most severe forms are open spina bifida, or *spina bifida aperta*, in which part of the spinal cord is actually exposed through the skin of the back. Infants born with spina bifida aperta require immediate surgery; in fact, a prenatal diagnosis can sometimes identify the problem well enough in advance for a prenatal surgery to correct it. In the situation of an open spine defect in an infant, it is generally possible to have a very successful surgical result from closing over the spine to prevent infection and to preserve most normal functions of the spinal cord. This problem, which had greater than 80 percent mortality thirty years ago, today is almost universally survived. Children born with open spinal cords, however, very often suffer some lifelong neurologic symptoms, such as difficulty with strength in their ankles and even bowel and bladder function abnormalities.

One condition associated with spina bifida is called a *myelomeningocele* (pronounced—my–elo-men-ingo-seal), which means that some of the membranes of the spinal cord are exposed and have emerged through the skin surface. These malformations are also repairable and actually have a lower risk of neurologic impairment or infection than in a truly open-cord abnormality.

A Tethered Cord

In normal development, the body grows much faster than the spinal cord does. Essentially, the bottom end of the spinal cord gradually moves up the spinal canal as you get taller. Although the bottom tip of the spinal cord can be in the mid to low lumbar spine at birth, it will have moved up the body to the very top of the lumbar spine, or the very low end of the thoracic spine, by the time you reach adulthood (see Fig. 8.2).

There is a condition related to spina bifida in which the spinal cord is at its correct depth below the skin, but instead of ending neatly as a closed set of nerves surrounded by fluid, it ends in a ball of fatty tissue and nerve tissue called a *lipomyelomeningocele*. This often presents few or no symptoms at all until adolescence or even adulthood, when the natural growth of the individual comes into conflict with the previously hidden condition. In abnormalities such as the lipomyelomeningocele, the spinal cord tip remains stuck, or *tethered*, in the low spine, and as the body grows, the spinal cord becomes gradually stretched. Symptoms of a tethered cord begin to appear just as the child is entering a growth spurt, as in the teenage years, when an otherwise perfectly normal young boy or girl starts to develop bowel or bladder problems or leg numbness or weakness.

It is often possible to release the tether surgically and to allow the tip of the spinal cord to move upward. Sometimes a tether is only a small, cord-like formation called a *filum terminale*, or it may be a very complex lipomyelomeningocele, which requires an elaborate surgical dissection to separate the fatty tissue from the functioning nerve tissue. The tethered cord is another area where the application of advanced technology can safely correct and relieve the effects of a congenital abnormality.

Figure 8.2 Spina bifida and tethered spinal cord syndrome. This individual was born with an abnormally formed lower spinal cord. The cord extends to the L5 lumbar level instead of terminating at L1, as in most people. The spinal cord was tethered, or attached, to the dura at this level. As she grew to adult height, she began to experience numbness and pain in the legs associated with the stretching of her spinal cord.

Arnold-Chiari Malformations

In a third class of major congenital abnormalities that are often associated with spina bifida and even with scoliosis are the *Arnold-Chiari malformations.* Just as spina bifida often pertains to the low end of the spine, Arnold-Chiari malformations pertain to the very top of the spine. Essentially, they are a set of conditions in which the low end of the brain is actually passed down through the top of the spinal canal.

Severe Entrapment of the Lower Brain in the Top Vertebrae

Arnold-Chiari malformations are categorized as grades 1, 2, and 3. Grade 3, the most severe, is a very rare, life-threatening brain and spine abnormality that sometimes requires urgent surgery at the time of birth or within one to two months afterward. The lower portion of the infant's brain becomes entrapped in the base of the skull and the upper cervical vertebrae. In this situation malfunctions in the ability to breathe or swallow can develop immediately or at a very early age. This is treated surgically by opening the upper spinal vertebrae and the base of the skull to allow room for the abnormally positioned brain to grow.

Grade 2 and grade 3 malformations of this type occur in about one of every 2000 births in the United States.

Milder Entrapment of the Cerebellar Tonsils in the Foramen Magnum

Much more minor Arnold-Chiari malformations occur when the *cerebellar tonsils* at the bottom of the cerebellum reach down through an opening at the base of the skull, called the *foramen magnum*. Over time and with growth, the presence of the abnormal cerebellar extension along with the cord in the foramen magnum leads to scarring of the *arachnoid* (a spidery, thin membrane) and interrupts the normal passage of spinal fluid from the brain to the spinal canal (see Fig. 8.3).

A grade 1 Arnold-Chiari malformation, or AC 1, may not lead to symptoms until mid to late adult life. It can cause severe headaches that characteristically reach up the sides of the neck to the ears and over the top of the head and are greatly aggravated by extending the neck. The condition can be diagnosed from a cervical MRI scan that shows the cerebellar tonsils at or passing through the

Occiput

Cerebellar tonsil

C1

C2

C3

Figure 8.3 Arnold-Chiari malformations. The lower part of the brain, or cerebellum, can be abnormally positioned so that it extends down through the foramen magnum, the opening at the base of the skull. If it crowds the spinal cord in this location, a variety of symptoms, including headache and neck pain, can result. Image published with permission of Joe Bloch.

foramen magnum. The treatment is actually relatively simple: surgically opening up the base of the skull and the top vertebrae and expanding the *dura membranes* at that site to provide more space in the canal for the cerebellar tonsils and spinal cord. This will often relieve the headaches and any other whole-body numbness or neurologic abnormalities, called a *foramen magnum syndrome*, that can arise from a C1 compression.

These malformations have been observed in about 1 percent of all brain MRIs obtained for various reasons. Of the individuals having the AC 1 malformation on their MRI scan, only about 15 percent seem to have symptoms related to it. Overall, this means that about one person in 600 will have headache and neck pain symptoms from this otherwise unobtrusive congenital malformation.

Syringomyelia

One of the possible consequences of an Arnold-Chiari malformation is that abnormalities of cerebrospinal fluid (CSF) flow dynamics at the base of the brain can force the fluid to run down the inside of the spinal cord, rather than flowing around the outside as it should normally. Running down the middle of the spinal cord is a central canal, which is usually microscopic in size; however, if an abnormality forces excess CSF into the central canal, it can expand very significantly, pressing and thinning the surrounding spinal cord against the walls of the dura in the main spinal canal. This condition, called syringomyelia, can cause a variety of progressively severe neurologic symptoms (see Fig. 8.4).

Syringomyelia has been a challenging problem for neurosurgery. One of the operations to treat it involves blocking a site called the *obex*, which is the entry point of the central canal into the fourth *ventricle* (fluid-filled chamber) at the base of the brain. It turns out that it is also often possible to relieve syringomyelia by expanding the foramen magnum, just as is done for the AC1 malformation. These procedures allow normal spinal fluid flow around the outside of the spinal cord to be reestablished, thereby enabling the *syrinx* (the abnormal fluid cavity in the center of the spinal cord) to shrink. A complex and less frequently performed type of treatment is to put a small *shunt* (tube) into the spinal cord to drain some fluid out of it. The other end of the tube may be inside the spinal canal or may actually be led into the chest to the pleural space around the lungs. This type of shunt placement poses significant risks, because the shunt can become clogged or dislodged, and there is the obvious possibility of injuring the spinal cord when passing the tube into the interior of the spinal cord from the outside. For these reasons an anatomical treatment that actually solves the problem is generally preferred.

Dura

CSF space

CSF fluid

Spinal cord

Figure 8.4 Syringomyelia. Accumulation of fluid inside the spinal cord can occur after trauma to the spinal cord, in the setting of some congenital abnormalities, and occasionally when there is spinal cord compression due to degenerative spine disease. Image published with permission of Joe Bloch.

Syringomyelia can occur spontaneously for no obvious reason and can be a small, stable fluid collection that never causes any symptoms or poses any risks. However, it can also occur when a degenerative change in the spine, such as a bulging disk with surrounding arachnoid inflammation, blocks the flow of spinal fluid in the spinal canal. A syrinx may form above the blockage. In this case, the syringomyelia can be treated by a very simple, routine spine operation such as a *laminectomy* (see chapter 14) to decompress the spinal canal.

Congenitally Narrow Spinal Canal

One of the more minor types of congenital spinal abnormality involves a disproportion in the shape of the bony canal around the spinal cord. The normal shape of the canal at the level of any vertebra is defined by the width between the *pedicles* (columns) that hold up the lamina, and by the height of the pedicles that essentially determines how high that roof is above the vertebral body.

Some people have spinal canals of extraordinarily large diameter. This brings to mind one of my patients, who managed to crash his airplane and had a severe neck fracture with essentially a 100 percent displacement of one vertebra relative to the one below it. Such an injury almost universally causes complete paralysis. This patient, having a very large spinal canal, however, suffered no neurologic symptoms at all because there was still room for the spinal cord even with an entire vertebra moved into the canal.

At the other extreme are individuals with a very narrowed spinal canal, for whom the slightest disk bulge or herniation can pose a significant risk of severe neurologic symptoms. A congenitally narrow spinal canal often doesn't cause any harm until some sort of intervening degenerative problem or traumatic injury brings the problem into sharp focus. Symptoms of spinal narrowing, or stenosis, more commonly develop in people in their sixties, seventies, and eighties; but for people with a congenitally narrow spinal canal, symptoms may develop in their twenties and thirties, because the canal is already so narrow that the slightest amount of degenerative change puts pressure on the nerves and spinal cord tissue inside. The presence of this condition is usually very apparent on an imaging test, and the treatment—opening up the narrowed canal to allow additional space—is often very routine from the point of view of spinal surgery.

A congenitally narrow cervical spinal canal is sometimes a concern in athletes, such as a football player who has a sudden, brief paralysis after a tackle. This phenomenon, called a "stinger;" is very terrifying to watch during an athletic event, when the player is unable to rise and experiences immediate paralysis and numbness, as though there has been a neck fracture; yet his symptoms clear up in a matter of days. When the congenital condition is discovered, it poses a huge problem: Can the athlete return to play? Is spinal surgery necessary to make it safe? Often, there is no generalized answer, and the decision has to be tailored to the individual. Fortunately, the type of surgery that will reduce the risk from the problem, a laminectomy, or a decompression from the back of the spinal canal, can often be carried out in such a way that the athlete can return to his usual activity after only a limited period of interruption.

Ossification of the Posterior Longitudinal Ligament

Some congenital abnormalities of the spinal canal do not affect the process of spine formation in the embryo, but rather affect the sensitivity of the spinal tissues to inflammation and the way in which degenerative change impacts the spine later in life. One of the most unusual of these is a condition called *ossification of the posterior longitudinal ligament* (OPLL; see Fig. 8.5).

Ossified posterior
longitudinal ligament

Figure 8.5 Ossification of the posterior longitudinal ligament (OPLL). The ligament between the vertebrae and the spinal dura is called the posterior longitudinal ligament. Ossification, or bone formation, in the ligament can compress the spinal cord. The existence of OPLL requires special planning for surgeries done from the front of the cervical spine. Image published with permission of Joe Bloch.

Inflammation Causes Abnormal Bone Formation

Within the spinal canal, the posterior longitudinal ligament lies behind the vertebral bodies but anterior to the spinal cord. It runs up and down the spine, helping to tie the vertebrae together and providing a smooth canal floor. However, in some individuals, because of their HLA type (a system of naming for genetic similarities that is a very elaborate expansion of the A, B, and O typing for blood) and other aspects of genetic ancestry, this ligament begins to calcify and thicken; with age, this *ossification* (conversion to bone) increases and the ligament becomes thicker and thicker, becoming a solid spike of bone within the spinal canal that gradually presses into the spinal cord.

The simple presence of OPLL does not necessarily cause symptoms. However, it does increase the risk of injury as, for instance, in the case of a rear-end motor vehicle accident producing whiplash, wherein the ossified ligament can fracture. There is relatively little room left in the spinal canal to allow the spinal cord to move out of the way of injury. Often, symptoms from OPLL turn up as the consequences of pressure on the spinal cord, causing a syndrome of myelopathy that affects balance and leg function.

A Surgical Surprise

OPLL is particularly common among the Japanese and continues to have a high frequency in Japanese people who did not grow up in or have never even been to Japan, so this condition appears to be genetic rather than environmental. It is therefore well understood by Japanese spinal surgeons but often surprises American surgeons, who may very rarely see it. The incidence is as high as 1.8 percent of the population in Japan, but only about 0.1 percent of the population who are Caucasian.

On first glance in some types of imaging, OPLL appears somewhat like a herniated disk, which is readily removed by routine, anterior spine surgery. However, if the surgeon doing the removal stops at the usual point, some calcification in the spinal canal may be left in place still compressing the spinal cord. Or if the surgeon encounters the calcification and doesn't understand what it actually is, an attempt to remove it will often remove the calcified and brittle dural membranes as well, which can lead to a very difficult spinal fluid leak or even an injury to the spinal cord.

Although it is possible, in some cases, to treat OPLL with a very elaborate anterior spinal surgery, as is done by some Japanese spine specialists, it is more common in the United States to treat it with an operation that opens up the posterior of the spine, a laminectomy, or a *laminoplasty*, which are described in chapter 14. These procedures essentially expand the spinal canal to allow room for the ossification to progress, in contrast to the anterior surgical approach, which is intended to remove the ossification completely.

Spondylitis, DISH, and Spondylolysis

Some other related types of congenital abnormalities develop with age and have some similarity to OPLL, but are less frequent.

One of these is *ankylosing spondylitis*, in which the vertebral bodies of the spine naturally fuse together, forming a long, rigid, bamboo-like bone. People with ankylosing spondylitis may develop abnormal spinal curvature. As the fusion takes place, the normal shapes of the vertebrae are not maintained and the neck may become curved over so the patient can only look down at the ground. People with extensive fusion from ankylosing spondylitis are also at high risk for spinal fractures from such minor events as a sneeze or a cough. Surgical treatment of a fractured spine in this situation is very difficult because of the very long lever arm across the fracture site. It's like surgically fusing two long bones rather than two small vertebral elements.

A related type of abnormality is *diffuse idiopathic spinal hyperostosis* (DISH), in which excess bone forms in a variety of areas around the spine. This is another

Figure 8.6 Spondylolysis. Separation can occur between the front and the back half of the lamina. The part of the lamina affected is called the pars interarticularis, so the separation is sometimes called a pars defect. The separation splits the vertebra into two parts; the first part includes the vertebral body, the pedicle, and the superior facet. The second part includes the inferior facet and spinous process. Stress across the separation line can cause back pain. This condition also can allow the development of slippage, or spondylolisthesis (see Fig. 6.5). Photo by Aaron Filler.

situation in which certain genetically determined tissue types lead to the ongoing deposition of excess bone around the vertebrae.

Spondylolysis is a congenital abnormality related to spine formation, which often becomes apparent only in later age. Spondylolysis reflects an abnormally thin formation in the part of the vertebra that links the main part of the vertebra lamina to the upper facet joint. The facet joint can actually become disconnected from the rest of the vertebra (see Fig. 8.6). When this happens, the affected vertebra can start to slide relative to the vertebra above it, causing a spondylolisthesis, or misalignment between the two vertebrae.

Abnormal Numbers of Vertebrae

Another type of congenital abnormality that can cause symptoms, or even lead to mistakes during surgery, is an abnormal number of vertebrae. The usual pattern in humans is to have seven cervical, twelve thoracic, and five lumbar vertebrae, followed by the sacrum (five naturally fused vertebrae ending with the coccyx, or "tailbone"). However, this is not always the case.

One abnormality in vertebral number that is most likely to cause symptoms is the presence of something like a rib on the seventh cervical vertebra. People with this condition are at a high risk for developing what's called a thoracic outlet syndrome, in which some of the nerves that go to the pinky finger or to both the fourth and fifth digits are pinched after they leave the spine. Thoracic outlet syndrome can also involve a pinch of the main artery to the hand (see Fig. 8.7).

Another common abnormality in vertebral number is having only eleven thoracic vertebrae instead of twelve. Also, a significant number of people have four or six lumbar vertebrae instead of five, leading to variations in the position of the *sacrum*. These abnormalities become very important during planning for spine

Figure 8.7 Cervical vertebral number abnormalities. The presence of a rib on the seventh cervical vertebra greatly increases the risk of developing arm and hand pain from thoracic outlet syndrome. This is a rare congenital abnormality. Frank Netter illustration reproduced with permission from www.netterimages.com © of Elsevier Inc. All rights reserved.

Figure 8.8 Lumbar vertebral number abnormalities. These lumbar X-ray myelograms show a comparison between a person with only four lumbar vertebrae and a person with six lumbar vertebrae. The great majority of humans have five lumbar vertebrae.

surgery. For instance, when an MRI report indicates that disk L4-L5 is herniated, the radiologist, counting down from the lowest rib, counts four normal lumbar disks and then correctly identifies the herniated fifth disk as the disk between vertebrae L4 and L5. But if the patient has six lumbar vertebrae, and if the X-ray taken during surgery shows only the pelvis and lower lumbar vertebrae, the doctor will see the sacrum and vertebra L6 but think that it's L5, and will end up operating on disk L5-L6, rather than L4-L5 as intended. A standard lumbar X-ray, therefore, should always show the position of the sacrum as well as the ribs, which will readily identify those rare patients in whom the number of lumbar vertebrae is abnormal (see Fig. 8.8).

9

Patterns of Nerve Pinches: From Shoulder to Toe

In order to answer the question of whether or not you need spine surgery you have to know the answer to one very key question: Is your pain coming from a pinched nerve in the spine or is it coming from a pinched nerve somewhere else in the body?

This may sound basic and simple, but every year as many as 100,000 spine surgeries fail because the doctor did not fully consider this question. The patient had a pinched nerve out in the body, away from the spine, but the doctor did a spinal operation. The spine operation was perfect, recovery went well, but the operation had no effect at all on the pain that led the patient to see the doctor in the first place!

How could this happen in this day and age? Not only can it happen but it does happen all the time. This mistake is one of the biggest threats to success that you face in your quest to get out of pain. This occurs because most spine doctors—whether orthopedic or neurosurgical—have little or no training in diagnosing and treating pinched nerves. It may sound puzzling to you as a patient. Why would a doctor treat sciatica if he wasn't considering both spinal and non-spinal causes. If your doctor isn't considering alternatives—how can you as a patient decide?

Once you walk into the spine specialist's office, the doctor makes an assumption that you have a spine problem. The doctor imagines that you were referred to him or her because another doctor believes you have a spine problem. However, your internist or family doctor or physical therapist or neurologists is really counting on the orthopedist or neurosurgeon to figure it out. It ends up being the patient's responsibility to make sure the surgeon fully considers peripheral nerve as opposed to spine as a cause.

Telling the Difference—Nerve or Spine?

There are two main differences between the symptoms from a spine problem versus symptoms from a peripheral nerve problem. First, you need to consider whether your problem includes pain in the neck or back. Second, your doctor needs to be aware in the differences in the pattern or layout of pains from spine versus peripheral nerve.

Spine problems often (but not always) come with pain in the spine. If you have midline low back pain and radiating pain extending down the leg, both started at the same time, and anything that aggravates the back simultaneously aggravates your leg pain—well that is probably sciatica caused by a lumbar spine problem.

However, what if you have only buttock and leg pain, but no midline spine pain at all? Well this could still be from the spine, but it also means that non-spinal causes need to be carefully considered. When a herniated disk in the spine pinches a spinal nerve, you often get a long strip of pain starting at the spine and extending all the way to fingers or toes. The pain usually follows the pattern of one single dermatome (see Figs. 6.4, 7.1, and 7.3). However, there are different patterns for peripheral nerve pains.

Carpal Tunnel Syndrome—The First Three Fingers

The most common and widely recognized nerve pinch starts in the wrist and affects the hand. This problem affects three fingers—the thumb as well as the index and middle fingers. The finger counting is critical. A herniated disk in the neck between C5 and C6 will affect two fingers only—the thumb and index finger. A herniated disk between C6 and C7 affects just one finger—the middle finger. When all three are affected together, carpal tunnel is more likely. This difference occurs because nerves that start out at C6 and nerves that start out at C7 join together as they pass through the body and both sets enter the hand mixed together in the median nerve.

Carpal tunnel pain affects the wrist, the palm, and those first three fingers. It may be worse when you extend your wrist—that is, when you bend it back to point your palm forward. It can be caused by *repetitive strain*—doing the same work related stretch over and over again thousands of times. Sometimes it is just a consequence of routine wear and tear.

What is happening in this condition is that the median nerve is getting pinched and irritated at the point that it crosses the wrist on the way from the arm to the hand. In the wrist, there is a group of bones that form the hard part of the carpal tunnel. They are assembled together into a broad, low U shape with the opening of the U pointed toward the front of the wrist (palm side)—this forms three of the four side walls of the tunnel. The open part of the U is covered by a ligament called the *flexor retinaculum,* the roof of the tunnel. When that ligament gets thickened, the space inside the tunnel starts to shrink. The median nerve, along with the tendons that operate the fingers all pass together through this tunnel.

Distribution of branches of median nerve in hand

Activities or medical conditions that increase contents and pressure within tunnel may result in nerve compression.

Sensory distribution of median nerve

Figure 9.1 Carpal tunnel syndrome anatomy and clinical features. A. The median nerve passes beneath the transverse carpal ligament (also called the flexor retinaculum) as it enters the wrist. When this ligament becomes thickened or when the nerve begins to stick to the ligament symptoms can develop. B. In cross section, the tunnel is shown to be made up of bones of the wrist on three sides, with the transverse carpal ligament providing the "roof." The median nerve, in the tunnel, is surrounded by the various tendons running out to the fingers. C. The thenar muscles at the base of the thumb may be come atrophied. D. Pain and numbness are felt on the palm side of the hand, primarily in the thumb, index and ring finger—the distribution (innervation area) of the median nerve. Frank Netter illustration reproduced with permission from www.netterimages.com © of Elsevier Inc. All rights reserved.

When ligaments or tendons expand, there is less room for the nerve and it gets squeezed. Also, the nerve has to slide and move as you move your hand around. Sometimes, the nerve gets stuck to one edge wall of the tunnel so that in certain positions of the hand, the nerve starts to pull against the point of attachment or adhesion and this also causes pain (see Fig. 9.1). Similar symptoms can also arise when the median nerve is entrapped higher up the forearm (see Fig. 9.2). When the pain is on the back side of the thumb, index and ring fingers, it can be from a radial nerve entrapment instead (see Fig. 9.3).

To treat carpal tunnel, the most common recommendation is to rest the wrist. Sometimes, workplace accommodations will help. If your carpal tunnel

Proximal Compression of Median Nerve

Pronator syndrome

Median n.

Hypesthesia and activity-induced paresthesias

Pain location

Provocative maneuvers

Flexion of middle finger against resistance

Compression by flexor digitorum superficialis muscle

Compression by pronator teres muscle

Pronation against resistance

Supra-condylar process

Ligament of Struthers

Medial epicondyle

Lacertus fibrosus

Pronator teres m.
Humeral head
Ulnar head

Flexor digitorum superficialis m. and arch

Flexor pollicis longus m.

Anterior interosseous n.

Compression by lacertus fibrosus

Flexion of wrist against resistance

JOHN A.CRAIG—AD

Anterior interosseous syndrome

Normal

Abnormal

Hand posture in anterior interosseous syndrome due to paresis of flexor digitorum profundus and flexor pollicis longus muscles

Figure 9.2 Proximal entrapments of the median nerve. Although carpal tunnel syndrome is the most common entrapment of the median nerve, there are other typical locations along the arm where this nerve sometimes becomes entrapped. When this happens, hand symptoms similar to carpal tunnel occur along with other symptoms coming from higher up the arm. Illustration reproduced with permission from www.netterimages.com © of Elsevier Inc. All rights reserved.

Radial Nerve Compression

Motor signs

Posterior interosseous syndrome

Proximal compression. Loss of wrist and finger extension

Sensory signs in radial tunnel syndrome

Pain and tenderness

Pain radiation

Paresthesia and hypesthesias

Radial n.

Recurrent radial a.

Posterior interosseous n.

Extensor carpi radialis brevis m.

Supinator m.

Provocative tests for radial tunnel syndrome

Supination against resistance

Resistive extension of middle finger

Provocative tests elicit pain over radial tunnel.

Superficial radial n.

Vascular leash of Henry

Fibrous arcade of Frohse

Posterior interosseous n.

Innervation of extensor mm.

Tendon of brachioradialis m.

Superficial radial n. at wrist

JOHN A.CRAIG—AD

Figure 9.3 Common entrapments of the radial nerve. Entrapments of the radial nerve can cause pain and numbness on the back of the hand as well as weakness of finger extension or wrist extension (straightening the fingers and lifting the had at the wrist). The major motor branch of the radial nerve can be entrapped at the "Arcade of Frohnse." This branch—is called the posterior interosseous nerve—can be entrapped where it enters the muscles on the back of the forearm just past the Arcade. Frank Netter illustration reproduced with permission from www.netterimages.com © of Elsevier Inc. All rights reserved.

syndrome seems to relate to holding your hand in an extended position while you type or use your computer mouse, then you may get a great deal of help from using a pad that holds your wrist up as you use the computer. This shifts the wrist into a more neutral position and gives the carpal tunnel a chance to heal. If rest, repositioning at work, splints worn to reduce movement, and medications all fail, surgery is sometimes advisable to open up the space around the median nerve, to get you back to normal.

Cubital Tunnel at the Elbow Affecting the Hand

Because carpal tunnel syndrome is so common and so well known, there can be a mistake made by thinking that all pain in the hand is carpal tunnel. The number two cause for nerve based hand pain is *cubital tunnel syndrome*—a pinch of the ulnar nerve at the elbow (see Fig. 9.4). The cardinal difference from carpal tunnel syndrome is that it affects the fourth and fifth finger—ring and pinky finger— and does not affect the first three fingers (thumb, index, middle).

Even more than carpal tunnel, cubital tends to weaken the hand and make it clumsy. This draws attention to two very different aspects of hand strength. The main strong power of the grip in our hands actually comes from the mass of muscles of the forearm (elbow to wrist) sending tendons to reach the finger bones. However, there are also dozens of small muscles within the hand itself that do the fine positioning and control work for the palm and fingers. These are called *hand intrinsic muscles,* and these are the ones most affected by problems with the ulnar nerve.

If you compare to the information on carpal tunnel, you'll recall that the C6 spinal nerve affects the first two fingers and the C7 affects the middle finger. You are right if you're thinking that the C8 spinal nerve affects the ring and pinky finger. But wait a minute—how can there be a C8 nerve if there are only seven cervical vertebral levels? Well, it so happens that the spinal nerve coming out between the C7 and the T1 (first thoracic) vertebra is called the C8 spinal nerve. However, unlike C6 and C7 it is extraordinarily rare for the C8 nerve to get pinched in the neck. It just is one of those things that almost never happens.

What else besides cubital tunnel can cause fourth and fifth finger pain with internal hand weakness? Well, the ulnar can get pinched as it enters the wrist near the carpal tunnel. However, the ulnar nerve doesn't go through the carpal tunnel. It gets into the hand via its own special tunnel off to the side near the pinky finger. This is called the *Guyon's canal* (see Fig. 9.4). Compared to cubital tunnel, the Guyon's canal syndrome is rare.

One more common nerve pinch that be confused with cubital tunnel is a squeeze that can occur between the neck and the shoulder in the brachial plexus nerves (see Figs. 7.4 and 8.7). One part of the brachial plexus—the lower

Compression of ulnar nerve

Figure 9.4 Common entrapments of the ulnar nerve. The two most common locations of ulnar nerve entrapment are at the cubital tunnel at the elbow and at the wrist at Guyon's canal. Symptoms often include numbness in the ring and pinky finger as well as weakness of the small muscles in the hand. Illustration reproduced with permission from www.netterimages.com © of Elsevier Inc. All rights reserved.

trunk—has got all of the relevant ulnar nerve components in it (traveling through the plexus on their way to form the ulnar nerve). However, it can be told apart from cubital tunnel because although it covers the fourth and fifth fingers for pain and sensation, it carries all of the movement nerves for the intrinsic muscles of the hand—those headed for the ulnar nerve, as well as those headed for the median nerve. Therefore a lower trunk brachial plexus problem causes more extensive weakness in the hand than cubital tunnel or carpal tunnel alone.

Thoracic Outlet Syndrome and Other Shoulder Nerve Entrapments

It is certain fact that everyone knows about spine problems, but almost no one knows about *thoracic outlet syndrome* (TOS). TOS is a very common cause of shoulder, arm, and hand pain. Surprisingly, there are almost as many surgeries done every year for TOS as for lumbar spine problems.

Where is the thoracic outlet? It is not the same thing as the thoracic spine—they are near each other, but they are two totally different areas with very different nerves.

The thoracic outlet refers to the opening at the top of the rib cage—the *sternum* is in front, the cervical and upper thoracic spine is in back, and the first rib rounds out the circle. The major blood vessels for the head and arms pass through the thoracic outlet as they travel out from the heart or return to it.

Most important for pain problems—all of the nerves for the shoulder, arm, and hand pass by the thoracic outlet and can be entrapped or pinched at this site. The symptoms are often similar to symptoms from a cervical spine herniated disk, and this is why mistakes in diagnosis between cervical spine and TOS are a very large problem that leads thousands of patients every year to have failed or unhelpful cervical spine surgery.

The most common symptoms from TOS are pain and numbness in the ring and pinky fingers (fourth and fifth digits), clumsiness in the hand, pain along the medial or inside edge of the *scapula,* and pain and weakness when the arm is raised. However, because all of the nerves for the shoulder, arm, and hand pass through the thoracic outlet area, almost any symptom of pain, numbness or weakness in the shoulder, arm, and hand (upper extremity) can be caused by TOS.

The term *thoracic outlet syndrome* actually includes several separate medical conditions that share the same general region of the body. There is vascular or vasogenic TOS, which affects primarily arteries and veins. In that condition, raising the arm overhead cuts off blood flow to the hand and leads to numbness and weakness due to the resulting vascular (blood supply) reduction. When veins get compressed, the result can be swelling and bluish discoloration in the arm.

The problem of pain, numbness, and weakness can also occur from nerve compression TOS (neurogenic TOS). In some patients with this condition, the shoulder, arm, or hand hurt all the time, but in others, the pain is triggered by certain positions—such as raising the arm. This is different from cervical spine problems that tend to cause pain with neck turning—although there is some overlap that the doctor has to sort out.

Neurogenic TOS also can come from several different problems that are near each other. The most common type involves the scalene muscles that are out to the side of the neck. The *anterior scalene muscle* and *the middle scalene muscle* form an upside down V (see Fig. 7.4) and all of the upper extremity nerves pass between the two of them or actually pass through the middle scalene muscle. They start on the cervical spine and attach to the first rib. When either or both of these muscles gets injured—a chronic muscle spasm problem can develop that can strangely last for years. The spasm of the two muscles results in pinching of the nerves.

The widely known problem of *whiplash* after a rear end motor vehicle accident is very often due to scalene muscle spasm. This causes neck pain (from the sore muscles) and can cause nerve symptoms in the shoulder, arm, and hand. In many cases, the injured person has X-rays or an MRI of the cervical spine that look normal. The doctor may mistakenly say there is nothing wrong—but he or she really means there is nothing wrong with the spine. The actual and very real problem is very often a scalene syndrome TOS problem that simply does not involve the spine but is just as painful and disabling as a spinal problem.

The nerves involved are grouped together in a structure called the brachial plexus. This is actually a group of more than a dozen different nerves. The C5, C6, C7, C8, and T1 spinal nerves emerge from the spine and then fuse, separate, fuse, separate, mix, and re-sort themselves as they pass through the brachial plexus and emerge on the far end as the median, radial, ulnar, axillary, or other nerves at the far end of the plexus. A nerve such as the median nerve—headed to the hand—could include some nerve elements from the C6 spinal nerve and some from the T1 spinal nerve. This is why the pattern of nerve impingement symptoms and TOS symptoms often form in complex patterns that are far different from the simpler dermatomal pain patterns caused by spinal problems.

To make matters even more difficult, the scalene spasm can lead to headache syndromes by pinching nerves to other neck muscles such as the *splenius* and *semi-spinalis*. Those muscles can then go on to irritate the occipital nerves and related nerves of the scalp—running all the way forward to the forehead. When the *sternocleidomastoid* muscle (SCM) gets involved—ear pain can result along with pain turning the head.

As the brachial plexus travels along its course from neck to shoulder—splitting and mixing along the way—in can also get entrapped as it crosses over the first rib and under the collar bone (clavicle), or as it approached the underarm (axilla). A doctor checking for TOS has to think about each of these possible locations of entrapment. Other shoulder symptoms can arise from a middle scalene syndrome affecting the long thoracic nerve (see Fig. 9.5) or from supraspinous capular nerve entrapment.

Figure 9.5 Entrapments of shoulder nerves. Pain between the shoulder and neck can be due to entrapment of the suprascapular nerve. The musculocutaneous nerve can be entrapped causing weakness of the biceps that affects arm flexion at the elbow. The long thoracic nerve is often subject to stretch or entrapment injuries that cause "winging" of the scapula and affect shoulder movements. The entrapment can occur in the middle scalene muscle or elsewhere along the nerve. Frank Netter illustration reproduced with permission from www.netterimages.com © of Elsevier Inc. All rights reserved.

Pain in the Chest or Abdominal Wall

When you have chest pain or abdominal pain, the most common causes are deep on the inside—heart, lung, stomach, gall bladder, intestines, bladder—and you have to get evaluated by an internist or even an emergency room doctor. However, sometimes all the tests turn up negative. The doctors tell you that everything is fine on the inside and you are safe. However, you may still have the pain. One reason this can happen is if you are experiencing pain due to a pinched nerve in the outer body wall of the chest or abdomen.

The intercostal nerves run along under each rib. These can get pinched or entrapped either as they emerge from the spine or as they run along the rib. A small muscle tear or injury to a rib or to the muscles around it can cause this kind of nerve pinch. The pain then can run around the body like a bucket handle—extending from the spine in back, then on around to the sternum or midline in front.

Similar issues apply to the nerves of the abdominal wall. A pinched body wall nerve can cause a half ring of pain or numbness reaching around to the front of the abdomen. Another type of puzzling abdominal nerve pain is one that affects the *rectus abdominis* muscle. This is a muscle that runs vertically from the lower end of the sternum (breast bone) and on down to the pubic bone of the pelvis. The upper half (above the belly button), the lower half, or all of the rectus abdominis can be involved in a nerve pinch pain.

Tarsal Tunnel Syndrome at the Ankle and Other Foot Pains

Foot pains are a very common problem and there are many problems that occur in the ligaments or bones of the foot or ankle that don't involve pinched nerves. A sprained ankle is something everyone knows about. Pain along the bottom of the foot can be an inflamed fascia (ligament layer) called plantar fasciitis—a condition that is often treated by podiatrist.

Nerves near the toes can get torn or swollen and this lead to a painful condition called a Morton's neuroma. The torn ends of the nerves can try to regrow and instead form into a ball of sensitive nerve tissue between the toes that get pinched when you stand or walk.

A herniated disk in the lumbar spine can certainly cause a pain that extends all the way to the toes—and in fact that is very common in spinal problems. However, when the spine is the cause of foot pain, there is usually also pain in the low back, buttock or leg. Also, when the pain originates in the toes them-selves—it is likely that it will hurt to put pressure directly on the pain generator in the toe. Spinal pains that reach the foot are typically radiating pains. You feel the pain in the foot, but it doesn't really affect the pain if you push on the painful area; the sensitive spot is actually far away, up in the back.

The most common nerve pinch problem in the foot is a tarsal tunnel syndrome (see Fig. 9.6). This is the foot equivalent of a carpal tunnel syndrome. The tarsal tunnel is on the inner ankle. There are two large bony bumps on the ankle—the one on the outer surface is called the lateral malleolus and the one on the inner surface (facing the other ankle) is the medial malleolus. The tibial nerve makes a turn around the medial malleolus as it descends from the leg and then heads out into the foot to form the nerves to the heel (calcaneal branch) and the nerves to the bottom surface and muscles of the foot and the toes (medial and lateral plantar branches). When the tibial nerve gets entrapped in the tarsal tunnel (taking its turn around the medial malleolus) you can get pain, weakness, and numbness in the ankle or throughout the foot.

Figure 9.6 Tibial nerve and tarsal tunnel syndrome. The tibial nerve is one of the two major nerves that result when the sciatic nerve splits in the lower thigh. After innervating the gastrocnemius in the calf, the tibial nerve curves around the ankle (medial malleolus) and reaches the bottom of the foot where it splits into medial and lateral plantar nerves. Entrapment of the tibial nerve in the tarsal tunnel causes pain on the bottom of the foot. Frank Netter illustration reproduced with permission from www.netterimages.com © of Elsevier Inc. All rights reserved.

Peroneal Pinches at the Knee

Some parts of the body are just more vulnerable to injury than others. There is no worse design and no better setup for trouble than the peroneal nerve at the knee. The sciatic nerve descends down the thigh and then splits into the tibial nerve and the peroneal nerve—both of which travel on the back side of the knee joint. The tibial nerve goes to the calf muscles and to the muscles on the bottom of the foot. The peroneal nerve, however, heads off to the side and wraps around onto the front surface of the lower leg. When it wraps around, there is a point where it is near the skin surface and is directly on the side of the body. At this point it also passes over the bone of the upper part of the fibula. At this point, a major nerve is just under the skin with no soft tissue below it that could give way to cushion the nerve. It is skin, major nerve, then hard bone (see Fig 9.7).

Because of this anatomical setup, a hard blow on the side of the leg—just below the knee, or even repeated pressure there—can lead to a peroneal nerve problem. The consequence is pain over the top of the foot and even worse—it can be the cause of a *"foot drop."* This is a situation where the foot does not move properly during walking.

Normally, as we walk the foot comes off the ground and the toes and ball of the foot get elevated so that it is the heel that strikes first at the next step. If the peroneal nerve is compressed severely enough, the muscles that lift the foot don't work properly and the front of the foot fails to come up as we walk. The consequence is an increased risk of tripping and falling, an odd foot slap as the foot comes down in a step, and significant difficulty running. This is actually a very common sports injury as well as problem of wear and tear of life that affects come people.

A foot drop can be due to a problem in the spine where the nerves that lead to the peroneal nerve first come out of the lumbar L5 area. However, if the symptoms of pain, numbness, and weakness start just below the knee and if the nerve is very sensitive as it passes over the upper part or head or neck of the fibula, then it may be a peroneal nerve entrapment. The pain runs down the front of the lower leg and onto the top of the foot.

Sciatic Entrapment in the Pelvis and Piriformis Syndrome

There has been controversy in neurology, neurosurgery, and orthopedics for over eighty years in trying to distinguish between sciatica caused by the spine and sciatica caused by a pinched sciatic nerve in the pelvis. Each of these two problems can affect a million people every year. Spinal causes of sciatica—pain running down the back of the leg and into the ankle and foot—include herniated disks and bone spurs in the lumbar spine. Doctors have been far more likely to diagnose these spine problems while missing or forgetting to check for the non-spinal causes. Mistakes on this point are thought by some specialists to lead to over 50,000 failed spine surgeries every year in the United States.

Common fibular (peroneal) nerve (phantom)

Biceps femoris tendon

Common fibular (peroneal) nerve (L4, 5, S1, 2)

Head of fibula

Fibularis (peroneus) longus muscle (cut)

Superficial fibular (peroneal) nerve

Branches of lateral sural cutaneous nerve

Fibularis (peroneus) longus muscle

Fibularis (peroneus) brevis muscle

Medial dorsal cutaneous nerve

Intermediate dorsal cutaneous nerve

Inferior extensor retinaculum (partially cut)

Lateral dorsal cutaneous nerve (branch of sural nerve)

Dorsal digital nerves

Lateral sural cutaneous nerve (phantom)

Articular branches

Recurrent articular nerve

Extensor digitorum longus muscle (cut)

Deep fibular (peroneal) nerve

Tibialis anterior muscle

Extensor digitorum longus muscle

Extensor hallucis longus muscle

Lateral branch of deep fibular (peroneal) nerve to Extensor hallucis brevis and Extensor digitorum brevis muscles

Medial branch of deep fibular (peroneal) nerve

Cutaneous innervation

Lateral sural cutaneous nerve

Superficial fibular (peroneal) nerve

Deep fibular (peroneal) nerve

Sural nerve via lateral dorsal cutaneous branch

Figure 9.7 Peroneal nerve entrapment. The peroneal division of the sciatic nerve curves around the outside of the head of the fibula and this is often the site of entrapments or injuries. A problem with the peroneal nerve causes a "foot drop"—difficulty raising the front of the foot (difficulty achieving toes up, heel down). Frank Netter illustration reproduced with permission from www.netterimages.com © of Elsevier Inc. All rights reserved.

Parts of the lumbar and sacral spinal nerves of L4, L5, S1, and S2 join together in the interior of the pelvis to form the sciatic nerve. The nerve then emerges from the pelvis by passing through an opening in the bone of the pelvis called the sciatic notch. However, the sciatic notch is stuffed with other structures passing from the inner pelvis to the posterior and, in particular, the largest structure in the notch is the piriformis muscle. The sciatic nerve takes up about 20 percent of the space in the opening, the piriformis muscle takes up about 75 percent, and the remainder is taken up by smaller nerves and blood vessels.

Like the scalene muscles in the neck, the piriformis muscle just happens to be one of those few muscles in the body that can go into chronic spasm that lasts over years. Unfortunately, the spasm can both stiffen and enlarge the muscle so that it begins to rub on and compress the sciatic nerve as two structures exit the sciatic notch together. This can result in radiating pain extending down the back of the thigh and into the foot.

Sometimes, the inflammation that occurs in this situation also causes scarring or fibrosis that makes the sciatic nerve literally become attached or adherent to surrounding tissues. Normally, the tissues of the body glide past each other into different relative positions as we move or shift into different postures. When a nerve adheres to a nearby muscle, bone, or ligament, it becomes fixated and cannot move normally. The consequence can be a positional pain. In piriformis syndromes this often means that a severe sciatica develops whenever the person sits down and then goes away promptly when the person stands up. Some men have developed or aggravated a piriformis syndrome by carrying a large wallet in their back pocket.

The piriformis muscle attaches to the top of the femur at a large bony bump on the side of the hip called the *greater trochanter*. The resulting *trochanteric bursitis* pain can be confused with hip joint pain. A mistake in diagnosing the cause of this has led some patients to get an unnecessary hip joint replacement!

Piriformis syndromes can often be resolved with a program of stretching of the piriformis muscle. In resistant cases, image-guided injections into the piriformis muscle are necessary to get it to settle down. In the worst cases, nothing can be done to settle it down and the only option is surgical removal of the muscle. Fortunately, this removal has no detectable effect on movement—even for athletes and performers.

One other nerve that can be entrapped where it goes through the sciatic notch is the *superior gluteal nerve*. This nerve can cause three different problems that cause huge confusion for doctors and patients. First, the main part of this nerve turns up after exiting the notch and innervates (goes into) the gluteus medius muscle. This muscle starts along the top edge of the iliac crest—the very top of the hip bone (see Fig. 9.8). Many patients—and doctors—will call this back pain even though it really is in the upper pelvis. This is important because a sciatic notch problem in the pelvis that causes this sort of pain is easily mistaken for a lumbar spinal problem. The superior gluteal nerve also reaches down to the side of the thigh via a muscle called the *tensor fascia lata*. This one is a bit confusing for doctors because sciatic pain is usually on the back of the thigh and this one is on the side. Even more confusing is that this muscle pulls on ligaments in the

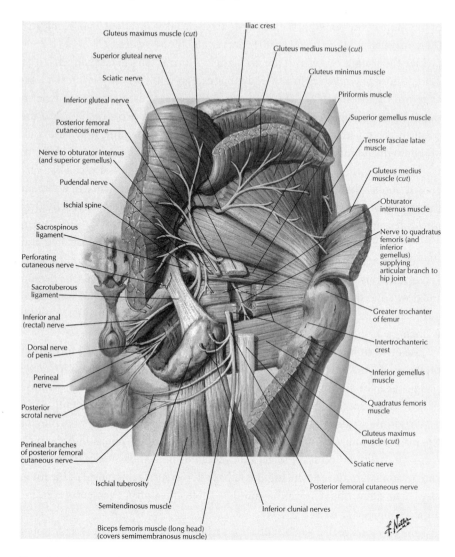

Iliac crest

Gluteus maximus muscle (*cut*)

Superior gluteal nerve

Sciatic nerve

Inferior gluteal nerve

Posterior femoral cutaneous nerve

Nerve to obturator internus (and superior gemellus)

Pudendal nerve

Ischial spine

Sacrospinous ligament

Perforating cutaneous nerve

Sacrotuberous ligament

Inferior anal (rectal) nerve

Dorsal nerve of penis

Perineal nerve

Posterior scrotal nerve

Perineal branches of posterior femoral cutaneous nerve

Ischial tuberosity

Semitendinosus muscle

Biceps femoris muscle (long head) (covers semimembranosus muscle)

Gluteus medius muscle (*cut*)

Gluteus minimus muscle

Piriformis muscle

Superior gemellus muscle

Tensor fasciae latae muscle

Gluteus medius muscle (*cut*)

Obturator internus muscle

Nerve to quadratus femoris (and inferior gemellus) supplying articular branch to hip joint

Greater trochanter of femur

Intertrochanteric crest

Inferior gemellus muscle

Quadratus femoris muscle

Gluteus maximus muscle (*cut*)

Sciatic nerve

Posterior femoral cutaneous nerve

Inferior clunial nerves

Figure 9.8 Entrapments of the nerves of the sciatic notch. Several of the nerves emerging from the sciatic notch of the pelvis are subject to entrapment when the piriformis muscle is in spasm. Pressure on the sciatic nerve causes pain down the back of the thigh and in the calf, shin and foot. The pudendal nerve can be entrapped affecting the urogenital system and the perineum between the legs. The obturator internus nerve can cause pain in the hip and groin when it is entrapped. The superior gluteal nerve causes pain reaching up towards the iliac crest in the low back by affecting the gluteus medius muscle and it also sends a branch down to the lateral thigh to innervate the tensor fascia lata muscle. Frank Netter illustration reproduced with permission from www.netterimages.com © of Elsevier Inc. All rights reserved.

knee and can actually be a cause of knee pain. The combination of upper buttock pain and lateral thigh pain with knee pain and pain in the sciatic notch sounds like a random collection of different problems, but a properly trained physician should be able to identify the underlying superior gluteal nerve syndrome.

Moving our focus lower in the pelvis—it is also useful to consider that the sciatic nerve can become entrapped at other sites in the pelvis. After leaving the area of the sciatic notch and piriformis muscle, the sciatic nerve passes through the ischial tunnel along the outer or lateral surface of the "sit bone" or ischial tuberosity. In the *ischial tunnel,* the sciatic nerve is crossed by the tendon of the *obturator internus* muscle. This muscle is very low in the pelvis and can also be associated with a sitting pain that includes sciatica. One frequent cause of this is a badly fitting bicycle seat used by a person who does a great deal of cycling.

The hamstring muscles of the posterior thigh are attached to the *ischial tuberosity.* A tear or injury at the attachment site of these tendons can cause an irritation or an adhesion of the sciatic nerve in the ischial tunnel. This is yet another cause of a positional pain, aggravated by sitting, that is associated with sciatica.

Front of the Thigh—Femoral Nerve and Its Neighbors

The main power for the kicking motion of extending the knee comes from four large muscles on the front of the thigh that are often called the quads. This is more formally the *quadriceps femoris.* All of these muscles attach to the patella and help extend the knee.

Entrapments are rare, but the femoral nerve can be caught in a pinch or adhesion as it crosses the *inguinal ligament* in the groin (see Fig. 9.9). It can also be caught up in a stretch or tear injury to the psoas muscle. The psoas is a long muscle that runs down the sides of the lumbar vertebrae, starting way up in the mid-back. It then runs down to the femur. It helps lift the thigh when you are lying flat on your back and it helps swing the leg forward when you are walking.

In the front of the thigh, a pain is possibly from a pinch of the femoral nerve and on the outer side of the thigh it can be from the tensor fascia lata (TFL). This leaves two more areas in the thigh that can be made painful by a common type of nerve pinch. The first of these is a strip of the thigh between the front and the side is the area of the lateral femoral cutaneous nerve. Because this nerve passes by a bony prominence in the front of the pelvis (the anterior superior iliac spine or ASIS), it can be compressed by an overly tight belt. There is a Latin/Greek name for this type of pain that remains in use—*meralgia paresthetica.* That's the ancient aspect of this condition—but the modern aspect is that an increase in occurrence of this pain has been blamed on the on the additional pressure that can be placed on the nerve by low-rise jeans.

Last in the list of the four nerves involved in anterior thigh pains is the *obturator nerve* (see Fig. 9.10). This nerve supplies the adductor muscles on the medial aspect of the thigh the muscles that pull the leg inward. Entrapments of the obturator nerve sometimes affect athletes but they can also be part of pulled groin muscle that sets off the entrapment.

Figure 9.9 Entrapments affecting the anterior thigh. The lateral femoral cutaneous nerve (LFC) can be pinched by a tight belt and causes pain in the antero-lateral thigh. Problems with the femoral nerve affect the ability to straighten (extend) the knee. The saphenous branch of the femoral nerve can cause pain along the medial portion of the leg below the knee. Frank Netter illustration reproduced with permission from www.netterimages.com © of Elsevier Inc. All rights reserved.

Groin Pains—Ilioinguinal and Genito-femoral Nerves

Pains along the crease of the groin are occasionally caused as a complication of lower abdominal surgeries such as hysterectomies and hernia repairs. The *ilio-inguinal* and *genito-femoral* nerves run in the crease where abdomen meets

Iliohypogastric nerve

Ilioinguinal nerve

Genitofemoral nerve

Lateral femoral cutaneous nerve

Femoral nerve

Obturator nerve (L2, 3, 4)

Posterior branch

Articular branch

Anterior branch

Posterior branch

Cutaneous branch

Articular branch to knee joint

Adductor hiatus

Note: Only muscles innervated by obturator nerve shown

L1
L2
L3
L4
} Lumbar plexus

Lumbosacral trunk

Obturator externus muscle

Adductor brevis muscle

Adductor longus muscle (*cut*)

Adductor magnus muscle (ischiocondylar, or "hamstrings," part supplied by sciatic [tibial] nerve)

Gracilis muscle

Cutaneous innervation

Figure 9.10 Entrapments of the obturator nerve. The Obturator nerve can be trapped or compressed where it passes through the obturator internus muscle inside the pelvis. In some athletes, it gets entrapped in the obturator canal. The result is weakness in the adductor muscles that pull the leg inward and pain in the medial thigh. Frank Netter illustration reproduced with permission from www.netterimages.com © of Elsevier Inc. All rights reserved.

the upper thigh. Surgical incisions that go a little too far out to the side can cause injury to these nerves. Scar tissue that forms after these surgeries can gradually entrap the nerves over the weeks following surgery as surgical healing progresses. The pain will be in the inguinal crease, but can also extend into the genital area.

Because these nerves are mostly sensory—they don't control any major muscles—chronic pain due to pinched nerves is sometimes treated by cutting the nerves out. This certainly leaves permanent numbness in the area supplied by the nerves, but it often fails to relieve the pain. Simple nerve release surgeries (see chapter 20) can often relieve these entrapment pains.

Pudendal Neuralgia and Nerve Pain in the Genital/Rectal Area

Almost anyone will admit to having back pain, neck pain, or shoulder pain, but having nerve pain in the areas between the legs is often very embarrassing to even talk about. Not only that, but so few doctors are knowledgeable about these nerve entrapments and the emotional aspects are so significant that patients with mechanical entrapments of the *pudendal nerve* often get referred to a psychiatrist rather than to a neurologist or neurosurgeon. Needless to say—this is not an area that orthopedic surgeons have much interest in.

The pudendal nerve is responsible for sensation in what is called the *perineum*—the area between the legs from just behind the anus and on forward to include the genital area. Because this nerve also plays a role in controlling the rectal and urinary sphincters (the conscious part of control) and because it also plays a role in sexual function, there is a great deal of crossover into urology, gynecology, gastro-intestinal issues, and yes—even psychiatry. It also plays a role in bladder function, so it can be a cause of lower abdominal pain and bladder pain as well.

The strange thing is that despite all the various body systems, sensitive structures, and emotional issues involved, it is still just a routine simple nerve entrapment—as long as the physician considers it and knows how to diagnose it. This sounds simple, but there are huge barriers to diagnosis that arise because GI doctors, urologists, gynecologists, and psychiatrists don't want to deal with nerve entrapments and conversely because neurologists and neurosurgeons don't want to deal with urogenital organs or rectal pain! The result is literally a medical "no man's land."

The pudendal nerve runs a complicated course that exposes it to several different potential sites of entrapment. The S2 and S3 sacral spinal nerves can pass through the piriformis muscle just after they exit the sacrum and as they pass through the lumbosacral plexus to form the pudendal nerves. Spasm in the piriformis muscle can result in pudendal pain along with sciatic pain, since both nerves pass through or near the piriformis muscle and both nerves exit the pelvis together through the greater sciatic notch.

The pudendal nerve then takes a sort of U-turn and goes back inside the pelvis through the lesser sciatic notch. A variety of types of entrapment can affect the nerve as it makes its U-turn.

After it reenters the pelvis, the pudendal nerve does something that few other nerves do—it runs in a dense covering on the inner surface of a muscle—the obturator internus muscle. The thickest part of this covering is called the *Alcock's Canal*. Build up of fibrous tissue in the Alcock's Canal or even muscle spasm in the obturator internus muscle can cause pain, numbness, and functional disorders in any area supplied by the pudendal nerve.

Pudendal nerve pains are often made worse by sitting, and in some unfortunate patients the pain is aggravated by lying down. Many, but not all, get relief by standing or walking. In some cases, physical therapy and stretching exercises directed at the piriformis muscle or the obturator internus muscle can help relieve the problem. Surgeries to release pudendal nerve entrapment are relatively new, but they have improved greatly in success rate in the past five years.

Small Nerves and Neuromas

Quite aside from the series of major nerve entrapment types described in preceding portions of this chapter—there are smaller nerves throughout the body that can be the cause of a pain syndrome. Even a very small nerve that normally provides sensation to a small patch of skin can be the source of a serious pain problem. This is because a severe pain can cause just as much distress regardless of whether it comes from a pinpoint, small area or from a much larger portion of the body.

If a small nerve is entrapped—it can be source of pain. In addition, very small nerves are more likely to be torn or severed by an impact. When a nerve is severed, it tries to regrow. In many cases, however, the growing end can't find its target and so it forms an ineffective—and highly sensitive—ball of nerve tissues near the damage point called a neuroma. Any contact over the neuroma or pressure on it can be extremely painful.

Small-area nerve pains of this type can be treated with radiofrequency heating by a needle probe or by freezing (cryotherapy). A complete destruction of the small neuroma or small entrapped nerve will only lead to a small numb patch. This kind of small neurological deficit is often quite acceptable if the numbness effectively and permanently relieves the pain.

10

Medical Imaging and Diagnostic Tests: X-Rays, Electrons, and Magnetic Spin

Underlying all of Western science is the basic paradigm or principle that first you observe and collect objective facts and then, based on consideration of what you see or find, you decide what it is that you've seen and what you're going to do about it. For Western medicine, this paradigm essentially dictates that the diagnosis and treatment follow the examination. The oldest forms of examination are still very important, from the physical exam or "laying on of hands" to taking a medical history and listening to what the patient says about his or her experience. But a variety of technologies can now extend the range of the physician's ability to discern a problem. In dealing with the spine, the most important of these technological extensions are *diagnostic imaging* and *electrodiagnostic tests*. Modern medical diagnostic imaging relies primarily on four types of technology that allow clinicians to see through solid tissues. The first and oldest type of medical imaging is the *X-ray*, a sort of high-energy light wave, with its original and classic use for seeing bones. The second, *ultrasound*, utilizes sound waves to detect shapes within the body. Although ultrasound is important in many areas of medicine and can be used to examine the spine, it plays a very minor role compared with X-rays and the third major type of imaging technology, which is *magnetic resonance imaging* (MRI), a technology that relies essentially on radio waves and magnetic fields. The fourth general category of medical imaging is termed *nuclear medicine*, and this relies on radioactive nuclear energy. This class of imaging technology also has fairly limited use in the spine.

Electrodiagnostic tests include various methods of either sending electricity into the body to activate brain, nerves, and muscles or monitoring electrical activity taking place in these tissues. The various versions of these tests continue to play a critical supporting role in diagnosis and treatment but generally are used only to support or elaborate on information gained from diagnostic imaging or from the physical exam.

X-Rays: Seeing Through to the Bone

There is a tendency to think about X-rays in terms of radiation protection, as X-rays can be produced by radioactive materials, but understanding how X-rays do what they do best is easiest if you think of them as an intense form of light. Essentially, the clinician shines the X-ray beam through the patient, and whatever tissue is most dense in the body, which tends to be the bone, blocks the beam from reaching an imaging surface on the other side of the patient (see Fig. 10.1). Although the X-ray is the oldest technological extension of the physical exam, it is still the best at providing a detailed view of the bones, and X-rays are always appropriate for getting a detailed look at the bony parts of the spine. A very large fraction of all spine problems involve the vertebral bone itself. Even when the bones are not an issue, it is often important for the surgeon to have bone images to assist in the planning of surgery.

Figure 10.1 X-ray fluoroscopy machine. The C-arm structure of this Siremobil system from Siemens allows the operator to easily obtain an X-ray from any direction by rotating the C-arm around the patient table. The images are captured in the fluoroscope and shown on a video screen in real time. This advanced Iso-C 3D model provides a significant new technical advance: It can actually make a single-slice cross-sectional image similar to the image from a CT scanner. Reprinted with permission of Siemens AG.

X-Ray Categories: Portraits, Movies, and Cross-Sections

There are three main categories of X-rays. First is the plain X-ray, which is very much like a standard snapshot with a camera: An X-ray source on one side of the patient is turned on briefly, and an image of the patient appears on a plate or a piece of film on the other side. The X-rays charge right through the parts of the body that are the least dense, such as the watery tissues of the lung, and expose the X-ray plate below, darkening it. Whatever is most dense appears white, as that area of the film has the least exposure to the X-rays, thus producing the white appearance of the bones on an otherwise black background.

A second category is *fluoroscopy*, which is similar to a plain X-ray but is more like shooting a movie than using a single-shot camera. Instead of an X-ray plate at the receiving end of the beam, a fluorescent screen lights up where the X-rays hit it. The more X-rays it receives, such as those passing through the air and water in the body, the brighter the screen shines; and where the X-rays are blocked by bones, the screen is dark. What is essentially a movie or video camera takes pictures of the fluorescent screen while the X-rays are turned on. As the body moves, or the surgeon moves an instrument inside the patient during surgery, a continuing moving image is collected, which is generally viewed in real time on a television monitor.

The third major category of X-ray is *computerized axial tomography*, which is called *CAT scanning* or *CT scanning* for short. In the world of normal light and cameras, there is really no equivalent of what this scanning does or how it works; X-rays are used to produce a "slice" or a cross-sectional view of what's inside the body. This is explained further in the next section of the chapter.

What Else Does an X-ray Reveal?

Although X-rays are very good for imaging bone, they do show some of the soft tissues as well, as gray shadows. There are a number of soft tissue features in addition to bone problems that the radiologist, neurosurgeon, or orthopedist looks for when evaluating a spine X-ray after an injury. For instance, careful examination can identify shadows showing evidence of blood expanding the soft tissues of the neck in front of the spine.

In addition to looking for degenerative changes and fractures, X-rays can also be a good way to survey for the presence of certain types of tumors. For instance, a trained radiologist's eye will examine all the shapes, margins, and edges of the bones, particularly the pedicles (the struts that reach around the spinal canal to connect the vertebral body to the lamina, or roof of the vertebra behind). When the pedicles are viewed in an X-ray from directly behind the body, they appear like little, round "owl eyes" in much of the spine. The radiologist looks for any difference between right and left "eyes" and for any evidence of loss of normal bone density, either of which can reveal the presence of a tumor.

X-rays are also helpful in evaluating osteoporosis. Of the specialized forms of X-ray that are most useful for this, one is *dual-energy X-ray absorpsiometry* (DEXA) *scan*, which measures how much X-ray energy is actually passing through the bone, and thereby gives a measurement of calcium loss.

The Spine Series: Seeing It from All Angles

Plain X-rays still play a very important role in spinal diagnosis because they are superb at giving the doctor an overall view of the spine: its general appearance, its curves, the relationships among the bones, and evidence of arthritis and bone spurs. They are also a very good way to put together a simple view for information about the way the spine moves. Imaging the spine usually involves a series of X-rays taken from several angles, called a *spine series*.

The most common of these angles is an *anterior-posterior* (AP) X-ray, taken from the front toward the back; in some situations, the reverse, a *posterior-anterior* (PA) X-ray from the back forward, is also taken. There is also usually a *lateral X-ray* taken from the side, and *oblique X-rays* looking through the spine at some particularly useful diagonal angles. In evaluating the neck, there is usually an open-mouth view as well. This is because the top of the spine is behind the back of the mouth, so your jaw can get in the way or your teeth can hide the vertebrae from other angles. One way to solve the problem and get a clear picture of the very top is to have you open wide and to shoot the X-ray straight through the back of your mouth.

Oblique X-rays must be taken from both the left and right in order to see both sides, which is almost always desirable, at least for comparison. This brings us to another feature of X-rays, which is that the part of the bone that is closest to the X-ray plate shows up best. When the left side of the neck is closest to the plate, the left side appears much more sharply and clearly in the image, even though the X-rays cross through both the right and left sides. In this way, one side or the other of a bone can be seen.

One set of oblique X-rays is taken of the cervical spine and another set of the lumbar spine. Cervical oblique views are targeted at the foramina, or canals through which the nerve roots and spinal nerves travel when they leave the spine and travel into the body, toward the head and arms. The cervical nerve canals don't point straight out to the sides of the vertebrae, but instead point slightly forward; so if you angle the X-ray just right, you can actually get a view "straight up the barrel" of the nerve canals. This is a great way to look at all the nerve canals on one side and to see whether any of them are narrowed. As you can imagine, because the front and the back of the bone will overlap each other in an X-ray taken directly from the front, it is very difficult to determine the degree of canal narrowing unless you are looking straight up the canal.

Oblique X-rays in the lumbar region are used for a slightly different purpose, because standard lateral views can show the lumbar foramina very well. Lumbar oblique views are very helpful for getting a good picture of the joints, particularly when looking for weaknesses or fractures in the part of the vertebrae, the *pars interarticularis,* that leads into the joints. A congenital abnormality or a traumatic injury to the spine can result in a condition called spondylolysis, which is a gap or break in the connection between the facet joint and the rest of the vertebra, and the oblique X-ray is a very good way to see this abnormality.

The Flexion-Extension Study: Checking for Slips During Movement

In addition to the routine cervical and lumbar views is the important *flexion-extension study,* which is a set of lateral views (shot from the side). It generally looks at the neck bent forward, then held in a neutral position, and then bent all the way backward, and similarly for the lower back. This study is a good way to check for several types of problems in the spine, but its main focus is instability.

Normally, as the spine moves from a point of being bent forward (*flexion*) to a point of being bent backward (*extension*), the ligaments between the vertebrae and joints allow the entire spine to bend as if it were an essentially solid but flexible rod that stays smooth while bending. However, if there is abnormal movement between two of the vertebrae, one of them may slide backward when the neck is bent backward, so that instead of seeing a smooth, bent cylinder on the X-ray, you will see a protrusion backward. Then when the neck is bent forward, that same vertebra may slip to the front of the one below it. This slippage demonstrates instability or abnormal movement in the spine; it can happen as ligaments, joints, or disks begin to degenerate, or it can be a sign of injury after trauma.

The first objective of obtaining an X-ray after a neck or back injury is to look for any fractures. But even if no fractures are found, the spine may not be safe or secure. When the patient takes off the neck collar and first bends his or her neck forward or backward, if there is a complete tear of the ligaments, the vertebrae may slide out of alignment and do tremendous harm to the nerves or the spinal cord. That's why two of the important steps in proving that the spine is not injured after a trauma ("clearing the spine") are first the plain X-ray spine series and then the flexion-extension study. Taking flexion-extension X-rays sometimes has to be delayed as long as two weeks after a neck injury because even if ligaments are torn, the neck muscles may be in spasm and may temporarily keep

Figure 10.2 The CAT computerized axial tomography scanner is in the form of a thin ring. It uses X-rays to make a cross-sectional image of the human body. A high-quality CAT scan typically takes only a few seconds to complete.

the vertebrae in line, with the risk that as the muscle spasm wears off, sliding may begin. Therefore, the specialists who see a patient after a neck injury may decide to delay or repeat the flexion-extension X-rays to clear the patient's spine as having no abnormal movement.

Computerized Axial Tomography: Seeing in Slices

The specialized form of X-ray called computerized axial tomography, or CAT or CT scanning, creates an image that is a slice through the individual. The root of the word "tomography," "tom," means "cutting." It is a little puzzling to understand how light will do that, but it essentially involves taking a number of pictures from a number of different views (see Fig. 10.2).

An early type of tomography was portrayed in popular culture in the movie *The Exorcist*: little Regan is held upside-down in a chair in a doctor's office while a strange X-ray device travels around her head. The overall image, though eerily appropriate for that particular movie, does represent how tomograms were carried out before they were computerized. For the most part, noncomputerized tomography is a relic of the 1960s and 1970s. It is still occasionally performed to obtain particular, complex views of problems in the upper cervical spine, but this sort of plain tomographic study is rare, and there are probably many major cities in the United States where it isn't even offered anymore. The advent of the newest "volume" CT scanners with advanced computer reconstruction technology has finally surpassed the old spinal tomogram for clarity and detail in the sagittal plane. So, in any case, don't worry—if you are ever sent for a tomogram, you will not have to hang upside-down in a chair.

Who Thought of Doing This? Hounsfield at Wimbledon

The idea of using computers to improve tomography was originated and fully developed by an engineer at the music record company EMI, Sir Godfrey Newbold Hounsfield, who was knighted and eventually won the Nobel prize for devising CT scanning. He took his idea to the Minister of Health in the United Kingdom, who sent him to the leading neurological hospital in England, Queens Square Neurological Hospital, where he was directed to the chief of neuroradiology. Hounsfield presented his idea of how to make cross-sectional images through the brain and spine. The chief radiologist became very upset, told him that he could already diagnose every condition perfectly with existing technology, and that there was no need for cross-sectional images. He threw Hounsfield out of his office and even called the Minister of Health, telling him Hounsfield was an eccentric and never to send him or anyone else like him to waste his time in the future.

Fortunately for the rest of us, Hounsfield figuratively picked himself up and dusted himself off, and went down the road to the next best neurological hospital in England, which was Atkinson-Morley's Hospital in Wimbledon, just up the street from the tennis courts. Although many British like to do things in the old, conservative way, they also tend to like an eccentric, and Jamie Ambrose, the chief of neuroradiology at Atkinson-Morley's, thought this was an interesting idea. Before long, Hounsfield was set up in a downstairs room with a dentist's chair, a pig's head, and a bunch of dental X-ray cameras. Soon enough, he produced the first cross-sectional X-ray image of a nonliving organism, and rapidly moved on to the first CT scans of the brain in live human patients. The rest, as they say, is history.

Spirals, Electron Beams, and Reconstructions

The idea underlying CT scanning is to shine a beam of light no wider than a pencil lead through the body and to put a detector at the other end to measure how much of the light was absorbed, thus measuring the total average density of the body through a single path. Then the light source is rotated on the detector a little bit to measure the average density at a slightly different angle, and then at another angle, and another, taking dozens and then hundreds of different shots through the body from slightly different angles. A computer can process all of this data, showing where the dense parts are and where the nondense parts are, and ends up producing an image of what the body would look like if you were to slice through it at a designated level. The body is then ratcheted past the light source and detector a few more millimeters to take another series of measurements, then ratcheted another few millimeters to take another series, soon resulting in a stack of slices showing the densities all through the body.

The very earliest CT scanner developed by Hounsfield probably took about ten or twelve different views, and then "sliced" the side of the head in five or six places, whereas the most modern CT scanner takes thousands and thousands of views at an extremely rapid pace. The technology of CT scanners has advanced so that multiple slices can be taken at the same time—this allows the possibility of getting thinner and thinner slices that show progressively more detail and do a better and better job of suppressing "metal artifact" when you are scanned after a metal implant has been placed in your spine. These advanced scanners are described by the number of scans they can take at the same time—4-slice, 16-slice, 64-slice scanners, and so on.

The whole process now only takes a matter of seconds and produces a spectacularly detailed internal view of the brain, the body, or a specific body part such as the spine. In fact, using advanced computer technology, it is possible to put together all those slices, reconstruct a full three-dimensional shape of the body, and then simulate a fly-through of the body's internal structures (see Fig. 16.8). One important aspect to keep in mind, though, is that this can result in a great deal of X-ray radiation—equivalent to the radiation from hundreds of chest X-rays taken all at once. The newest scanners have improved X-ray detectors or receivers so that lower doses of X-ray will produce an image that is just as effective.

So, in the nearly forty-five years since Hounsfield first had his idea, the CT scan has gone from being a crude first view into the interior to being a dramatically advanced and incredibly sensitive tool that looks at very fine structures such as tiny plaques in the arteries. Continuing advances are directed at reducing the radiation dose required for the excellent imaging. Among different imaging techniques, the CT scan provides an excellent way to see the bony details of the spine.

Contrast Agents to Extend the Capabilities of X-rays

Although X-rays and CTs have a very great range of helpful uses, they can accomplish even more when they are aided by the administration of contrast agents. The prototypical contrast material in X-ray is based on iodine. The iodine atom is very high up in number along the periodic chart, and that is what it takes to block X-rays efficiently (carbon has an atomic weight of 12, calcium is 40, and iodine is 127). The iodine is held by a biologically safe molecule that carries it through the body dissolved in a fluid that can mix safely with various body fluids. The earliest iodine-based contrast dyes were later discovered to cause serious nerve irritation in some patients, but modern "non-ionic" iodine agents are extremely safe. Nonetheless, some patients are allergic to them so they are always given with careful monitoring and adequate medical backup available.

When iodine contrast agents are injected into the bloodstream, it is possible to make an X-ray of the blood vessels, or an *angiogram*. Contrast in the spinal fluid allows the X-rays or CT scanner to show where the nerves are floating and to confirm some types of spinal nerve root compression, a process called *myelography*. Contrast injected into the intervertebral disk space can be used to generate a *discogram* that shows fine details of the interior of a disk. Angiograms are used only in unusual and rare spinal disorders involving abnormal blood vessels and tumors. Myelograms and discograms, however, are still very commonly used in spine diagnosis.

Myelography: An Old Technique That Won't Go Away

Because of the density of the element iodine, which has many protons and neutrons in its nucleus, effective contrast effects are produced even in low concentrations. By injecting a small amount of iodine contrast agent into the spinal fluid, you can make the fluid appear on an X-ray as even more dense than bone. This is the basis of myelography, which involves inserting a needle into the spinal fluid and injecting a dye of iodine in a carrier molecule of some sort. On a *myelogram*, the dye will outline any pinches of the *dural sac* (enclosing membranes) around the nerves and will also give a view of how the nerves and spinal cord take up space with in the fluid. The image provides initial insight into the internal anatomy of the spine and its neural structures. Once the dye has been put in, you can obtain both a plain myelogram with a regular set of X-rays taken in different positions and then a CT myelogram, which actually requires far less dye and can be taken a while after the initial injection.

Despite the general safety of modern contrast agents, myelography is still an invasive test with risks: Spinal fluid can leak from the point where the dura is punctured by the needle, possibly causing headaches, or dye can go into the wrong space, possibly causing some pain or interfering with the utility of the picture produced. If enough dye leaks upstream and around the brain, some patients may have reactions to the dye and occasionally even seizures. In the 1960s and 1970s it was common to use myelogram dyes that had another risk—a chronic inflammation of neural tissue inside the dura membranes called arachnoiditis. Modern contrast agents greatly reduce this risk. So although myelography is still a very useful tool and can be conducted safely, it certainly bears risks beyond those of exposure to some X-rays.

X-ray radiation itself does pose a small risk, and it is always best to minimize this. Nonetheless, except in situations such as pregnancy, a small amount of X-ray radiation is felt to present a low enough risk that myelography continues to be considered as a method of getting diagnostic information about the spine. It is increasingly possible, however, to get much of this information from more modern studies such as MR neurography, which requires no contrast agent and involves no X-rays (see Fig. 10.3).

Myelography was very common before the widespread availability of MRI, and now it is a specialized test used when other tests fail or because of unusual aspects of the underlying problem that the doctor is trying to diagnose. Plain and CT myelograms are especially important for patients who have metal instrumentation in the spine. Metal implants cause quite a bit of distortion in the magnetic fields used to produce an MRI scan, so reliance on the CT scan becomes necessary. In addition, fine details of the interactions between bone, nerve, and spinal dura sometimes cannot be seen in adequate resolution on an MRI because the MRI doesn't depict calcium and bone very well. With the occasional limitations of other imaging techniques and the unique aspects of myelography, there is still a place for myelograms.

Figure 10.3 Myelogram and neurogram. The myelogram image on the right (B) is obtained by injecting an iodine dye into the spinal fluid space. It provides precise detail about the shape of the dural lining of the spinal canal. The magnetic resonance (MR) neurogram on the left (A)—showing the same patient—provides similar information but also shows the spinal nerves after they exit from the dura. Both images show normal anatomy at the asterisk (*), but the Neurogram shows a nerve pinch (n). The MR neurogram does not require any injection.

Discography: Revealing Painful Rips

Another important use of injection-contrast agents is for detailed study of the disks. The procedure of *discography* involves using X-ray or fluoroscopic guidance to put a needle into the disk space between vertebrae and inject medication, such as an anesthetic and steroid combination, along with a contrast agent directly into the disk. It is then possible to see on the image, called a discogram, if there is any tear in the retaining ring, or annulus, of the disk. There is usually a plain discogram and a CT discogram, done in sequence at the same imaging session, and this gives a very nice picture of any tears within the disk space.

Discography carries a risk of infection because the disk space itself doesn't have its own blood supply and is not very well protected. The procedure can also be painful, particularly if it is difficult getting the needle in place or if the disk is extremely sensitive, in which case even injecting anesthetic may actually cause more pain than pain relief. Discography to demonstrate annular tears is still an essential study for many types of spinal pain and is used in a number of specialized types of spinal pain treatment, such as *intradiscal electrothermy* (IDET; see chapter 12 for an explanation).

As with myelography, the discogram still carries with it the risks of iodine reaction and significant exposure to X-rays. In my own clinical work, I've developed and have considerable experience with MR discography (see Fig. 12.2). For this test, there is no radiation, and the contrast effect is provided by the water in the local anesthetic. An MR discogram provides excellent detail and is also less painful for the patient because of the accuracy of needle placement. This is a new procedure, however, requiring specially configured interventional MRI scanners, which are not widely available.

Ultrasound, Nuclear Medicine, and Holograms

Although the vast majority of all spinal diagnostic imaging involves X-rays or MRI scanning, there are some situations in which ultrasound or nuclear medicine can play a role. The principal limitation of ultrasound for spinal imaging is that the imaging effects of ultrasound are blocked out by the hard tissue of spinal bone. Nonetheless, during a surgery directed at the interior of the spinal canal, ultrasound can play an important role. Once the spinal lamina has been removed, the ultrasound can look through the spinal dura to locate a tumor precisely. Ultrasound can also be helpful in young infants who have relatively little bone formation and who have very high risk from X-ray exposure. It also can play a critical role in diagnosing serious spine abnormalities in the unborn fetus as part of prenatal imaging.

Nuclear medicine involves placing controlled nuclear reactions inside the human body. For X-rays, ultrasound, and MRI, the image requires directing some energy into the body and then observing what comes back out. For nuclear medicine imaging, however, the actual source of the energy is placed inside in the form of various radioactive elements. One application sometimes useful for spinal diagnosis is the bone scan. In this test, a radioactive compound is injected in a chemical form that will distribute itself into bone in a fashion that can reveal injuries and abnormalities in the bone.

The quality of the image resolution in nuclear medicine, however, is generally quite low. The emerging gamma rays are detected with a flat camera or in a tomographic system called SPECT, which stands for *single-photon emissioncomputed tomography*. A slightly higher resolution can be achieved with certain types of nuclear reactions that lead to matter-antimatter annihilations; these are detected by a process called positron emission tomography (PET). At present, PET is used to detect tumors with high growth rates assessed by oxygen consumption or metabolic rate.

One other image technology bears some mention, and that is the *hologram*. This is really a means of viewing medical images rather than a means of obtaining them. A hologram uses an optical phenomenon called interference to generate a shimmering three-dimensional image that appears to float in space in front of the viewer. In the future, this sort of viewing technology may help surgeons understand some of the complex shapes of the abnormal spine as part of the surgical planning process.

Magnetic Resonance Imaging: "Tuning In" to the Body's Water

Once Hounsfield had introduced the medical world to the value of cross-sectional imaging with CAT scanning, the search was on for ways to obtain even better scans without the X-ray exposure. Another area of physics came to the rescue with the development of magnetic resonance imaging (MRI). Difficult as it is to conceive of how shining a tiny beam of light through the body results in a cross section, the trick to understanding MRI is perhaps even more complex.

Magnetic resonance images essentially show the presence of water in the body, rather than looking at density, the way X-rays do. The fundamental property in magnetic resonance is in the realm of magnets and radiowaves. One of the basic physics experiments many of us saw in elementary school showed that moving a magnet can produce an electric field and that moving an electric field can produce magnetism; an MRI is based on those principles.

Spinning Hydrogen Nuclei in a Magnetic Field

A critical aspect of MRI is the magnetic field of a single proton, which is essentially the nucleus of a hydrogen atom (the H in the formula H_2O for water). The nucleus of a hydrogen atom spins around on its axis just like the earth does, and it also has a magnetic orientation. If you put a hydrogen atom inside a big, strong magnet's magnetic field, the magnetic axis of the hydrogen atom will align with the axis of the larger magnetic field. As the nucleus spins, it generates an electric field in the form of a fluctuating radiofrequency signal. The nucleus of a hydrogen atom, like any other type of atom, has a very precise rate at which it prefers to spin. This rate is based on arcane aspects of nuclear physics, but it does vary exactly in proportion to the strength of any magnetic field surrounding it.

When you beam specially tuned radiowaves into water, it can add energy to the spinning of the hydrogen nuclei, at their exact resonant frequency. This is the same principle as the sympathetic vibration of a tuning fork in response to a sung note of the appropriate frequency (when a singer sings the note C in front of a tuning fork tuned to C, the tuning fork will receive some of the energy and then transmit it out again by actually humming the same note itself).

Gradients to Give Every Spot in the Body a Different Spin

The idea of creating an image by using a magnetic field was one of those classic inventions written out on a napkin in a moment of desperation and inspiration by Paul Lauterbur. The result of his invention, Magnetic Resonance Imaging, has completely transformed medicine and is continuing to do so as the capabilities of this technology continue to expand. Ironically, the technology assessment specialists for the State University of New York decided not to go forward with a patent on the invention on the basis that they did not think there was much commercial value in it. In 2003, Paul Lauterbur was awarded the Nobel Prize for his contributions-along with those of Sir Peter Mansfield and Raymond Damadian, among others-that helped to lead to the development of MRI scanning.

The MRI Scanning Process

An MRI scan usually takes anywhere from three to ten minutes to complete. Usually, an MRI scanner is able to look at a volume of only about one square foot in the center of the magnet.

MRI scanners vary in quality because design differences affect their ability to perform on a number of fronts. They have magnets of various strength (super-powered 3 Tesla imagers, on down to 0.1 Tesla) and also differ in a number of other technical aspects. All of these features affect how good the picture will be and how long it will take to complete the imaging process.

MRI Sees the Soft Tissues: Information and Complexity

Although CT scanning is good for looking at bones, MRI is good for seeing soft tissue such as the disks in the spine, the spinal fluid inside the dura, and the nerves inside the spinal fluid, which show up as dark shadows. MRI can also visualize bone, in that a lot of bone is made up of blood and fatty tissue. Very solid, hard cortical bone contains very little water and is essentially black on an MRI; that's why bone spurs don't show up well other than appearing as black or empty spaces displacing soft tissues. Nonetheless, MRI is usually the most comprehensive way to see herniated disks. It is very good for imaging fractures, narrowing of the spinal canal, tumors, and a wide variety of tissues (see Fig. 10.4).

An MRI is often the first place to start a search for a diagnosis because it does not involve any risky exposure to X-rays. Scientists have never been able to find any symptoms that are due to the effects of the magnetic and radiofrequency fields used in standard MRI, so it is very safe, and there is also no need for a spinal needle puncture as with a myelogram. Sometimes it is necessary to administer a contrast dye, usually intravenously, in trying to distinguish on an MRI between a recurrent disk herniation and the formation of scar tissue. The contrast agent used in MRI is not iodine but the element *gadolinium* (chosen for its magnetic properties rather than its density).

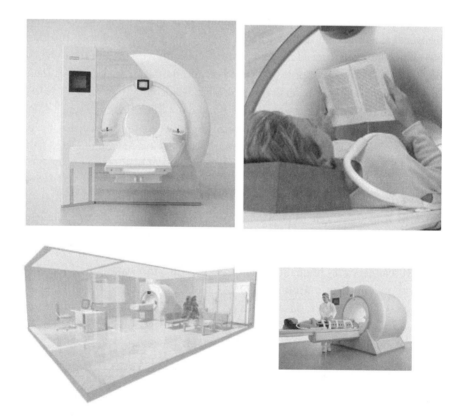

Figure 10.4 MRI scanners. The best MRI images are produced in imagers that are shaped like long tubes. As the technology advances, the tubes have become shorter. The whole imaging study may take anywhere from fifteen to forty-five minutes. Harmony and Symphony MRI Systems illustrations reprinted with permission of Siemens AG.

The free-floating atoms of gadolinium do have some toxicity and don't dissolve in blood. To use the gadolinium, each atom is mounted in molecular carrier called a chelator (based on the Greek work for teeth). The name of the chelator molecule is a true mouthful: diethylene triamine pentaacetic acid (DTPA). Each molecule has five electrically charged points on it that point toward the center of the molecule. The atom of gadolinium is electrically trapped as it floats at the center point surrounded by these five electrical teeth. The whole complex of gadolinium-DTPA is very safe, dissolves well into the bloodstream, and is separated very efficiently by the kidneys to be excreted into the urine after the imaging test is complete.

Good MRIs and Bad MRIs: Caveat Emptor

This leads to the question of whether all MRIs are the same. Out there in the clinical world, top-quality MRI magnets are usually 3.0 or 1.5 Tesla and usually require the patient to be positioned inside a tube. Unfortunately, the closed tube of high-performance MRI scanners may lead to an experience of claustrophobia in some people.

In fact, many people have no idea that they have claustrophobia until their first MRI scan. Some people can manage it by having their eyes closed or by wearing special reflector glasses that let them look out the end of the tube. Some need a little anti-anxiety medication, and others simply can't tolerate an MRI without being made completely unconscious through medication. This sort of sedation for MRI can usually be arranged if the MRI is absolutely essential; however, the image center must also have MRI-compatible equipment for monitoring vital signs during the scanning process for sedated patients. Lower-field magnets, such as a 1 Tesla magnet, may also entail being in a tube and produce a slightly lower quality image.

The reason for the closed tube is the electric coil that generates the magnetic field: It wraps around the tube, and the electricity flowing around in it is kept going with supercooled fluids in the magnet chamber. There are, however, a variety of types of open MRI scanners, such as electromagnets that are two flat disks with magnetic fields between them; the patient lies on a bed or sits in a chair between the two disks (see Fig. 16.9). There are also a few other configurations for the magnetic fields that give the patient the experience of being in more of an open room. The space that you are in may be important to you: In CT scanning, the whole study may take a matter of seconds, whereas for an MRI, each sequence may take three to ten minutes, and the whole study may take up to an hour.

MRIs definitely vary in quality. Some show tremendous detail, some are virtually unreadable. Open MRIs, in general, don't have as good a quality as closed MRIs. A high-field system with a 1.5 Tesla magnet and special advanced antenna coils called phased array coils gives the best possible image. It is interesting that for a top-of-the-line, fully equipped magnet or for a very simple low-field, poor-quality magnet, the cost is actually the same to the patient and to the insurance company. So it is always worthwhile for the patient to consider that for the same price, why not get a high-quality image in fifteen minutes instead of a low-quality image that takes forty-five minutes to complete.

One circumstance that may warrant having an open MRI would be a significant problem with claustrophobia. Other factors are simply the size or weight of the patient or what MRI machine happens to be available in the community. Also, insurance companies such as HMOs sometimes try to pay a very low price, and because the open, low-field magnets may be much less expensive, they are more likely to offer their services to low-cost HMOs.

MR Angiography and MR Neurography and DTI: A First Look at the Vessels or Nerves

In addition to the basic type of MRI, there are a couple of special types. One is *MR angiography*, which gives a special view of the blood vessels; this is only occasionally important in diagnosing a spine problem. Another is *MR neurography*, a technique that I invented. Until the advent of this technique, none of the imaging methods provided any means for imaging nerves after they left the spinal column to travel through the body. MR neurography provides a detailed view of the nerves and is sometimes important in diagnosing spinal disease as well (see Fig. 10.5).

Figure 10.5 Magnetic resonance neurogram of the neck. Unlike a standard MRI, a neurogram shows the nerves including the dorsal root ganglions (d), which are important sensory processing points outside the spinal cord. An injured or compressed nerve may show up as hyperintense (h), or abnormally bright. An MR neurogram also shows where spinal nerves (s) are bent out of their normal straight course by an entrapment.

One reason that neurography is important for spinal diagnosis is that it is very effective for showing compressions of the spinal nerves as they travel through the spinal foramina. This part of the spinal nerve is difficult to see well on standard MRI and can't be seen in a myelogram. An MR neurogram also includes an *MR myelogram* (see Fig 10.3), which provides a view of the spinal fluid sac without having to have the needle puncture. MR neurography is also important in identifying problems with nerves outside the spine that may otherwise be mistaken for spinal problems. Because of its emphasis on the nerve itself, the view in a neurogram sometimes helps to distinguish unimportant bumps, spurs, or lumps from those that actually are important because they are compressing, flattening, or irritating a nerve.

DTI stands for *diffusion tensor imaging*—a new type of MRI that is now used prior to virtually all brain surgery in United States and is increasingly used for evaluation of head injuries. It is becoming more important in evaluating spinal cord injuries and is also used to evaluate more subtle nerve impingements and spinal root compressions. DTI (which I also invented) provides a view of the neural fibers themselves. This is particularly striking in the brain where it has allowed surgeons to see the critical pathways that must be avoided during surgery. DTI is very sensitive for detection of subtle damage to nerves and neural tracts that don't show up in other types of MRI. It detects a special property of nerve axons in which water diffuses up and down the length of the nerve (anisotropy) instead of diffusing in all directions (isotropy) as in most other tissues. This property of neurons is affected by mild injury so DTI's ability to detect this is expected to further extend the sensitivity of nerve and spine diagnostics just as it already has for the brain.

Electrodiagnosis: Shocks Through Needles

Quite apart from the use of medical imaging, it is often necessary to study the electrical behavior of nerves to determine the nature of a patient's problem. A typical situation where this is valuable occurs when it appears from an image that a disk is pinching one of the nerves to the leg. The patient tells the doctor that there is pain, numbness, or even weakness. The electrodiagnostic tests can objectively verify what the patient is describing.

Electrodiagnostics can also help to distinguish among various suspected problems. One example of this would be the use of these tests to help to confirm the doctor's impression that the patient is experiencing symptoms from a single nerve root. Sometimes an electrodiagnostic test can pinpoint the location of a nerve pinch, and sometimes it just shows details about the affected muscles that are difficult for the patient or the doctor otherwise to identify reliably.

The drawback to any electrodiagnostic test is that it generally involves sticking needles into the patient and administering an electric shock; this, as you can imagine, is not always the most pleasant experience. The more needles inserted, and the more electric shocks given, the better the diagnostic information that is provided to the physician-which all sounds like a pretty bad deal for the patient. Nonetheless, these tests do play an important role in spinal diagnosis.

Electromyography: Objective Evidence from the Muscles

Electromyography (EMG) is based on putting needles into muscles and evaluating how the muscles react to being activated or electrically stimulated. Electromyography shows how a muscle is affected when the nerves that innervate it are dying off or when regrowing axons are finally arriving at the muscle after a nerve compression has been relieved. An EMG provides evidence of an abnormality, such as a nerve irritation that underlies muscle spasm, when otherwise all that can be seen is the patient experiencing subjective pain. This may be very helpful when an objective test is needed to confirm a patient's claim, such as in workmen's compensation litigation. Another area of use for an EMG would be where the findings from diagnostic imaging are uncertain, and the physician wants additional information in order to plan treatment.

Nerve Conduction Velocity: Speed and Site

Together with the EMG, a test of *nerve conduction velocity* (NCV) is very good for spotting pinches of the nerves out in the body and extremities: in the wrist at the carpal tunnel; in the elbow at the cubital tunnel; in the leg near the head of the *fibula* bone and the *peroneal nerve*; and in the ankle at the tarsal tunnel. Basically, in an NCV test, a needle sends an electrical signal into the nerve in question, an electrode picks it up when it passes by, and a timer measures how long it took for the signal to travel that distance down the nerve. In a pinched nerve, the signal travels more slowly than it otherwise would. By taking measurements at different segments in the nerve, NCV tests can actually locate the site at which the slowing of the signal occurs.

Evoked Potentials: Protection During Surgery

The third type of electrodiagnostic test, which is often used during surgery for protective monitoring, is called *evoked potentials* (see Fig. 10.6). This includes checkups on your sensory nerves, or *somatosensory evoked potentials* (SSEPs), as well as checks on your motor system, *motor evoked potentials* (MEPs). The SSEP is a way to send a signal into a part of the body such as the hand or foot and then to measure the signal's travel time and strength as it makes its way through the

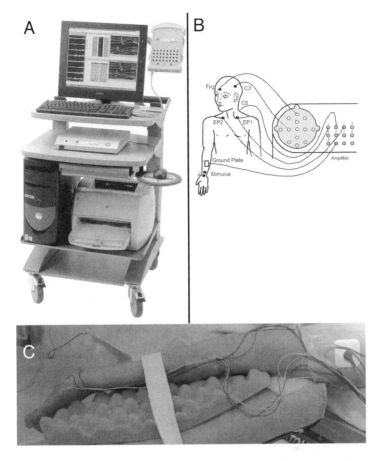

Figure 10.6 Intraoperative electrodiagnostic monitoring. For some surgeries, the surgeon will monitor electrical function of the nerves and spinal cord during the course of the operation. The SSEP (somatosensory evoked potential) waveform on the screen (A) monitors sensory function. The motor side of the nervous system can be monitored with EMG (electromyography). (C) Electrodes from the scalp and limbs are connected to the monitoring equipment (B). Cascade monitoring device photograph reproduced with permission of Cadwell Laboratories Inc.

nerves and spinal cord to reach the surface of the brain. The MEP starts with a magnetic stimulus over the surface of the scalp and ends up causing a tiny twitch in your hand or foot.

The signal that arrives in the brain after a quick SSEP stimulus to the hand or foot is a very tiny, very faint bit of electrical activity, masked by the hundreds of millions of other cells firing all around it as the brain goes about its normal activities. The idea of an evoked potential is to use a computer-based strategy to detect and to enhance the incoming signal.

The strategy has two components. The first is *time locking*: This means that the computer looks through its electrodes on the scalp to find an arriving signal at a precise predicted time delay, or *latency*, after the triggering stimulus in the hand or foot. The second component is repetition: The signal is repeated identically hundreds of times. By adjusting the latency, the technician then locates the incoming signal and the computer summates the hundreds of identical *cortical responses*. Everything else coming in from the cortical surface tends to vary constantly in wave form, timing, and intensity, while the SSEP signal always arrives at the same instant, same strength, and same waveform.

If, during surgery, a nerve becomes pinched or the spinal cord becomes subject to excessive pressure, the SSEP or MEP computer will detect this. The signals will start arriving later, they will vary more in their arrival times, and the overall intensity will start to drop off. The technician can warn the surgeon of the change. This gives the surgeon a chance to move a retractor or reposition an instrument in such a way to relieve a pressure on a nerve that otherwise might not have been noticed.

Knowledge and Power: A Good Diagnosis Is the Key to Good Treatment

The last thing any patient wants is "exploratory surgery" in which a surgeon digs around inside the body looking for some clue as to what might be wrong with the patient. This is why a complete and definitive diagnosis—knowledge of exactly what is wrong—really should be in hand before any sort of aggressive or invasive treatment is considered. Fortunately, modern diagnostic science has advanced tremendously. Through the various elegant methods described here, it is usually possible for your doctor to know with a great deal of precision exactly what is causing your problem. The more precise the diagnosis, the more precise the repair, and the greater the chance of successful treatment.

11

Recovery and Repair in the Nerves and Spinal Cord

When any of your nerves are subjected to irritation, compression, trauma, or restriction of movement or in any other way find themselves in an abnormal surrounding, you may experience symptoms as a result. The very first symptoms of a nerve irritation or injury will usually be some kind of pain. With more severe pressure on a nerve, you may notice numbness, tingling, or some altered quality of sensation. The numbness may progress to be more and more complete, and as the pressure becomes more severe, the nerve's signals to its target muscle may be interrupted or disrupted so that weakness occurs.

Any of these symptoms—pain, numbness, weakness, or loss of normal function—lead people to seek medical help. A doctor's diagnostic plan is intended to identify the cause of the problem, and the chosen treatment is intended to relieve whatever is bothering the nerve. But what goes on inside the troubled nerve itself? Further, how likely is it that repairing a nerve will allow it to return to normal?

How Nerves Recover from Injury

The overall message of this chapter is that nerves do have a great potential to regrow and to recover function. For this reason, it is always worthwhile to consider treatment when nerve function is disrupted. The way a nerve conducts signals is somewhat like the way electricity is transmitted in a wire; however, it is also somewhat like the way water moves through a pipe. Therefore, both the liquid contents and the outer casing of a nerve must be properly intact for it to convey an electrical signal. This situation is unique in comparison to almost anything in the mechanical world around us and is critical to the transmission of nerve impulses in biological systems. To understand the way that nerves are organized, it may also be helpful to consider their similarity to wires inside of a conduit. In electrical engineering, a conduit is a piece of tubing installed in a wall or other structure through which wires are passed to help them reach their destination and also to protect them from being struck by nails during construction. This is somewhat like the way conduits in the body help nerves to go where they should during nerve regrowth.

Pressure and Scarring

To understand the potential for nerves to recover, it is helpful to outline the ways in which nerves are affected by adverse surrounding conditions. In response to conditions such as nerve compression, irritation from a nearby tissue injury, or an *adhesion* (abnormal attachment) that causes a nerve to rub or to be pulled in the course of normal activity, the body produces inflammatory chemicals called *bradykinins*, which lead to swelling at the site of the problem. Apparently, the chemical events associated with inflammation impair the normal function of the affected nerves, and the brain often perceives this impairment as pain or potentially as numbness or weakness. This kind of interruption of nerve function is usually relieved very rapidly once the local irritant is gone.

A slightly more significant level of pressure is comparable to what all of us have experienced when a leg or arm "goes to sleep." This occurs when a pressure mechanically deforms a nerve sufficiently to interrupt its biophysical processes temporarily. The resulting weakness, numbness, and tingling resolve very rapidly as soon as the pressure is removed, taking a few minutes at most. But when a deforming pressure is maintained for a long enough time, certain types of more lasting breakdown begin to occur.

One problematic aspect of nerve compression is the potential for scarring to develop around the nerve. The medical word for scarring, *fibrosis*, describes the activation and function of *fibrocytes*, which are cells that produce fibrous tissue. The natural and correct purpose of fibrosis is to fill in and close any open wounds in the skin and deeper tissues. Unfortunately, when excessive new fibrous tissue is laid down around an injured nerve, it can impede the nerve's recovery later. Nerves normally glide with body movements; but when fibrous tissue causes an adhesion that prevents a nerve from gliding properly, movement results in small and possibly painful tugs on the nerve. In cases of more severe compression, fibrous tissue can actually form inside the nerve *fascicle* where the effects of scarring can be virtually irreparable. A fascicle is a collection of dozens or hundreds of nerve fibers that travel together to their destination. Most nerves are made up of a collection of fascicles separated from each other by fatty padding tissue within the overall bundle that makes up the nerve (see Fig. 11.1).

For the most common types of spine problems, such as pinched nerves, herniated disks, and narrowed nerve canals, the prospects for recovery of normal function are very good. In general, symptoms will improve immediately within a few hours of corrective surgery or, at worst, within a few weeks. Mild

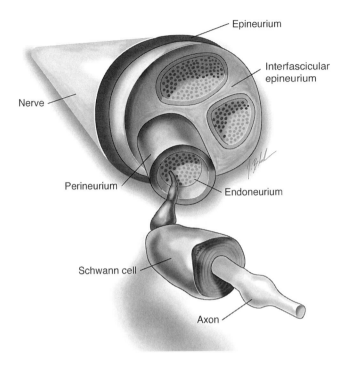

Figure 11.1 Nerve structure. A nerve is usually made up of a variety of fascicles. Each fascicle is encased by perineurium. Inside the fascicle are a group of axons bathed in endoneurial fluid. Each axon has an insulating lining of myelin, a fatty material inside the Schwann cells. Between the fascicles is a fatty material called the interfascicular epineurium. The nerve is then wrapped in the main epineurium. Even if the sensitive living extensions of the nerve—the axons—are damaged, the conduit made up of epineurium and perineurium will often survive and provide a pathway for regrowing nerves. Image published with permission of Joe Bloch.

compressions that cause only pain and a little numbness are sometimes even allowed to persist without surgical treatment in hopes that they will resolve on their own. More severe and lasting nerve injuries do occur, however, and some problems become more and more intractable the longer the pressure remains on the nerve. For this reason, severe compressions that result in actual weakness are generally viewed as warranting surgical *decompression* (removal of the pressure on the nerve) without extended delay (see chapters 14 and 20).

Demyelination and Loss of Insulation

To keep the electrical charges where they need to be in order to transmit information, most nerve fibers require their own individual insulating lining made of a fatty material called *myelin*. Myelin is formed inside a type of cell, called a *Schwann cell*, that wraps around the outside of a nerve cell to provide a layer of myelin insulation. Pressure on a nerve causes *demyelination*. The myelin coating

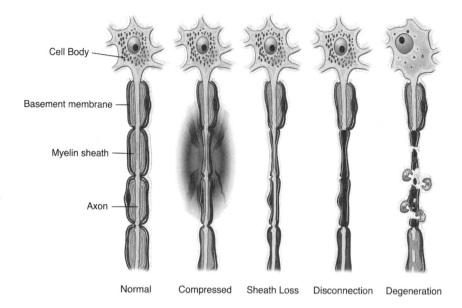

Cell Body

Basement membrane

Myelin sheath

Axon

Normal   Compressed   Sheath Loss   Disconnection   Degeneration

Figure 11.2 Types of nerve damage. When a nerve is compressed or injured, a variety of injuries can usually be found; each has its own time course for recovery. A simple compression will recover very rapidly; if the sheath is destroyed, then weeks may be required for a new insulating lining to be rebuilt. If the axon itself is disrupted, then a replacement must be grown from the cut point all the way on out to the skin or muscle at a rate of one to four millimeters per day. If the conduit itself is destroyed, then a regrowing nerve may never find its way past the point of injury. Image published with permission of Joe Bloch.

begins to wear away and break down, and with inadequate insulation, the nerve won't transmit signals properly.

Once the pressure is relieved, surviving Schwann cells that lost their myelin need time to regenerate their insulation, and new Schwann cells need to migrate to the site to fill in any gaps. This process takes a few weeks at most, and once the insulating lining is completely restored, the nerve returns to normal function. More severe and prolonged pressure, however, may lead not only to destruction of myelin but also to the disruption of the nerve cell itself (see Fig. 11.2).

Broken Nerves Need Open Conduits

It is possible to put sufficient pressure on a nerve that the *axons*, the fibers of nerve tissue that travel from the nerve cell body to the target tissue and conduct electrical signals, are fully disrupted and actually break down. When this happens, everything "downstream;" or beyond the point of injury, is gravely affected: The entire portion of the axon extending from the point of disruption to the axon's normal end at the muscle or skin dies off and becomes permanently unrecoverable. Back "upstream:" however, the cell body of the nerve survives, and so does the intact portion of the axon running from the cell body to the point of injury. Fortunately, the ending of a broken nerve has a tremendous potential to regrow.

Although a nerve is inherently able to recover, regrow, and reconnect, it can do so efficiently only when two conditions exist. The first condition is that the conduit or bulk mechanical *nerve tube* in which it travels is still intact. The growing *nerve cone*, the tip of a regenerating nerve, will simply progress forward along the conduit and continue all the way to its normal ending, where the nerve will then regrow its attachment to the muscle, skin sensor, or other organ.

When the conduit itself is interrupted, however, the regrowing nerve has to find out how to get through the body to get where it is going, and most such nerves immediately become hopelessly lost. If the nerve end is near its target, it may pick up the chemical signals that will help to tell it where to go, but if it is at any significant distance from its target, it may go to the wrong target or simply fail to progress at all. That is why the end of a disrupted nerve with no preserved conduit will form a ball of abnormal nerve tissue called a *neuroma*, which may be very painful.

In addition to having a preserved conduit, the second condition is that the interior of the conduit must be sufficiently open to allow the growing nerve to travel through the area of injury. The reason that nerve regrowth doesn't always work is that the conduit may become filled with scar tissue. Scar tissue is often impenetrable for a regrowing nerve ending, which will again come to a halt in a useless ball of nerve tissue.

Nerve regrowth is slow, taking place at a rate of about a millimeter per day. For example, a severely injured nerve with axon die-off starting at the level of your knee could take months to regenerate all the way out to your toe. Nonetheless, if the conduit is intact and is not blocked by scar tissue, regrowth of the nerve will occur.

Fixing Damaged Nerves and Conduits

When a nerve is fully severed and its conduit is completely disrupted, or the conduit is intact but completely filled with scar tissue, it is generally quite unlikely that the nerve will grow back to its target, and the only potential for recovery is through surgery. To reconnect the nerve, the surgeon either replaces the missing or scarred segment with a nerve graft or inserts a synthetic material to restore the conduit, allowing the regrowing nerve to travel through it to its ending. The process of reconnecting nerves often includes waiting until scar tissue has finished forming inside the damaged ends of the nerves so that the scar can be cut out and fresh, open nerve can be used for the graft or for the entubulation process.

Obstacles to Reconnection

As already mentioned, one limitation on the recovery capability of nerves is the problem of assuring that regrowing nerves reach the right targets. This can be difficult even when the nerve conduit can be reconstructed, because there may be dozens of smaller conduits inside a main nerve conduit and there is really no way to match them up in fine detail.

The other big obstacle has to do with the working end where the nerve connects with, or *innervates,* its target. Once a muscle has been without any nerve input for six to twelve months, it becomes unreceptive to *reinnervation* (reconnection with the nerve). So even when everything is done right to help a disrupted nerve grow back to its target muscle, if it takes as long as a year for the nerve to arrive, reinnervation may not succeed after all because the muscle may no longer receive the incoming nerve.

This time constraint on nerve repair is an important issue. It is often difficult to know whether a nerve is going to grow back on its own, and therefore some time may be allowed to elapse after symptoms of nerve injury or irritation appear. After a month, if there is no recovery of function or cessation of pain, it can be assumed that the problem is not simply a matter of compression affecting the nerve's myelin sheath. Magnetic resonance neurography imaging may make it possible to determine directly whether the nerve is intact or disrupted, and if it is disrupted, then surgical nerve repair can be considered.

The Promise of Grafts and Entubulation

A *nerve graft* (a piece of a nerve that is spliced in at the site of injury) can be made in several ways. The most common source is a transplant from the patient's own body. Nobody really has an "extra" nerve, but the one most commonly used for this purpose is the relatively expendable sural nerve. The *sural nerve* starts behind the knee, runs all the way down into the foot, and may be eighteen inches long, but provides sensation to only a small patch of skin on the outer surface of the ankle. So if the surgeon takes your sural nerve, you get quite a bit of graft, and the only loss you'll experience is a numbness in a limited area, which is often safely protected by a shoe. There are also some small nerves in the arm that can be used. These grafts from yourself, called *autografts,* avoid all of the problems such as donor matching, rejection, and transmission of disease that may be associated with donor grafts, or *allografts.* In addition, a number of active research efforts are presently directed at developing synthetic sources of nerve grafts.

The use of *entubulation* conduits, which are synthetic tubes that secure a regrowing nerve and provide a framework for a new neural sheath, is now proving to be very effective in patients with severe nerve injuries (see Fig. 11.3).

Figure 11.3 Surgical nerve repair with synthetic graft tube. A 20-year-old young man suffered a severed peroneal nerve when a piece of a shattered plate glass window pierced the skin behind his knee. A & B—At surgery, the ends of the severed nerve were identified and drawn into line. C—Goretex sheeting is placed behind the segments and the outer nerve linings are sutured to the Goretex to provide strength against "pull-apart" forces during healing, and the crushed end surfaces of the two ends are trimmed. D—A synthetic collagen based NeuroGen tube from Integra is sutured into place to reconstruct the nerve and provide a passage through which regrowing nerve ends can grow. Photos by Aaron Filler.

The two ends of the cut nerve are put in the opposite ends of the tube. A suture or glue can be used to hold the nerve in place. The internal surface of the lining of the tube is bioengineered to promote the efficient growth of nerves. This area of biotechnology is based on the remarkable discovery that the texture of a surface may do more to promote efficient nerve growth than the presence of various biochemicals or nerve growth-promoting molecules (*trophins*). The nerve fibers will travel down the synthetic conduit, and gradually the normal nerve conduit will grow into it. Schwann cells will migrate into the tube and provide linings for the individual axon nerve fibers, and other types of cells will provide the new outer sheaths for the fascicles and the nerve. These entubulation surfaces are even better than some of the biochemical nerve growth factors that have been produced. The use of these new types of nerve conduits, such as NeuroGen and Neuro Tube products, have reduced the need for the use of grafts to reconnect nerves.

Spinal Cord Injury

The situation for recovery from spinal cord injuries is more complex than the situation for recovery of *peripheral nerves*. Some of the same principles apply, but the tissue of spinal cord is different from the tissue of nerves out in the body, or the periphery. The differences in design and architecture between these two tissues make their potentials for regeneration very different.

The key difference between peripheral nerves and spinal cord is that in the spinal cord there are essentially no conduits, only nerve cells. That means that when any nerve tissue in the spinal cord is disrupted, there is no existing guide to help it find its way again. Nerves do grow and travel in response to their surroundings, and they will tunnel their way between existing nerves to some extent, but there are very few natural processes in place that allow a regrowing nerve axon in the spinal cord to find a proper path to a target. Therefore, although nerve cells inside the spinal cord have the potential to regrow, they have a very difficult time finding where they should grow to.

The problem of scar formation blocking neural growth is much more serious in the spinal cord than in peripheral nerves. It seems that scar formation is somewhat more exuberant and rapid in the spinal cord. Further, repair in the spinal cord is not nearly as straightforward as reconnecting peripheral nerves, because instead of dealing with a small number of nerves having a small number of targets, the spinal cord at any given location has tens or even hundreds of thousands of individual nerve fibers traveling to a variety of very specific destinations.

Another restriction on surgical repair of the spinal cord is the complexity of mechanical access to the cord. If any part of the spinal cord is damaged, there are very strict limits on what can be done in reaching into the spinal cord to remove scar tissue and allow the damaged nerve fibers to regrow. Disrupting other nerve fibers around the initial injury will also lead to severe consequences that affect nearby nerve cells that might not already be injured.

Gray Matter and White Matter

The spinal cord is different from peripheral nerves in another important way, which is that virtually all of the portions of the spinal cord contain two distinct types of nerve tissue. One type, the *spinal gray matter*, is made up of nerve cell bodies, each of which has thousands of connections to its neighbors. The second type, the *spinal white matter*, is made up of axon fibers that carry nerve signals over long distances (see Fig. 11.4).

Both the fibers and the cell bodies are living nerve tissue, but the cell bodies with all their many connections are far more complex than the long fibers

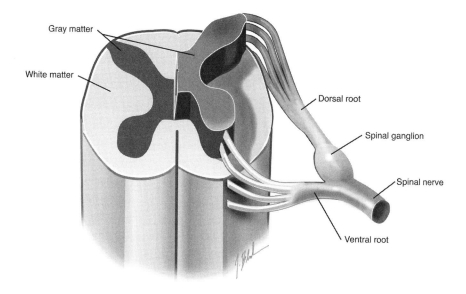

Gray matter

White matter

Dorsal root

Spinal ganglion

Spinal nerve

Ventral root

Figure 11.4 Spinal cord structure. The spinal cord has two major types of tissue. The gray matter contains the nerve cell bodies and all of the many thousands of connections between nerves. The white matter is more like a freeway composed of nerve axon fibers traveling long distances between the spine and the brain. The ventral root carries motor axon fibers from cells in the gray matter out to the muscles. Incoming sensory signals pass through a connection, or synapse, in the dorsal root ganglion and then follow the dorsal root into the gray matter. Image published with permission of Joe Bloch.

that simply have a single direction and carry a single signal per nerve. When you think of the connections in the gray portion in the center of the spinal cord, each nerve cell has hundreds or thousands of connections to hundreds of nerve cells around it. The same nerve cell, if you examine its axon, or long transmitting portion, has just one signal traveling in one direction. Peripheral nerves out in the body are made up almost entirely of the axons carrying single individual signals. Injury and repair of peripheral nerves simply don't involve the level of complexity that exists in the gray portions of the center of the spinal cord.

This dual nature of spinal cord tissue poses an interesting question for the objectives of spinal cord repair. It would be excellent, of course, to be able to repair and rebuild all of the injured areas of the spinal cord. However, shouldn't it be easier to fix the white matter than to fix the gray? Can't a segment of the gray be given up for lost while the white is rebuilt? This might mean, for instance, abandoning the bit of gray matter in the spinal cord of the neck that manages the detailed control of the fingers so that you could restore communication between the brain and the legs.

In fact, this concept does underlie a lot of what is being developed in attempts to repair the spinal cord. The important step seems to be to prevent extensive scar formation that will prevent the axons from traveling to their destinations, and also creating a condition in which the regrowing nerve fibers are allowed to enter and travel among the other cells to their destination beyond the point of injury. There still are no solutions immediately in sight, but this does help to lay out the terrain that still needs to be covered.

Stingers and Bruises

Just as with peripheral nerves, there are various degrees of injury in the spinal cord. For example, the spinal cord can suffer a very brief injury that leads to a complete but temporary paralysis that resolves rapidly. This is the frightening event that football players call a "stinger." It leads to the surprising situation in which a player who was found paralyzed on the field after a tackle is playing again by the next game or later in the season.

The stinger appears to mirror some of the milder forms of nerve injury. For one thing, the spinal cord apparently can be "stunned" by a brief sharp blow. This is the kind of event that resolves in hours or a few days. A slightly more severe compression may affect many of the axon fibers traveling past the point of impact so that they lose their myelin sheaths. These impaired axonal fibers may be recoverable over a period of weeks. The myelin sheaths around the axon fibers in the spinal cord will regrow, and then, as the weeks and months pass after an injury, recovery of function will take place.

Very mild injuries in the spinal cord also can cause the release of the inflammatory chemicals, such as bradykinins, that interfere with nerve function. As the tissues of the spinal cord cleanse away these irritating chemicals, normal function can recover over days or weeks. In a spinal cord bruise, there probably is some degree of full disconnection and breakdown of nerve fibers. However, if scar formation in the spinal cord is not too dense, some of these bruised nerve fibers will regrow. Gradual recoveries over one and two years are occasionally seen, a result showing that some interrupted nerve fibers in the spinal cord are indeed capable of regrowing through the site of injury and reaching their destination to restore normal function.

A number of times, I've had an experience related to this issue that is something like seeing a ghost. A patient I haven't heard from in two years walks into my office and thanks me for making it possible to walk again. Often the last time I saw the patient was as he or she left the hospital heading off to rehab, completely paralyzed after a car accident. I've always had a policy of doing urgent surgery to decompress and repair spine fractures no matter how severe the paralysis. In the days after surgery there may be little or no sign of any recovery. Yet clearly, in some cases the spinal cord does recover when given a chance. No one really understands the details and mechanics of this, nor can we reliably identify in advance which patients will recover, but it does document not only the basis for hope but also the very long times required for the process to take place.

Swelling, Damage, and Severe Disruption in the Spinal Cord

Despite the recovery of the spinal cord from minor injury, the overall picture for regeneration and recovery in the spinal cord is far more gloomy at present than it is for peripheral nerves. A peripheral nerve can almost always be repaired to some extent, but severe damage to the spinal cord can only rarely be repaired.

The main hope for regeneration and recovery after a spinal cord injury is the possibility that there has been no complete disruption of the spinal cord itself and no disconnection of the nerve fibers. Any pressure on the spinal cord from fractures in the vertebrae around it, of course, has to be relieved immediately. The best possible conditions for regrowth should always be established at the outset. Then the hope is that some or all of the loss of function is due to the loss of myelin sheathing without actual disconnection of the nerve fibers. As long as this is the case, there may be eventual recovery gradually over time.

Unfortunately, at present, the best types of medical imaging available really cannot always completely distinguish among the various severities of spinal cord injury. This is why, after injury, there is always hope and there are certain steps that are always wise to take. These include treating any instability from surrounding fractures and moving or removing anything that is causing pressure on the spinal cord as soon as possible (see Fig. 11.5).

Two other steps must also be taken after a spinal cord injury. First, because blood pressure can drop, it has to be supported with specialized types of medication used only for this precise situation. This is critical to maintain good blood flow to the spinal cord. Second, sometimes the weakness from the injury makes breathing impossible or at least inefficient. Obviously, insufficient oxygen will make a bad situation even worse, so there must be careful attention to breathing during the hours and days after a severe spinal cord injury.

High-dose steroid medication can reduce the harmful effects of the spinal cord's own inflammatory chemicals. This type of medication may also help to limit the severity of harmful scar formation in the injured spinal cord. For this reason, after spinal cord injuries of any severity, it is extremely important that a precise type and dose of steroid medication be given intravenously starting as soon as possible within hours of the injury.

Injured
spinal cord

Fractured
vertebral body

Figure 11.5 Spinal cord damage. An injury that causes a fracture of one of the vertebrae of the neck can result in pressure on the spinal cord. To provide the best possibility for recovery, the pressure on the spinal cord is relieved using either traction or open surgery to pull the bone fragments away from the spinal cord. Image published with permission of Joe Bloch.

Biotechnology: Hope on the Horizon

At present, the only drug in use for treating spinal cord injury is a type of steroid medication, methylprednisolone, developed decades ago. Thousands of laboratory studies have proven that there may be a chance in the future for just the right medication to swoop in and rescue some of the most serious spinal cord injury patients.

Other technology being applied to the problem of treating spinal cord injury comes from the field of bioengineering. Here the idea is that in many cases, recovery of the neural tissues just can't happen or won't happen. The signals for movement are generated in the brain, travel down the spinal cord, reach the site of injury, and halt. So the idea is that it may be possible to use electronic detectors to learn what the brain is trying to do, capture those signals, and then transmit them on to do their useful work. Similar considerations apply to detecting the environment with sensors and then communicating what is going on back to the brain.

Drug Development: Neuroprotection and Regeneration

New drugs are being developed to mount a successful attack on a problem called *secondary injury*. These are injuries caused by harmful cellular chemicals released inside the spinal cord during the hours after the initial injury. In some cases, the secondary injury may be as bad or worse than the original injury. The idea is that nothing can be done after the fact to stop the initial mechanical injury. However, with the presence of *neuroprotective agents*, at least the secondary injury can be halted. There is a tremendous effort to discover effective neuroprotective medications that can halt the progress of this destructive cascade. Some of these drugs are intended to limit scar formation or to provide optimum conditions for recovery and regrowth.

Aside from the problem of limiting the initial damage, there are also widespread efforts to discover medications that can encourage nerves to regrow more aggressively, tunnel through scar tissue, and be more sensitive to the cues and clues that may lead them back to their original targets. Another focus of research is to find ways to encourage the spinal cord to be receptive to forming new connections, if and when cells regrowing nerve fibers finally reach back to their old, abandoned destination territories.

Even now, these types of effects can sometimes be accomplished in the laboratory under controlled situations, but none of these new drugs has yet been made usable for patients. Some failures have occurred in the laboratory and after large-scale trials involving actual spinal cord injury patients. So far, only the high-dose methylprednisolone steroid treatment has shown any real beneficial effect.

Drug Delivery in the Spinal Cord

In addition to finding compounds that will have the desired useful effects, there is also a great problem in delivering these compounds to where they are needed. Simply taking an oral medication to get a drug into the bloodstream does not guarantee that the medication will reach all the way into the center of the spinal cord. Spinal cord tissue is protected by a kind of chemical barrier from what would otherwise be toxic chemicals that get in the bloodstream.

The blood-brain barrier, the blood-nerve barrier, and its spinal cord equivalent involve tiny cells that line the blood vessels and block any undesired chemicals.

However, this innate design for protection may also prevent useful medications from reaching into the interior of the spinal cord. One focus of drug-delivery design is compounds capable of penetrating the barrier and carrying other drugs across. Medication delivery and design are important frontiers where progress is steady but frustratingly slow.

The various approaches to drug delivery include both mechanical and advanced biomolecular designs. The mechanical approaches involve developing gels and *polymers* (elongated drug-carrying molecules) that can deliver growth-promoting factors into the spinal cord tissue. Some mechanical approaches along these lines involve pumps and catheters as well. On the more biological front, a process called *axonal transport* can carry a medication from an intact nerve ending in the muscle or skin, up the axon, and into the cell body in the spinal cord, where the medication is then released or allowed to diffuse into neighboring spinal cord tissues (see Fig. 2.1).

Implanting of genetically modified cells that produce growth factors and even the use of stem cells are being explored, but so far, the best progress seems to be coming from neuro-electronics.

Bioengineering: Sensors and Chips for Restoration

There are two approaches to designing sensors for reestablishing functional neural connections. One of them is to try to pick up signals from the surface of the brain. These sensors essentially monitor in fine detail what the person is thinking or intending to do. Parts of the brain are specifically involved in controlling motion. Even more specifically, some parts can trigger some very particular movements. By monitoring these, it may be possible to capture the intention to movement. This is a technically complex problem from a number of points of view, but may prove to be the basis for at least some movement and recovery sometime in the future.

Another avenue being explored is the possibility of actually putting fine microchip sensors into the damaged segment of the spinal cord. In this way, although the damaged nerves can't physically reach their intended destination, they can reach into a chip and activate a set of transistors. The signals can be captured, and an output data set can show which nerves are firing. This data can be sorted, analyzed, decoded, and then transmitted back into a robotic system to activate and drive a robotic limb. Alternately, the output from the system may even be used someday actually to activate nerves in the lower spinal cord so that the body's natural capabilities can be used to restore motion. Even if the original nerves' signals can't be sorted out correctly, the injured individual may learn over time to operate his or her own electronic output system.

Electroneural Interfaces: Making Use of the Signals

These bioengineering approaches are still largely in their early stages when it comes to walking or using the hands. Simpler devices that help to activate patients' breathing muscles, however, are already in use. Active research programs in major universities and scientific laboratories are directed at *electroneural interfaces* for detecting nerve function. One positive result of the Iraq War has been a tremendous effort—with significant results—toward developing advanced robotic systems that injured soldiers can actually use for complex activities. Some of these are now working at a level of efficacy that is actually astonishing to watch—like seeing the Luke Skywalker/Star Wars hand repair occurring in real life!

For larger movements that use a robotic frame for movement, a constant energy supply is needed. Robotic frames have also advanced dramatically during the course of the Iraq War. Methods for using this electronic output to drive or to activate muscles without a direct connection from brain to nerve to muscle are also being explored. If the person's own muscles can be used, then the body's own energy supply can be used.

Similar capabilities are also being developed to restore lost sensation by detecting signals traveling along in nerves. After a spinal cord injury, the information in these signals can't reach past the injury to inform the brain. However, new advanced methods for using electronic methodology to present the information to the nervous system for processing have proven very effective for restoring the essence of perception—an essential aspect of information needed by the brain for the control of fine motion.

Structural Framework for Repair

Aside from all the promise and possibility of neural repair, there has been tremendous progress in development of the tools and capabilities for locating, repairing, and reconstructing the damage to the mechanical structures of the spine. The ability to understand the physical aspects of the spine and neural tissues has to precede the advance into biotechnology that will be needed for spinal cord repair to become a reality.

» Part II «

Spine and Nerve Surgery

Without an Incision: Percutaneous Procedures for Diagnosis and Treatment

In the past, any mention of spinal surgery suggested large operations with liters of blood loss and long, bedridden recoveries. However, not only is spinal surgery being performed through smaller and smaller incisions with more and more rapid recovery, but in many cases, open spinal surgeries are being replaced with procedures that are carried out through the skin, or in a *percutaneous* fashion. These procedures include a variety of injections as well as percutaneous therapeutic treatments involving electrical and other stimuli. In addition there are a variety of tools including lasers, high-powered ultrasonic devices, and very small mechanical instruments that can be operated at the end of a long wire, through the skin, with the surgeon's vision replaced by other imaging technology.

Diagnosis and treatment in the spine now rely very heavily on injections, and there are a number of reasons for this. Most important is that imaging of the spine usually does not provide specific proof that any of the abnormalities seen in an image are actually causing the pain that the patient is experiencing. *Anesthetic* and *anti-inflammatory* injections can provide a critical diagnostic link between the findings on an imaging study and the actual symptoms experienced by the patient, and in many cases the injections can also have a therapeutic effect, which can delay or even eliminate the need for spine surgery.

In essence, most of these methods achieve a final precise diagnosis by testing the response to a little bit of treatment. If applying a small amount of short-acting anesthetic to a suspect spot in the body can relieve the pain, then that spot is a good target for more substantial treatment. If some steroids injected at that spot provide a few days or weeks of relief, then the diagnosis is even more convincing. Overall, a grand technological search is under way to find ways of using the same percutaneous methods to achieve definitive cures rather than temporary "diagnostic" responses to short-term treatment. There is still a long way to go before that hope becomes a reality. Perhaps someday we'll be injecting a gene therapy agent or a microscopic nanomachine that can provide the definitive treatment.

Nonetheless, these confirmatory tests are crucial to optimizing the success rates of the more invasive treatments available currently, such as open surgery.

Injections for Diagnosis and Treatment

It is safe to say that MRI scans and X-rays of the lumbar spine are 99.9 percent *false positive. That means that a vast majority of findings in the radiologist's report on a lumbar X-ray or MRI have nothing to do with the symptoms the patient is experiencing.* This poses a huge problem to the spine specialist trying to treat the patient.

Abnormalities such as bulging disks, narrowing canals, and bone spurs can all be seen on an image without causing any symptoms, now or even in the future, for a given patient. In fact, 60 percent of patients who have never had any significant back pain or leg pain will show many of those abnormalities in an image of the spine, meaning that 60 percent of imaging studies are going to be falsely positive independent of what they reveal. Therefore, it would appear that most findings from diagnostic imaging have no significance. With the vast majority of information being false and misleading, you might reasonably wonder why it is worth doing these tests at all. It turns out that having fourteen wrong leads and one correct one is better than having no leads at all and a thousand equally plausible causes. The image provides a limited number of precise findings, each of which can be carefully considered for its likelihood of being the cause of the problem.

The neurologist, neurosurgeon, or orthopedist who orders imaging and other tests based on the patient's history and physical examination will have particular questions in mind and will be looking for specific findings. If those bulges and bumps then turn up in the scan, it is a reasonable bet that they really are causing the problem. Still, it is often necessary to inject some anesthetic at the spot that looks like it is irritating things to see whether numbing it makes the pain go away. First, this helps prove that the observed abnormality is causing the symptoms; and second, if simply putting an anti-inflammatory there makes the problem go away for an extended period, then there certainly may be no need for surgery at all. That is why image-guided injections of anesthetics, steroids, and other anti-inflammatory agents play a critical role in the diagnosis and treatment of spine conditions.

Epidural Injections: A Calming Flow

The most calming of these types of injection is an epidural injection. As a nonspecific treatment that places a medication close to the spine, epidurals rarely provide much proof as to any surgery that might be needed; however, in many cases, they can relieve significant pain problems. This procedure essentially

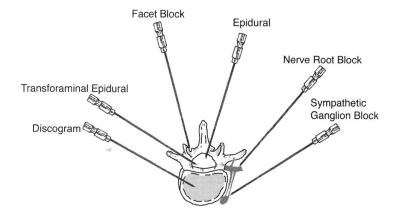

Figure 12.1 Epidurals, nerve root blocks, and facet blocks. The precise cause of spine or limb pain can often be tracked down with anesthetic injections. Image guidance is crucial during spine injections because small differences in location of the needle tip results in tests of very different parts of the spine. Drawing by Aaron Filler.

amounts to floating a big pool of calming steroids out over the spine and nerves in the involved region (see Fig. 12.1).

Very often after a disk herniation (breakthrough of disk material into an abnormal location) or other small amount of trauma, there is a great deal of inflammation that can be relieved by a steroid injection. Epidural steroid injections are often given in a series of three. They are usually done in the lumbar or cervical regions and occasionally in the thoracic region, and they may or may not require image guidance for placement of the needle.

One of the most appropriate uses of epidural steroids is for spinal stenosis, in which an arthritic process causes the joints of the spine to enlarge over the years so that the spinal canal itself gets increasingly narrower. As the space becomes critically tight, the nerves within the shrinking canal become irritated by rubbing on its edges and begin to swell. Then, as the nerves swell larger in an already small canal, the problem gets worse and worse: The nerves get more pinched, and they swell more. The typical symptom from this kind of stenosis is pain in the legs that is aggravated more and more as the individual walks farther and farther. In this situation, administering epidural steroids at the right location, by inserting a needle between the lamina of the spine and floating the medication into the general vicinity over the dura membranes, can relieve the swelling. If the nerves settle down and become small enough to fit in their reduced space, then spine surgery for the stenosis can be completely avoided.

Another type of epidural is called a *transforaminal epidural*. This is done to obtain some diagnostic information by sending the needle in from the side, through the foramen, parallel with the most involved nerve root, rather than from the back of the spinal canal. When appropriate, this technique can help assure that a good portion of the dose of the medication will be distributed over the one spinal nerve that is most involved.

Two things can go wrong in any epidural injection. First, it may be painful if the needle strikes or scrapes the bone on the way in; second, a puncture of the dura membranes may lead to leakage of spinal fluid. A leak occasionally will cause headaches and may require the doctor to go back and put in a "blood patch" (an injection of some blood outside the spinal dura to help to block the leakage). Although there is a small risk of injury to spinal nerves during a posterior epidural injection, the risk is slightly higher in a transforaminal epidural, particularly if the foramen or nerve canal is quite tight around the nerve root; when that's the case, the posterior epidural is often a better choice.

One other type of epidural is a *caudal epidural*, which involves passing a *catheter* (a small tube) through the sacrum. This can enable the epidural steroid to be introduced at even lower spinal levels, but poses additional risks of nerve injury because of the complexity of the course that the needle and catheter have to navigate.

Epiduroscopy: Lysis of Adhesions

There is a theory that some types of spinal pain are due to adhesions, or sticking points that form between the dura membranes and the surrounding vertebral bones. This would be particularly problematic in the case of an adhesion affecting a nerve root that's exiting through a foramen, because the vertebral elements around the foramen include parts of the spinal joint that should move during normal activity. If the nerve root, or dura, is adherent to the bone, then normal movement will produce unusual or unacceptable tugging on the dura membranes. Normally, fatty material around the dura separates it from the bone, thus allowing for normal sliding and gliding; but after an injury that leads to bleeding in the spine, when there is inflammation or following surgery, this gliding layer may be filled in by adherent scar tissue.

With *epiduroscopy*, a doctor can inspect the area and find any adhesions. Epiduroscopy is somewhat similar to an epidural injection, except that a catheter is placed to provide some video-guided vision and directability to the operator. Adhesions can be broken up mechanically, or destructive materials can be introduced for *lysis*, that is, to help dissolve them. One lytic agent is vitrase (or hylenex), which includes an enzyme called hyaluronidase that can dissolve some types of adhesion. The value of epiduroscopy, however, is not fully agreed on. It is not clear how many symptoms actually result from such adhesions, and the introduction of the dissolving agents can certainly cause complications, particularly if the agents leak into the wrong space and get too close to the nerve elements themselves.

Nerve Root Blocks: Zeroing in on the Pain

One of the types of injection treatment most helpful in resolving a diagnosis is a *nerve root block*. Here the objective is fairly simple. A needle is placed near the exit of the nerve root from the spine, and an anesthetic is injected to numb or "freeze" the nerve root. This is not usually a therapeutic action, but rather is diagnostic. It is most useful when there is some question about whether a pinch of one single nerve root is causing all of the back and leg pain a patient is experiencing.

If numbing that one nerve root makes all the pain go away, then you can be sure that it is involved in the "pain generator." With this confirmation, the doctor can confidently ignore other abnormalities appearing on an imaging test in order to focus on the problems affecting that individual nerve root. If a nerve root block does not produce numbness in any particular distribution, then it probably just wasn't successful. This is possible if there are too many bone spurs for the doctor to get the needle close enough to the nerve root or if a fatty layer prevents the anesthetic from reaching the nerve.

Another technique involves injecting steroids in the same fashion as in an anesthetic nerve root block. Sometimes nerve roots in narrowed nerve canals become inflamed and swell. Introducing steroids can make the swelling go down and allow the problem to be resolved for many months or even years.

Facet Blocks: Looking for Joint Pain

Among the different types of back pain, and even pain radiating into the buttock and thigh, are pains that originate in the small facet joints (joints along the posterior part of the vertebrae) along the lumbar spine. This can be suspected in a mechanical back pain that's aggravated by movement, particularly when the movement is arching backward or extending the spine.

To test for this, the doctor needs to use X-ray, CT, or MRI guidance to place a needle precisely within the joint and inject both anesthetic and steroid medication. The small nerve leading into the joint may also be blocked. This *facet block* can be done at several joints at once if the idea is just to settle down a *multiple joint facet syndrome*, which often occurs, or at a single joint if it is believed that just one joint is the cause of the pain and the purpose of the injection is to track it down. In both cases, the anesthetic is used to prove the diagnosis and the steroid is used to achieve some treatment effect.

Discograms: Keys to Identifying Disk Pain

Injections into the disk space are one of the most important types of image-guided spine injections. These often fall under the category of discography (disk imaging), but can sometimes be called anesthetic disk injections. They are intended to identify patients for whom the source of the pain is a tear in the annulus (retaining ring) of a disk. They may also be used when there are bulging disks at several levels and it is suspected that one of them is the cause, or there is an overall question about whether the patient has generalized muscle strain or if the back pain is really *discogenic*, or disk-caused pain.

A common injection test of this type that actually increases your pain is called a *provocative discogram*. The idea here is to inject fluid (such as saline) into the disk space and stretch the annulus hard, and see how much back pain results. The patient then has to say both yes, it hurts and yes, the pain is the same as my usual pain for the result to be considered a *concordant* response. A provocative discogram is very helpful when the result is clear; but for a patient with a lot of back pain, it may be very difficult to determine whether the induced pain is the usual back pain or a different one.

Putting the needle in can be very painful itself, so many doctors give a lot of anesthetic and sedation in order to do the discogram, which may then lead to a confusing result because the patient can't really remember whether the usual pain is the same as that from the injection, is slightly different, or hurts more or less. This is why many specialists have abandoned the provocative discogram and instead rely on the *anesthetic discogram*. Here the idea is simply to inject an anesthetic to numb the disk with the torn annulus, and if that makes the back pain go away, then it proves that the tear was the cause of the pain. Also, injecting steroids into a disk space can occasionally lead to very prolonged relief of low back pain, and that's why this is also typically a part of the anesthetic discogram procedure. This also a key step toward achieving some therapy or relief as opposed to simply diagnosing the problem.

At the time of a discogram, it is also usual to put in some kind of *contrast agent* unless the discogram is done in an MRI scanner, in which case the injection alone will provide sufficient fluid contrast. The goal is to visualize the tear in the annular ring, which will fill up with the contrast material. Injections done under MRI guidance in a specially equipped open MRI scanner avoid any exposure to X-rays and generally allow for a smoother and more comfortable process of advancing the needle into the disk (see Fig. 12.2).

Disk injections carry a slightly higher infection risk than most other injections because the disk space itself has relatively little blood supply. If a few bacteria get into the area of an epidural injection or a joint injection, they are likely to be gobbled up immediately by the body, but bacteria that get into the disk may grow in a protected space without the body reacting to fight them and may lead to a very serious disk infection. For this reason, it is frequent practice to give

Figure 12.2 Open MR discogram. The use of open MRI scanners (see Fig. 16.8) for guidance of injections is a relatively new development. It avoids X-ray radiation and allows the physician to see nerves, blood vessels, and other soft tissues along the way that are not seen with X-ray fluoroscopy.

intravenous antibiotics during the course of a disk injection or oral antibiotics for a few days following the injection.

Morphine Pumps: Trial and Implant

Another type of pain-relieving injection actually involves an implant and is very similar to the way an epidural is done, except that the needle is actually passed into the spinal canal, and a catheter is passed into the spinal fluid and led under the skin to an external access point. The doctor can then inject morphine or other drugs directly into the spinal canal through the access point. Normally, drugs are administered orally or intravenously, so they distribute through the whole body and only a little bit of the total dose ultimately gets into the spinal canal. However,

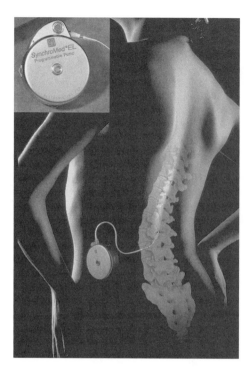

Figure 12.3 Morphine pump. These pumps are implanted inside the skin. The physician can refill the pump by directing a needle through the skin and into the port in the center of the pump. The catheter running away from the pump is placed inside the spinal fluid space. The pump rate can be controlled by an external telemetry device. SynchroMed illustrations reprinted with permission of Medtronic, Inc.

with a catheter of this type, it is possible to place the entire dose inside the spinal canal immediately next to the nerves most affected by the pain, greatly reducing the amount of the drug that goes to the rest of the body (see Fig. 12.3).

A test trial is carried out first, because this sort of treatment doesn't work for many patients. The trial is done by introducing the catheter through a needle and then injecting the medication into the spinal canal. If all other methods have failed and the trial is successful at reducing the patient's pain, then the surgeon or pain specialist is likely to recommend the implantation of a permanent pain medicine infusion system.

The implanted pump has a port under the skin, through which a doctor can place a needle to refill the pump. A buried catheter then leads from the pump device, under the skin, and down into the interior of the spinal canal. The battery is usually good for several years, although there is a continuing risk of pump malfunction, displacement or clogging of the catheter, and infection. In addition, having the pump may make it risky to have any further MRI imaging. The metal in the pump can heat up in an MRI, and the electronic control of the pump speed may be affected.

Electronic Pain Relief

Aside from medication, a number of electronic devices can be used to try to relieve spinal pain. One common method is a *radiofrequency* (RF) treatment. At the desired location, a specialized and complex probe is guided into place so that the tip is in contact with the nerve most involved in the pain. The specialized needle has an outer insulating coating, an electronically conducting shaft, and a specially designed tip that converts radiofrequency signal energy into heat. In addition, the needle incorporates a *thermistor*, or temperature sensor.

As an oscillating RF signal is passed down a wire to the needle, the tip of the needle begins to heat up; by using the temperature monitor, the doctor can control the temperature of the tip. This system allows a very thin needle to deliver very precisely controlled heat to a very specific spot, and this has several useful applications.

Radiofrequency Lesions: Shooting the Messenger

In a nerve, there are individual fibers, or axons, that have different jobs. Some are involved in creating movement by operating muscles, some are involved in sensing the position of muscles, and some are involved in different types of sensation such as light touch, temperature, sharp touch, and, of course, pain. The technical word for a pain-sensing nerve is a *nociceptor*, where "noci" is similar to the root of the word "noxious," describing a pain or other unpleasant stimulus.

Controlled heating can be helpful for pain control because of a particular biological fact about the nature of nociceptors. Most nerve fibers are intended to conduct signals at a very high rate of speed, and that conduction relies on thick insulation around the nerves. But many of the pain nerves transmit their signals very slowly and don't have the same kind of myelin insulation that coats other nerve types. This biological oddity is taken advantage of in RF treatment. When a certain amount of heat is applied through the RF needle, the thick insulation around most nerves protects them somewhat from its effects; the pain nerves, however, don't have a thick outer lining and are very sensitive to heat. Because of this, it is possible to use precisely controlled heat to destroy the endings of the pain nerves without affecting the movement nerves and other sensation nerves. Nevertheless, RF is used with great caution and generally only in areas where there are no major nerves that might be injured.

One of the most common and very successful uses of RF is in the case of a patient for whom a facet block, described earlier, has proven that most of the pain is coming from the facet joints. The RF needle can be put into place, and the nerve that goes to a facet joint can be *lesioned*, thereby destroying its pain-sensing fibers. Although the joint abnormality itself hasn't been fixed, the patient can no longer perceive the pain from the facet joint because the pain nerves have been destroyed by the RF treatment. The joint does have some general sensation nerves that help to tell its position, and if the heat is not applied perfectly, these could be burned along with the pain nerves. In the case of a facet joint, this could lead to some additional problems, but in general it would have no noticeable effect.

RF treatments are often very effective for patients with discogenic pain syndromes. In a patient who has had temporary but near complete relief of back pain from an intradiscal anesthetic injection, an RF treatment for the annulus is often recommended. A patient typically experiences immediate pain relief lasting for months or longer, and there is no special recovery period.

A major nerve such as the L5 or S1 nerve, which leaves the spine and runs down toward the leg, presents a different situation. It would be nice if an RF lesion could be done near the foramen and burn only the pain nerves; however, if the heating were not perfect, then you could end up with major numbness or weakness in your leg, making it impossible to walk. For that reason, there is great hesitation about using RF in the vicinity of major motor and sensory nerves. The newer technology of pulsed RF treatment, however, has made it possible to reduce the efficiency of pain fibers inside major nerves such as the exiting spinal nerve roots, so that RF with the proper, advanced equipment has a place in the treatment of entire nerve roots.

Intradiscal Electrothermy: Can Your Annulus Be Healed?

Another use for heating involves even higher temperatures than RF. The high temperature is not directed at silencing nerves but is actually used to attempt to repair damaged tissue. This type of treatment has worked well in the treatment of torn ligaments in the knee and is now being used to repair torn disks (see Fig. 12.4).

The annular tear is a difficult problem, as it may cause pain over a period of years and may be treatable only with a fusion surgery. In *intradiscal electrothermy* (IDET), a wire is placed into the disk space and positioned to run just below and along the area of the tear. Then, a very high heat is applied through the wire, which melts the proteins in the annulus, or *anneals* them, so they are reformed and strengthened, repairing the tear.

This sounds like an excellent solution that can be used in place of a lumbar fusion surgery, for instance, but IDET has certain risks and problems. First, although inserting the wire can be extremely painful for the patient, the manufacturer of the device recommends that the patient not have any anesthetic during the procedure. This is because anesthesia could mask the fact that the wire is positioned near a major nerve root, and if this were the case, then the very high heat could cause a severe nerve injury. This can make IDET

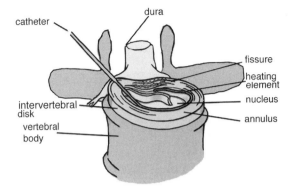

Figure 12.4 Intradiscal electrothermy (IDET). This procedure is done to repair tears in the annulus fibrosus. A needle is threaded into the disk space and a wire is then advanced into position near the tear. The wire is then heated to try to achieve a repair. Image reproduced with permission of Smith & Nephew.

extremely painful if the risk of nerve injury is to be minimized. Further, it is not always successful. Only a fraction of IDET patients achieve a lasting benefit, and even for those who do, the benefit is only partial: the pain is not completely relieved.

Although the success rate for IDET is very, very low compared with fusion surgery, having a needle and a wire put into your spine rather than enduring an extensive surgery through your abdomen and your back, with months of subsequent brace wearing, is certainly an attractive alternative. Nonetheless, after an IDET treatment, there is often significantly increased pain for weeks, and extensive physical therapy is required, so the pain may actually be worse for a while after the treatment. This scenario is very different from an RF treatment of a disk, in which the pain is usually relieved almost immediately. Some patients who seem to benefit a small amount from IDET may actually have improved only because the severe pain from the IDET kept them off their feet for a few weeks and allowed the back to recover.

Epidural Stimulators: Trial and Implant

A completely different use of electronics for pain relief involves a low level of electronic stimulation with a sort of alternating "buzzing" that is perceived by the nerves. This serves as a distracting stimulus, so that your body is more aware of the buzzing than of the pain. For patients who have multiple failed spine surgeries, and in whom the exact cause of their pain cannot be found, this electronic stimulation can be a huge benefit. Some patients have a fantastic response and find that it completely eliminates their awareness of their back pain (see Fig. 12.5).

Figure 12.5 Epidural stimulator. The electrodes of an epidural stimulator (C) are placed either through a needle or during open surgery. If the signals block the patient's pain during testing, then a generator (B) is implanted to send signals to the electrode. The system can be controlled and adjusted with an external controller device (A). Illustrations reproduced with permission of Medtronic, Inc.

Although *transcutaneous electroneural stimulators* (TENS) can be applied to the skin, the *epidural stimulator* has to be implanted internally. It is put in through a needle very much like the one used for an epidural injection. The electrode travels inside the needle and is passed down into the space between the dura membranes and the bones surrounding the spinal canal. Usually the patient is given short-acting anesthesia and then awakened once the stimulator is in place. Occasionally an open surgery is required to place the electrode.

The stimulator is a panel of three, four, or even six electrode disks. The doctor moves the disks around to find out whether a good location can be achieved to block the patient's pain. The stimulator is usually placed over the dura membranes in the low thoracic spine for relief of leg and low back pain. It can also be placed in the neck for arm and neck pain, but very few specialists actually perform the neck placement because it is considered more difficult and risky.

If the trial is successful, then a small surgery can be carried out to implant a generator below the skin that will drive the stimulator. The generator can be turned on and off or adjusted by a radio-control device, and has a battery that needs to be surgically replaced every three to five years. As with the morphine pump, having an epidural stimulator in place may rule out any future MRI scans.

Discoplasty: Knifeless Surgery for Disks

In some cases, the cause of back pain is apparently the bulging disk itself even though there is no real herniation or nerve pressure and no annular tear. In these patients it may be helpful to reshape or reduce the size of a disk with procedures that require only a small puncture through the skin or other tissues, thereby removing the pressure created by the bulge without resorting to open surgery.

Lasers

In the laser method of knifeless surgery, a needle is inserted into the disk space, just as for a discogram. The doctor then advances a fiber-optic laser that travels through the needle into the disk. When the laser is at the center of the disk, it is turned on and actually vaporizes some of the disk material, or nucleus pulposus, which can then be sucked out through the needle as smoke. Thus, the disk is reshaped from the inside, and as the central part evaporates, the hope is that the bulge will settle back in, reducing the internal pressure on the disk. *Laser discoplasty* is effective only in a limited variety of situations. Nonetheless, it has the attraction that the laser is being used not near the spinal nerves, but rather at the center of the disk, a safe distance from the surrounding nerves. The technique has not come into wide use but certainly is a potential treatment for the future. As with any laser, the greatest risks seem to be the unimpeded reach of the beam, which can cause tissue damage if the strength of the laser is too great or if its positioning is not perfect (see Fig. 12.6).

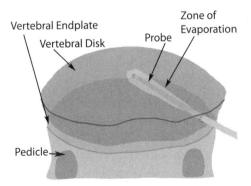

Figure 12.6 Nucleoplasty. A bulging disk can sometimes be treated without open surgery. This involves passing a probe into the disk. The tip is then heated to a very high level so that the solid tissue of the disk actually evaporates.

Radiofrequency and Coblation

Just as with laser discoplasty, a radiofrequency-type needle can also be used at a very high heat to evaporate central disk material and thereby reduce disk bulges. One manufacturer uses the term *coblation* to describe this process and distinguish it from the more common uses for RF heat treatment of pain nerves, which are sometimes termed *ablation*. This method provides somewhat more control than the laser, because RF can be counted on to act only in the immediate vicinity of the needle. A laser can travel an additional distance, and as tissue evaporates, the laser may go farther and farther and might evaporate or damage a tissue that the doctor did not intend to treat.

Endoscopy: Blind Alleys and Sympathetic Ganglia

It may be possible to conduct other, more extensive types of spine surgery largely through the skin in percutaneous fashion, with the help of *endoscopy*: inserting a tube that contains a video camera into the body and inserting a second tube through which the doctor operates special instruments.

Endoscopy has been very successful in the abdomen and pelvis—for instance, for gallbladder, appendix, and gynecological surgeries—but hasn't reached its full potential in the spine for two important reasons. First, in the abdomen, there is a large open space that can be filled with air and lit up, thus providing freedom of movement for both the video camera and the surgeon's endoscopic tools. Near the spine, there is only solid tissue, so the surgeon can't see very far and can't move the devices once they are in place. If there is any bleeding, the blood can immediately blind the surgeon in spinal endoscopy, while it would just run out of the way in the large working cavity of abdominal endoscopy. While vision is obscured, using suction and electrocautery to try to stop the bleeding presents an unacceptably high risk of injury to small nerves. Also, when introducing catheters large enough for cameras and instruments, there is a significant risk of hitting the nerves that exit the spine. These are several of the concerns that explain why neurosurgeons generally do not use endoscopy.

Another factor against using endoscopy in the spine is that the open incisions for many spinal surgeries completed with the surgical microscope may be only an inch or so in length. But the incision needed to introduce the endoscope may be nearly as large as the routine open microsurgical incision. The situation in the abdomen is much different, since the mobility of tissues requires much larger incisions for open surgery.

Nonetheless, opportunities for spinal endoscopy may increase over time as the technology improves.

One important potential advance will be to use images from MR neurography as part of an image-guidance system to help the doctor insert the endoscope and devices precisely as desired, dodging the nerves on the way. Then, if the equipment is brought to exactly the right location at the spine, the work can be done without full surgical exposure, as in abdominal endoscopy.

An area of spinal surgery in which endoscopy is playing an increasingly important role concerns the thoracic spine. Because this spinal region is surrounded by the open cavity of the lungs, it is possible to do several types of endoscopic surgery around the thoracic spine, including disk removal by using a variety of instruments such as mechanical grasping devices or even lasers under endoscopic control or radiofrequency devices under direct vision. Endoscopic thoracic spine procedures are attractive because the alternative may be a full open-chest surgery through very large incisions (see Fig. 18.1). Nonetheless, these endoscopic surgeries continue to be very risky because of the difficulty of achieving fine control of these devices inside the disks in the thoracic region. For this reason, thoracic endoscopic surgery is offered by only a very few specialists.

Another type of endoscopy relevant to the spine is the surgical treatment of sympathetic ganglia, the nerve clusters that are involved in some pain syndromes such as *reflex sympathetic dystrophy* (RSD) or *complex regional pain syndrome* (CRPS). It is possible to use an endoscopic approach to identify and expose the sympathetic ganglion that may be involved in the pain and to cut or lesion it. This *sympathectomy* surgery is still not a widespread procedure because it may have the complication of making the pain worse, and because epidural stimulators are often successful for treating patients with these pain syndromes. However, in patients for whom all else fails and a sympathectomy is recommended, an endoscopic procedure can avoid the need for major surgery to carry out the treatment.

Open MRI Guidance for Hyaluronidase Treatments

One additional type of treatment of that is of growing importance for nerve entrapments, and that may become more important for spine as well, is increased focus on the role of a crucial natural molecule in maintaining and improving movement around the spine and nerves. The natural molecule is called *hyaluronate* or hyaluronic acid or hyaluronan. It is based on a modified type of sugar or carbohydrate that is called a "glycosaminoglycan" because each unit or monomer has the amino group usually found in proteins. In many ways, hyaluronates serve as the lubricating oil of the body. Just like oils, the hyaluronates come in varying viscosities. Most of the variation has to do with the number of monomers linked together in a chain and whether there is any cross linking among chains. The length of the chains can include thousands or even millions of molecules, with the viscosity increasing with longer molecules. Cross linking can effectively congeal the hyaluronate.

Because of these properties, injectable high-viscosity hyaluronate has been used to help lubricate joints and also for plastic surgery applications—creating thickened lips by injection of Restylane or Perlane, which have various lengths of hyaluronate polymer. These agents may also be used in the future for lubrication functions in spinal joints or as crosslinked gels in efforts to help regenerate the intervertebral disks that have become dehydrated.

Another important aspect of hyaluronate medicine is the use of *hyaluronidase enzymes* to dissolve or shorten hyaluronate polymers. Hyaluronidase has been in use in many areas of medicine for decades, but its potential for treating spine and nerve disorders has been explored only more recently. Among the most important uses reported in formal studies is placing hyaluronidase around nerves, via Open MRI guided injections, that have become irritated due to adhesions—that is, due to becoming stuck to adjacent structures so that the nerves get unnaturally pulled, tugged, and irritated with movement. The hyaluronidase can break up the adhesions and relieve the pain. Similar uses have been explored to break down adhesions around the dural membranes and spinal roots that are thought to be the cause of spinal pain in some patients.

Hyaluronidase has been manufactured from various animal sources. For many years, the principal version was a bovine product called Wydase, but current products are sheep derived—Vitrase—or actually made from human recombinant DNA genetic engineering (Hylenex from Baxter). Hylenex was recalled in 2010 because of glass flakes in the vials—but became available again for a variety of uses beginning in 2012.

For nerve entrapment problems such as pudendal nerve entrapments, sciatic entrapments after surgery, and entrapments of the brachial plexus nerves in the distal plexus (between clavicle and underarm), *MRI guidance* is very helpful because of the need to inject very close to the involved nerve to get the maximum effectiveness. Guidance with ultrasound and electroneural stimulation or guidance by CT scanning may be effective in some situations. X-ray fluoroscopy is not generally helpful for guidance near nerves but is an effective way to administer hyaluronidase or hyaluronate near the spine because of its good bone visualization.

The most exciting aspect of this area of technology is the ability to take advantage of the excellent three-dimensional visualization of nerves and other soft tissues under MRI to navigate precisely inside the solid tissues of the body. The non-surgical, precise access is then used to apply an advanced, genetically engineered human enzyme to accomplish something—a nerve release surgery or neuroplasty—that requires open surgery for most patients at present.

13

Surgery—Before, During, and After: Common Elements You Should Know About

Independent of all the planning and diagnostic work and treatment considerations, the events immediately surrounding your surgery—what happens in the days and hours before, the surgeon's steps at the very beginning of the operation, and the choices at the end—can all have a tremendous impact on the success of the whole process and the nature and quality of your long-term outcome. A number of details that are common to many types of operations are important for any surgical patient to know about, particularly in the case of spine surgery. Some are in the realm of paperwork, and some have to do with small differences in the way surgeons perform procedures or in the choices that they make to optimize the results, speed the recovery, and minimize the risks of surgery. It may be helpful for you to be aware of all of these things in advance so that you have an opportunity to discuss them with your surgeon and get the best advice on how the various issues will be addressed.

Informed Consent: What You Need to Know

For every surgical procedure, an agreement between the surgeon and the patient documents, at the minimum, the fact that the patient has given the surgeon permission to touch him or her and to carry out the surgery. Aside from granting the surgeon the basic permission to do something, most informed consent procedures also use the *consent form* as a means of ensuring that everyone agrees on what's going to take place, that the patient understands the plan, and that there is no confusion about what is going to be done.

The major aspects of the surgery, any possible additional aspects, and any unusual or specialized steps should be listed in the consent form. If the condition and/or the surgery is on the left side or the right, that fact needs to show up on the consent form, too. Very commonly, your surgeon may plan to do something that is experimental or not specifically approved by the FDA (Food and Drug Administration); this will often show up on the consent form as well. Usually, the language on the consent form also allows for the possibility that emergencies may occur and the surgeon may have to make changes to the original plan during surgery. The form should indicate that you are aware that the surgery has risks and that you are willing to take those risks.

Consent to surgery is meant to be informed; that is, you sign the form after having the risks and benefits of the surgery, as well as the alternatives, explained to you. You often have the choice of signing a line on the form to indicate that you didn't want to know the risks, benefits, and alternatives, but the vast majority of patients want all of that to be explained. Typically, you have a talk with your surgeon or your surgeon's staff in advance of the surgery, which leads you to understand what procedure he or she is going to do and why that choice was made over the possible alternatives.

Risks and Benefits, Options and Indications

In a vast array of activities in our daily lives, we make choices based on risks and benefits. A good example is driving a car. We all know that tens of thousands of people get killed driving their cars every year, and far more get hurt, yet we continue to drive, well aware of the risks. Putting on our seat belts and having air bags give us some protection, but no one is under the illusion that there is perfect safety in a car. Yet we know the benefits of car travel, we understand the risks, and finally we make the choice. Surgery needs to be undertaken from the same point of view: we know why it's being done and that risks are involved.

Some of the concerns can be considered to be *general risks* of all surgeries. This includes problems such as excessive bleeding or infection, which could happen at any time in surgery and are known to occur with a certain frequency, particularly infection. The general risks of surgery even include a very tiny chance of death from anesthesia—just as you might die crossing the street in the morning or going to work. We understand, however, that the doctor will take measures to prevent or reduce these known risks.

There are also *specific risks* of any particular surgery that are worth being aware of. Some are common problems with the operation that the surgeon knows well and takes specific measures to avoid, and others are negative outcomes that result from the operation with a certain frequency no matter what is done. A good example of a specific risk has to do with the variable course of the nerve that goes to the vocal cords, which passes near the course that is taken by the surgeon for an anterior cervical spine surgery. There is a certain frequency, perhaps two or three out of 100 patients, who experience fairly severe hoarseness after such an operation, and there is really no good way to eliminate this risk completely. This fact should be factored into the surgical decision and consent. For many patients, a small risk of temporary hoarseness is no big concern, whereas for a patient who is a singer or other voice professional, that type of surgery may present an unacceptable level of risk. Thus, the significance of a specific risk depends on the individual.

Finally, there may be some catastrophic risk with very rare occurrence. For instance, it is possible to become permanently paralyzed during surgery near the cervical spinal cord. However, this would require some extraordinary catastrophic event and has an occurrence in the range of less than one in 100,000—possibly as low as your risk of being struck by lightning. Nevertheless, it is a conceivable risk of the procedure.

It is generally considered appropriate to mention these special catastrophic risks in part because many patients focus on these and will not entirely trust the surgeon who doesn't want to discuss them. Other patients, however, consider the risk to be so low that they would just rather not be frightened by something of little concern to them in advance of a surgery they must have anyway. This issue is somewhat cultural. In the United States, somehow it never seems to be wrong to provide all warnings directly to the patient, no matter how ill; doing so may even tend to build everyone's confidence in the physician. But in the United Kingdom, for example, this kind of warning may be seen as a kind of cruelty to the sick patient.

Risks of surgery are also judged by expected benefit. If you have a very mild back problem and could choose to take care of it or not, you may not be willing to take any risks in its treatment. If the problem is severe and life-threatening or if you have a risk of paralysis without treatment, you may be willing to undertake much greater risks and a more difficult recovery. All of these issues should be discussed in advance, and it's also traditional to review them just prior to surgery, often with the operating room nurse if not directly with the surgeon.

The concept of alternatives and indications can be illustrated by the following example. Your doctor has identified that you have leg pain, determined that the leg pain is caused by a nerve being pinched at a certain location, found that a protruding disk at that location is pinching the nerve, and planned a particular surgical approach to remove that disk. He has also explained to you that there might be an option simply to wait and do nothing or to do a different laser surgery, but he has doubts about its potential for success. He has therefore recommended that he do the open surgery because it has the best expectation, in his opinion, of success and rapid recovery.

Arbitration and Assignment: Legal Matters

Signing a consent form doesn't mean that you surrender any legal rights in case you have a complication or in case there is medical negligence, which might lead to a malpractice lawsuit. Hearing what you need to know to give informed consent and signing a consent form are important steps, but they do not relieve anyone of the responsibility to provide excellent and appropriate care.

One additional document that is sometimes provided before surgery is an *arbitration agreement*. With this document, both parties, patient and doctor, agree that in the case of an adverse outcome—something unexpected or negative that takes place in the course of surgery or recovery—the patient's recourse will be to arbitration instead of medical malpractice litigation. Arbitration is a legal proceeding that is usually simpler, faster, and less expensive to carry forward than a malpractice suit.

Usually, there will not be a jury involved, and the arbitration decision will be made and imposed by a judge based on the facts presented. For many patients, arbitration provides a safe and low-cost way of pursuing a disagreement; for others, maintaining the free right to sue is more important, so that is always provided as an alternative.

Another form that is often presented for signing in advance of surgery is an *assignment of benefits*. This is really an insurance matter and has to do with whether the insurance company is to pay you for the medical bill or whether the payment is to go directly from the insurance company to the doctor. Many hospitals and physicians insist on an assignment of benefits. A scenario that shows the effect of this is as follows. The insurance payment for the hospital bill and surgeon's fee comes to $20,000. If the patient personally gets an insurance check for $20,000, the doctor and hospital may then have to pursue collections against the patient for the entire amount to get any payment. Because the amounts of money are large and the payment is essentially from the insurance carrier to the provider with no specific intention to provide money to the patient, use of assignments have become standard. In this fashion whatever portion of the bill is covered by insurance will be paid directly to the doctor or the hospital, as appropriate, and only the remaining patient portion of the bill, if any, is to be addressed by the patient personally.

Measures for Heading Off Problems

Once you have moved beyond the business of paperwork to the actual medical procedures, there are a number of steps that can be taken before surgery begins or during surgery to reduce some of the routine risks and effects of the operation.

Getting Ready for the Operation

Most surgeons will provide some preoperative instructions so you know where to go, when to arrive, and what to expect. There are also a few general rules that can be a surprise. You usually have to stop taking anti-inflammatory medications such as aspirin or Motrin. These medicines have the side effect of interfering with the natural clotting mechanisms of your blood. It takes a week or more for the body to repair the effects of these medicines, so you usually need to stop taking them at least a week in advance.

A day or two prior to surgery, many surgeons require that you go for a visit with an internist who has "privileges" in the hospital where you're having your surgery. This means that the internist—who may or may not be your regular doctor—has approved credentials accepted by that hospital. The idea of this visit is to make sure that there are no general medical surprises—no heart problems, new blood sugar abnormalities, or any other medical issues. It also assures that while you are in the hospital for your operation and immediate recovery, there is a medical specialist available who has a recent and detailed knowledge of your full medical history and who is available to help with any medical problems immediately the moment they arise, such as high blood pressure after surgery, a reaction to a medication, any infection, or pneumonia. Usually, this internist has to give "medical clearance" for your surgeon to be allowed to proceed. If any specialty consultations are required, such as cardiology or endocrinology, this internist will work with your regular doctor and help to arrange them for you.

On the night before surgery, you're usually advised to have nothing to eat after midnight. This recommendation comes about because it's always better to have anesthesia on an empty stomach. You are generally allowed to take your usual medicines with small sips of water. However, this usually means that you'll have to skip your usual cup of coffee on the morning of surgery.

For some reason, many operations start at 7:30 in the morning. Because of this you may have to be at the hospital by 6:00 in the morning. Be sure to bring along any relevant X-rays you've been holding onto at home. If any friends or relatives are planning to wait at the hospital, be sure they bring plenty of reading material.

Preemptive Anesthesia

The first and most obvious concern about surgery may be postoperative pain. Surprisingly enough, it is often possible to keep this to a very tolerable minimum. A wide variety of medications are available to treat pain after surgery, but some things can also be done ahead of time to simplify the pain problems you will experience in the course of your recovery. Among these is the concept of *preemptive anesthesia*. Even though you will be under a general anesthetic, the idea here is to give additional numbing medication in the surgical region, helping to prevent the pain-sensing neural circuitry from becoming activated and to reduce the severity of your eventual pain.

Preemptive anesthesia can include special intravenous medications such as strong anti-inflammatory agents, but there is a plus and a minus to this practice. Anti-inflammatory agents do act as blood thinners and put you at more risk of bleeding after surgery, so they must be used judiciously. It is also the case that some anti-inflammatory agents may reduce the success of any fusion surgery, which becomes a consideration for those operations as well. Nonetheless, preemptive anesthesia is an important part of many surgeries, particularly those conducted on an outpatient basis.

Prophylactic Antibiotics

Although the skin is prepped during surgery and the instruments and gloves are sterilized, there is always the potential for some bacteria from the skin to get into the surgical wound. This is natural, and in normal tissue, the immune system and white blood cells will rapidly activate and destroy any stray bacteria. It is usually only in the setting of damaged tissue, a large amount of contamination, or the stray introduction of a particularly aggressive bacteria that the worst infections commence. However, some infections occur even when all precautions are taken.

A significant measure of safety is gained by one of the most common preoperative steps: administering intravenous antibiotic medication prior to making the surgical incision. It is also typical for a layer of antibiotic-coated or iodine-coated sheeting to be placed over all the exposed skin. The incision is made through the sheeting so that any remaining bacteria on the skin are sealed out of contact with the wound, the instruments, and the surgeon's hands. It is also common for the wound to be irrigated several times during surgery and particularly at the end with an antibiotic solution to wash out and fight any bacteria that may have come into contact with the surgical site. Even with all these measures, a certain number of infections still take place. However, preemptive or *prophylactic* antibiotics given intravenously, as a wound wash, and on the skin are fairly standard and effective means of controlling the risk of infection.

Antiemetics in Advance

Finally, one of the common risks of general anesthesia is postoperative nausea. For many types of surgery, having a lot of nausea and vomiting immediately afterward can really make the experience much more unpleasant than it needs to be. There are now very strong antinausea or *antiemetic* medications, such as Granisetron or Anzemet, which can be given preemptively at the start of anesthesia to minimize or reduce the risk of nausea after surgery. Careful selection of the anesthetic agent can also make a difference in some individuals with prior history of experiencing nausea after anesthesia.

Meeting the Operating Room Staff

The routine just before surgery varies considerably from hospital to hospital, but there are a few general guidelines. Once all the consents are signed, you're in your hospital gown on a gurney, and your intravenous line is started, your operating room (OR) nurse will generally go through a checklist with you. The OR nurse will be with you from start to finish, and it is his or her responsibility to make sure that a number of crucial details are taken care of.

First, there should be an ID check—are you the correct patient for the correct operation? Second, do you understand why you are there? It seems odd at this late stage, but the nurse will ask you to explain in your own words what you think is about to happen. This is actually a great way to head off some serious misunderstandings. She will take note of any special requests: "Be careful of my left wrist, please be sure the doctor calls my husband afterward"; and so on. Third, the OR nurse will often take out a pen or marker and write on your skin whether there is a left-sided or a right-sided problem (not always an issue in spine surgery). If a bone graft is going to be taken from your hip, the nurse can write on your hip bone whether you'd prefer right or left. It is also the OR nurse who usually makes sure that any special orders such as special stockings have been put on prior to surgery.

You will of course meet and talk with the anesthesiologist before the surgery starts. There are other team members who may or may not get a chance to say hello—this includes any assistant surgeon, the technologist who may be doing electronic monitoring of your nerves, an X-ray technician, any manufacturer's representative there to help the staff with implants, and a nurse or technician who will be scrubbed in along with the surgeon to help handle the various surgical instruments.

Care in the Incision: What Makes a Difference

Now, with all the paperwork done and all the initial medications delivered, you are asleep and the operation is ready to start. There are a number of choices that the surgeon can make at this point that will affect your recovery, so you may want to discuss them in advance.

Small versus Large Incisions

After a spine surgery, much of what you have to recover from is really the surgeon's approach to the actual problem. To get to the nerve pinch, the surgeon has to cut through skin, muscle, and other tissues, including bone, just to get close to the exact point of the problem. Removing a pinch on a nerve may make you feel much better, but the whole process of *exposing*, or surgically reaching into the right spot, and then closing it all up is what causes most of your postoperative pain and trouble.

In general, the size of the incision represents a trade-off. An older approach to surgery uses a very large incision for lots of exposure. This gives the surgeon a very good view of everything, but perhaps involves more blood loss and certainly a longer incision to close. Bigger incisions may also mean a longer time for opening and for closing. They can also leave larger scars and be more painful for you. The advantage is that once the exposure is complete, the surgeon has an excellent view and plenty of working room.

At the other extreme, using a very small incision—working through a keyhole, as it were—may make the operation more technically difficult for the surgeon because the view, exposure, and room to maneuver are so restricted. However, if there is enough space for the surgeon to get the job done, and get it done safely, then your recovery will be far simpler.

A one-inch incision hurts a lot less than an eight-inch incision, and there actually can be variations that great in incisions by different surgeons doing essentially the same spine surgeries. Some of the aids to vision, such as *endo-scopes* (video-assisted surgical instruments passed into the body through a small tube) and advanced types of *tubular retractors* (devices that spread outward in a circular fashion from an initial needle pass), can help the surgeon work through a smaller opening. Also, the use of the *operating microscope* can enable the surgeon to do fine manipulations without sacrificing good light and good vision. In all of these ways, the best medical technology helps your recovery by allowing the smallest appropriate incision for the surgery.

Skin Lines and Nerve Courses

Another aspect of surgical exposure is the cosmetic effect: That is, how well your scar disappears after surgery depends on exactly the way the incision was made. For incisions along the back, the surgeon almost always cuts up and down right along the midline of the spine. Other than the length of that incision, there aren't too many choices to be made in this case. However, for other types of surgery, such as an anterior cervical spine procedure, placement of the incision within an actual natural skin fold in your neckline may help the incision seem to disappear once it is healed. Additional incisions, such as in your hip to get some bone graft material, can be designed to fall in a natural skin line as well.

Incisions also have to be designed with attention to the course traveled by some of the small nerves that transmit skin sensation. An incision perpendicular to this course may cut many of those small nerves, leaving a numb patch on the skin, whereas an incision that runs parallel to their usual pattern may preserve normal sensation around the area of the cut. It is often unavoidable to cause some numbness right around the area of an incision, but sensation will often fill in gradually over the months after surgery.

Sides and Levels

To keep a surgical incision small it is important that it is made in the correct place. The two critical features in identifying the right place to cut for a spine surgery are the side of the body and the level of the spine. This is why the nurse should see that the correct side is marked on your skin before you start receiving any medications.

Once the patient is anesthetized and can't answer questions, there can't be any ambiguity. This is important in case some of the paperwork is wrong or the X-rays are displayed upside-down or backward—the patient, while awake, has already indicated the correct side and it has been marked on the patient's body, so the misleading medical information can be proven to be incorrect.

It is essential to perform a spine surgery at the correct level. That is, if the target is the L4-L5 disk, the approach is not supposed to be made at the level of L3-L4 or L5-S1. As you can imagine, simply looking at the skin surface and dissecting through the body does not guarantee that the surgeon is at the correct place. For accuracy, X-rays are typically taken during the surgery. The first X-ray is usually taken before a fresh skin incision is made in order to place the cut directly over the area of interest. If the incision is made by general body landmarks and an X-ray shows that it is not high enough or low enough, then the incision will have to be extended to bring the surgeon into the right line of exposure.

During the course of the surgical approach, X-rays are often repeated in order to be sure that the instruments didn't slide at the last minute over a ridge of bone either too low or too high, leading the surgeon astray. It is certainly very unfortunate if a whole operation is completed and then it is discovered, during surgery or even in the weeks or months afterward when the expected improvement does not occur, that the level was wrong and the surgery has to be repeated. Taking the time to shoot and evaluate the right number of *intraoperative X-rays* is the best guarantee of avoiding this type of complication.

Some Details of Surgical Technique

The whole surgical progression from the skin incision down to the spine can be done in a variety of ways. Some of these are faster, some are slower, and some are more or less protective of the tissues that the surgeon encounters.

Advances in Getting to the Surgical Problem

Between the skin and the entrapped nerve, the surgeon will encounter the various tissues of the body such as muscles, blood vessels, nerves, and bones. Much of modern surgery is designed around helping the surgeon get to the target with a minimum of unnecessary trauma to these intervening tissues.

Despite the availability of a wide array of mechanical, electronic, and laser-based surgical tools for dissection, the best means of making progress through the body may be very simple. Essentially, it is generally best to gently follow the planes of natural separation (e.g., muscle-splitting rather than muscle-cutting approaches) in the body rather than cutting anything that doesn't absolutely have to be cut.

Once a safe, gentle path to the target is developed, the surgeon can place retractors to hold the tissue out of the line of site while the surgical work is going on. When all this works well, all the surgeon has to do at the end is to remove the retractor, allow the various tissues to slip back into their normal positions, suture up any structural layers that were cut, and then close the skin.

Planning in Advance for Blood Loss

During extensive fusion surgeries, there can be very significant blood loss—as many as two, three, or even more units of blood—so a device called a cell saver is often used. As suction tubes clear blood away from the surgical field, this machine captures the blood that is suctioned up, washes the blood cells, and then allows them to be transfused back into the patient to minimize the need for additional blood transfusion. For most large fusion surgeries, you are encouraged to donate your own, or *autologous*, blood in advance so you don't need to receive someone else's blood. In an emergency, typed, cross-matched, and tested blood can be given, and for the most part this is extremely safe.

There can be quite a bit of variation in blood loss that has to do with particular details of a surgery, as well as individual features that vary from patient to patient. Most spinal surgeries can be accomplished with little or no blood loss. Occasionally, however, there will be enough routine blood loss that a transfusion is needed. This is to be expected and is not a special cause for concern or alarm.

Achieving Closure from Inside to Outside

After everything is done at the surgical site and all bleeding is controlled, the final steps involve washing the area with antibiotic solution, putting medication near the nerves or in the muscles to help reduce postoperative pain, and maybe using an antiscarring agent in and around the nerves. Then the surgeon proceeds through several layers of closure.

Pain Control Following Surgery

In addition to the more standard measures used to prevent pain after surgery, other steps can be taken at the time of closure. These include putting an anesthetic paste containing narcotic and anesthetic agents on the nerve roots, as well as placing steroid agents directly over the nerves. Another method that is sometimes used is to insert a thin catheter through the skin down to the nerves to pump anesthetic medication into the spine during the day or two after surgery. The negative aspects of catheterization are the risk of infection and the possibility of putting too much fluid into the wound, causing leakage or pressure on the nerves; the positive side is that a large amount of strong medication can be delivered precisely to the surgical site. Usually, measures such as catheters are reserved for treating patients with unusual, specialized pain problems.

Antiscarring in the Spine: Preventing Stuck Nerves

Many patients simply don't form much scar tissue around the nerves, but some produce enough to make the surgery fail. For this reason, measures are often taken in closing to minimize nerve scarring. There are a few choices of *antiscarring agents*. One, called Adcon-L, was a gel material that proved to cause problems with healing and was withdrawn from the market. Another resorbable antiscarring product more commonly used in the abdomen and in nerve surgery is Seprafilm. There are also types of Gore-Tex membrane that are placed near nerves, although sometimes these are more complicated for the surgeon to use. An older technique is simply to layer excess fatty tissue in and around the nerves to help minimize the risk of excessive scar formation.

The Use of Drains in Surgery

If there is any small amount of continuing bleeding at the end of surgery, the surgeon may choose to leave a small drain through the skin surface, typically through a separate puncture away from the surgical incision closure line. This is to help to prevent blood from accumulating close to the nerves. Such a drain is usually removed one or two days later, and antibiotic administration is often continued for as long as the drain is in place. However, drains are not usually used after smaller spinal surgeries.

Closing Fascia

The major constructive step of surgical closure in the lumbar spine and the back of the neck is to close the *fascia*, the very heavy ligaments to which all of the muscles are attached. Cut or damaged fascia are closed with very heavy-duty sutures that are tied very tightly and help to restore strength to the muscle layers. If any of the *fascial sutures* break and the fascia start to separate, this tends to promote the development of muscle spasm after surgery. Eventually, the fascia will heal closed, but delayed healing of the fascia tends to delay and lengthen the whole course of recovery.

Staples, Stitches, Glue, and Tape

Above the fascia, there is usually a deep closure of the skin and then a super-ficial closure (see Fig. 13.1). The types of skin closures used include staples, which go in quickly and come out easily, but often leave many little two-point scar marks along the incision line. For some patients, this is of no concern at all, but for others this is a great concern. Anyone concerned with the appearance of an incision should try to discourage the surgeon from using staples.

One option is to use buried, or *subcuticular,* stitches that hide below the skin and often give the best cosmetic appearance. The different varieties of stitching material for beneath the skin include absorbable sutures, which never need to be removed, and nonabsorbable sutures, which are often nylon and have to be removed a week or two after surgery. It is worth noting, however, that patients vary considerably in the speed and efficiency with which the absorb-able sutures are dissolved. This can lead to nonabsorbed suture knots poking through the skin surface weeks after surgery. Once the nonabsorbed absorba-bles are removed, the healing process can then proceed to completion.

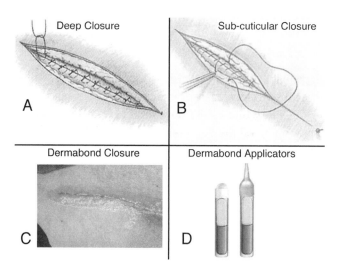

Figure 13.1 Skin closure methods. Closing the skin after a surgery is done in layers. The deep closure involves a series of separate stitches and knots, or interrupted stitching (A). The outer layer of the skin can be drawn together with a single running subcuticular or "buried" stitch that disappears below the skin as the closure progresses (B). Dermabond (D) is very similar to a superglue. It can provide both an outer closure layer and a simple wound dress-ing that does not require bandages (C). Illustrations reproduced with permission of Ethicon/Johnson & Johnson.

Another important advance in wound closure is the use of special glues, such as Dermabond, which is based on the cyanoacrylate super-glues. Applying this glue along the wound surface creates an immediate occlusive dressing. It is actually safe to go ahead and get the wound wet immediately, because it is sealed. The glue seal provides a very safe environment for the skin to regrow and heal, also preventing the passage of bacteria into the wound. The super-glues tend to wear off after a few days, but they are very helpful right after surgery.

Finally, particularly when subcuticular stitches are used, little tapes called Steri-Strips are often applied with some adhesive, which helps prevent the wound from widening. When there is stretching across the incision line, the space between the two separating edges of the wound often fills in with a bright red scar tissue, which makes the incision more prominent. If the skin edges can be perfectly aligned and kept closely together during the course of healing, the smallest possible scar results. Steri-Strips are often left on for as long as a couple of weeks.

Dressings and Braces

Finally, a dressing is usually placed over the closed incision, including some gauze and some sort of protective cover such as tape or Tegaderm, which is a clear, thin plastic. The gauze soaks up any small amounts of ooze from the wound and makes it possible for the nurse and doctor to see any leakage readily without necessarily giving bacteria a route into the body through the wound. For most clean, dry incisions, the dressing is left on to seal the incision for several days and then removed, but some surgeons expect more drainage and routinely change the dressings on a daily basis after the surgery. This is really a matter of the individual surgeon's preferences.

Braces of some sort may be applied in addition to the dressing. These include neck braces, lumbar braces, soft braces, and hard braces; the particular selection depends on the type of surgery that was done and the preferences of the surgeon. Braces are almost always recommended after a fusion surgery (see chapters 16 and 19), although with sufficient internal instrumentation such as screws and plates, an external brace is often not essential or is at least less critical to the recovery (see Fig. 13.2).

Final Touch-Ups for Wound Appearance

There are some products that can help achieve the most cosmetic possible result after a surgery. This is most often of greatest concern with an incision on the front of the neck. Several companies sell small silicone pads that can be placed over the healing wound beginning around two weeks after surgery. These help

Figure 13.2 Braces: cervical collar. After a fusion surgery, many physicians recommend that a patient wear a brace to hold the spine in place while the bone grows into the fusion site. For neck surgery, a collar is often worn for four to six weeks. After some lumbar surgeries, a brace may be needed for three to six months.

remind the skin to flatten out to its normal smooth contour. There are also bleaching creams such as Nuquin that can help equalize the color of the scar in some patients. Ask your doctor to recommend appropriate products if scarring is a concern.

Ideally, when all measures are taken, many surgical incisions can virtually disappear completely. However, for the most part, you should expect some sort of visible permanent scar line to remain after a spinal surgery. One hopes that this lasting mark will be a reminder of a successful treatment.

14

Surgery to Take Pressure off the Neural Tissues of the Spine

The essence of decompressive spinal surgery is the art of trimming away bones, ligaments, disks, joints, tumors, and any other surrounding tissues that are irritating or compressing neural tissue. Whether surgery is needed, when it is needed, how to get to the spine, how to finish up and get out are all covered in other chapters of this book. After accurate diagnosis, the success of the surgery will be measured by how well the surgeon approached the squeezed nerve and removed tissue to do the decompressive work, leaving enough space for the nerve to move freely. The work must be completed without damaging the delicate nerves nearby, and it must ultimately leave the spine able to function as the strong, flexible skeletal component that it needs to be (see Fig. 14.1).

One critical element for understanding the advice a surgeon gives and for being able to discuss the plan with him or her is to know something about the language of spine surgery. This will also help you to understand the operative report, if you should ever need to look at that, and even the billing of the surgery.

The beginning of the name for a surgery step or procedure generally comes from the specific part of the spine that is being treated. Among the most common of these terms are *lamina*, which is the roof over the back of the spinal canal; *facet*, which refers to a joint between vertebrae; *disk,* the cushioning spacer between vertebrae; *foramen* or *foramina*, the opening through which a spinal nerve exits the spinal canal to reach its target muscle or organ; and *vertebra*, or *corp*, meaning the main structural body of a vertebra. Next, the terms for the major types of spine operations usually have an ending such as "ectomy," "otomy," "plasty," or "lysis." When you do an "ectomy" on something, you remove it; when you do an "otomy" on something, you cut it; when you do a "plasty," you reshape something; and a "lysis" means to lesion, to remove, or occasionally to separate something. These beginnings and endings can thus be assembled as needed into surgical terms that indicate precisely what is being done:

Figure 14.1 Surgical instruments. Modern spine surgery employs a mix of old and new surgical instruments. Access to the spine through a MetRx tube system greatly reduces the invasiveness of surgery. A conventional root retractor and a tissue biting instrument called a rongeur can be used along with an endoscope. Illustration reproduced with permission of Medtronic. Inc.

laminectomy, corpectomy, foraminotomy, facetectomy, or vertebroplasty, and so on—the core operations of spinal surgery.

Discectomy: Battling the Bulge

One of the most common types of spinal surgery is the removal of a herniated disk, a process called a *discectomy*. In fact, in the past it was common for spinal surgeons to try to remove the entire disk; however, this posed certain severe complication risks and several major problems. If the disk is removed completely, then the vertebra above sits directly on the vertebra below. Such a bone-on-bone contact can result in grinding and bumping that can cause more back pain—obviously an undesirable outcome. Also, in attempting to scrape the entire disk space completely clean through a small opening, there is a significant risk of passing through the front of the ring and damaging one of the large blood vessels in the abdomen, such as the aorta, which can have disastrous consequences. For these reasons, spinal surgeons more commonly remove problematic disk fragments rather than an entire herniated disk.

The reason for trying to get a complete disk removal is to try to prevent one of the most common undesirable outcomes from discectomy, which is recurrence. Essentially, the original problem of a nerve pinch is caused because part of the interior of the disk has bulged out or escaped from the disk space. If only the fragment is removed, the concern is that another fragment will emerge and pinch the nerve again. However, it turns out that even when surgeons attempt to remove the entire disk through an opening of fairly significant size, a little bit is almost always left behind. Therefore, even with an attempted complete discectomy, there is still a significant risk of recurrence despite all the effort and additional risks involved, including the increased risk of causing bone-on-bone back pain.

Microdiscectomy

For the most part, complete discectomy is not done for routine disk bulges. Instead, the surgeon removes just the offending fragment and perhaps a little bit of disk from below it. This still leaves about a 5 percent risk of recurrence from reherniation. This is considered acceptable because the benefit is that the surgeries can be done through a very small incision, and the most severe risks of precipitating complete disk collapse or of injuring a large blood vessel in the abdomen are almost completely avoided (see Fig. 14.2).

To reach a disk fragment that is pinching a nerve, the surgeon uses a comparatively small opening. One of the big advances that allowed surgeons to reduce the size of this opening was the advent and further development of the surgical microscope. The microscope makes it possible to carry out a *microdiscectomy* by providing excellent three-dimensional visual detail and illumination down a long, deep hole with a small opening at the top.

For a microdiscectomy, the surgeon ideally makes an incision in the skin that is just about an inch long. A muscle-splitting approach can be used rather than actually cutting through muscle, and a very small laminotomy, or cutting of the edge of the lamina, can be carried out on the inferior (bottom) edge of the vertebra above the herniated disk and the superior (top) edge of the vertebra below it. This leaves just enough of an opening, probably about one-half to three-quarters of an inch in circumference, through which the surgeon can work using a stereomicroscope. The thick, overlying *ligamentum flavum* (an elastic ligament that runs from the lamina of one vertebra to the lamina of the next vertebra) between the laminar edges is removed, and the surgeon then moves the nerve root care fully out of the way; a device is used to seal any small veins nearby. The annular ring is then cut, and the offending disk fragments are then removed.

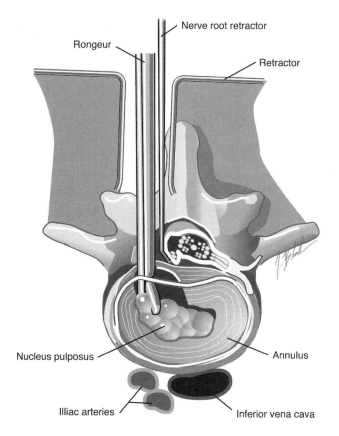

Figure 14.2 Microdiscectomy. For a conventional spine approach, the retractors retain the back muscles that have been peeled off of their attachments to the vertebra. Using an operating microscope to enhance visibility, the surgeon can use a nerve root retractor to move the nerve roots out of the way manually so that a rongeur can reach into the disk space to remove part of the nucleus pulposus. Image published with permission of Joe Bloch.

Microendoscopic Disk Removal

Having made an approach for a microdiscectomy, it is possible to use a *microendoscope* (a very small version of the video-assisted surgical equipment) to get a close-up view; however, the microendoscope takes up a lot of the space needed for surgical maneuvering. Microendoscopy has still not proven to be popular among surgeons for this operation, because it reduces the surgeon's tactile input and flexibility and doesn't really allow for any decrease in the size of the incision. Also, small veins near the disk will sometimes bleed during surgery. Although the amount of blood they lose is very small, in the tiny space under the illuminated end point of a microendoscope they appear to fill the field completely with blood. The surgeon has to withdraw the instrument and go back to a microscope under direct view in order to stop the bleeding and continue with the operation. For these reasons, use of the microendoscope for disk removal has not gained widespread popularity among surgeons. However, with further technical improvements, these devices may come to play a more important role in various aspects of spinal surgery.

In fact, there have been many attempts to design alternative operations with different equipment or approaches from other angles to improve on open microdiscectomy. The problem has been that the microdiscectomy as currently practiced is so safe and effective and typically has such a speedy recovery that it is hard to beat. Any additional complications or failures due to the new technology tend to override any small benefit provided. This may change in the future, though. In essence, spinal surgeons are committed to making the microdiscectomy operation into an outpatient procedure with minimal recovery time.

Nucleoplasty: Hot Wires and Lasers

Yet another possibility is to use the open surgical approach but then to apply a hot wire or a laser under direct vision. The device is introduced into the disk space and used to evaporate the disk, rather than biting and pulling pieces out of the disk space. Although this might be a helpful technique, there are very few disadvantages to direct mechanical removal, and the mechanical removal gives the surgeon the best direct feel for the tissues being removed. Also, with a laser there is always a possibility that if it is turned on within the disk space, it may penetrate the disk more rapidly then the surgeon realizes and pass out of the other side of the disk space. This could injure some other tissues such as the blood vessels in the abdomen. Therefore, the mechanical method of disk removal is still the most widely used among surgeons carrying out open-disk surgery.

The laser and heat methods were intended to simplify the work of disk removal but present their own problems because they increase the risk of accidentally causing damage outside the disk space. Keep in mind that just outside the disk space is the aorta. The Medtronic nucleotome shaver uses a high-speed blade within a thin probe that has a blunt end. This reduces the risk of pushing or cutting through the annulus. The device trims the disk into fine particles that can be washed and suctioned out of the disk space. The intended effect is to increase the surgeon's sense of being able to feel the confines the disk space.

Laminectomy and Laminoplasty: Roof Remodeling

An even older type of spine surgery that still has a variety of important uses is removing the very back of the vertebra, the lamina, which sits behind the dura. This operation is called a laminectomy if the lamina is removed completely or a *laminoplasty* if it is removed only partially.

Undoing Spinal Stenosis with Laminectomy

It is possible to remove the back of the vertebra—that is, the spinous process and the lamina that together form the roof over the spinal canal—without significantly affecting the strength of the spine or the safety of the nerve tissues in the canal. There is a very thick mass of back muscle behind the nerve tissue, and short of the rather uncommon event that someone sticks a penetrating object through your back into your spine, the loss of the laminar protection will really have no meaningful effect on you (see Fig. 14.3).

The advantage of removing the roof like this may be to increase the space within the spinal canal. However, if the abnormality that's squeezing the nerves is coming from the front, from the area of the disk, it is often preferable to remove the offending problem from the front rather than just removing the lamina.

Laminectomies are commonly done for patients who have stenosis, or narrowing of the spinal canal at multiple spinal levels. This is a situation in which arthritis causes the joints of the spine to expand and the ligaments, particularly the thick, elastic ligamentum flavum, or "yellow ligament," to become overgrown and gradually to squeeze the nerves of the spinal canal. In normal function, the ligamentum flavum provides elastic tension between the lamina of the

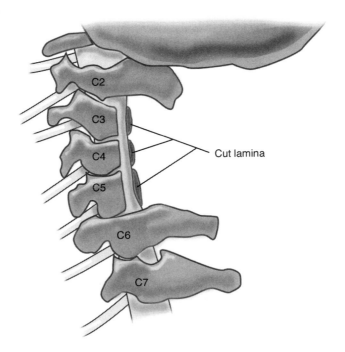

Figure 14.3 Cervical laminectomy. To increase space around the spinal cord, the lamina and spinous processes can be removed. Image published with permission of Joe Bloch.

vertebrae—it is stretched when you lean forward and relaxes or folds when you lean back.

The best surgical treatment for stenosis due to this type of overgrowth of ligament and bone is laminectomy. Removal of the lamina at multiple levels then allows the spinal dura to expand and takes the pressure off the nerves. A *hemilaminectomy* that removes just the right or left side of the lamina may also be a good alternative in the lumbar spine. This preserves much of the spinal musculature and reduces the scale of the opening. Working at a low angle, the surgeon then reaches across from the open side, below the untouched spinous process, to remove most of the ligamentum flavum and overgrown bone in the joints on the opposite side so that both right and left sides are opened up with an approach and exposure from one side only.

Bone Stitches, Wires, and Microplates for Laminoplasty

Laminoplasty opens up the spinal canal by raising the bony roof rather than by removing it. This is most commonly done in the neck because of the problems that can occur after a laminectomy when it's needed in the neck. Unlike the lumbar spine, removing the lamina in the cervical spine, particularly if the joints are affected, causes a risk of losing the normal curvature of the neck so that the head begins to fall forward. The general term for the situation in which the spine bends forward when it should bend backward is a *kyphosis* or *kyphotic deformity*. This is a potential complication of having a multiple-level laminectomy in the neck, which then has to be corrected by its own surgery such as a fusion.

A laminoplasty is done in the neck to reduce this risk, particularly in patients who are not yet in their 60s or 70s who need a cervical laminectomy. In the lumbar spine, laminoplasty is generally indicated only in the rare situations in which young children need laminectomies. The hemilaminectomy described above for the lumbar region cannot be safely used in the cervical region because of the shape of the spinal canal and the sensitivity of the spinal cord in the cervical spine.

The most common way a cervical laminoplasty is done is to make an incision in the outer surface of the bone on one side of the spine and to cut through completely on the other side of the spine. Each lamina is then opened and lifted up, like a door swinging open: the partially cut side acts like the hinge, and the fully cut opposite side lifts up and away from the spinal cord and dura. To hold the lamina in its lifted-open position, wires or sutures may be placed on the partially cut side, or *microplates* can be used to hold the laminoplasty open. The bone eventually grows into this modified shape, and the new spinal canal that solidifies is much larger in diameter than the previous one (see Figs. 14.4 and 14.5).

Until recently, laminoplasty was done only infrequently, but increasing understanding of the value of decompressing the spinal canal without requiring a fusion

Figure 14.4 R Laminoplasty plate. A—As an alternative to a laminectomy, the surgeon may elect to expand the spinal canal by repositioning the lamina in a *laminoplasty* operation rather than removing it completely in a *laminectomy*. On the right side of the illustration, the lamina has been cut through and opened. On the left side, the lamina has been scored and folded back. In this case, small metal plates are used to help the lamina heal in its altered configuration. Image A is published with permission of Joe Bloch. B—Medtronic provides specialized laminoplasty plates that improve the effectiveness and ease of placement for the surgeon. The plate holds the lamina open at the laminoplasty site. Image B reproduced with permission of Medtronic, Inc.

has led to wider use of this operation. One sign of this is the appearance of new specialized types of laminoplasty plate systems from several spine implant manufacturers. These improve the effectiveness and reduce the duration of the operation. They are designed to be secured by screws to the heavy lateral lamina of the cervical vertebra, with a forked portion that captures the elevated lamina. This holds the elevated lamina in place while small screws are placed to hold the laminoplasty open.

Laminoplasty is particularly helpful in patients who have a narrowed spinal canal at multiple levels in the cervical spine. In general, the same situation in the lumbar spine can't be treated with laminoplasty in adults because of the size of the bone elements and the forces involved; however, laminoplasty in the lumbar

Figure 14.5 Laminoplasty cervical spine result. This drawing shows Medtronic laminoplasty plates in place in a five-level laminoplasty including C4, C5, C6 C7 and T1. This procedures relieves stenosis pressure on the spinal cord. Notice that the plates at C5 and C7 hold small bone graft bridges to help the lamina regrow in the new configuration with an enlarged spinal canal. Image reproduced with permission of Medtronic, Inc.

region is often feasible in the rare situation in which young children require a surgery of this type.

The occurrence of a narrow spinal canal in the cervical spine in an adult can result from extensive degenerative change and arthritis, as in the lumbar region. But in the neck the condition may also be due to an abnormal variant carried along since birth or earlier—a congenitally narrow spinal canal—or due to progression of one of the conditions that causes ossification (bone formation) inside the spinal canal, such as ossification of the posterior longitudinal ligament.

Interspinous Spacers for Lumbar Canal Stenosis

An entirely novel method for decompressing the spinal canal has come along in the past five years that can dramatically reduce the scale of surgery needed to treat lumbar spinal canal stenosis. Lumbar canal stenosis affects the spinal roots and causes claudication—leg pain and weakness with walking. This is different from stenosis of the foramina or nerve canals.

Lumbar spinal stenosis generally affects older patients in their late 60s, as well as patients in their 70s or 80s. It is challenging to treat these patients because the risk of surgery increases significantly in older patients. The stenosis is generally due to three simultaneous issues. First, the intervertebral disk is dried out so it loses height. This leads the surrounding annulus to bulge backwards into the spinal canal. Second, the facets become overgrown with arthritis and bulge in from the sides. Finally, the ligamentum flavum in the back of the spinal canal bulges in due to the loss of intervertebral height as well.

Many patients with this condition find that they can relieve the symptoms by leaning forward. Often this means holding onto a shopping cart or wheeled walker. What is happening is that when two lumbar vertebra in this condition are flexed relative to each other, the axis of rotation shifts to the front of the vertebral body. This results in an opening up of the back of the intervertebral space, which pulls the annulus taut so that it pulls away from the spinal canal and back toward the disk. The same thing happens—but to an even greater degree—for the lamina. They spread apart and the ligamentum flavum is pulled taut thus lifting itself back up out of the spinal canal. However, once the person stands up straight, all these advantages are lost and the spinal stenosis resumes.

The technical advance that takes advantage of these mechanics is the interspinous spacer. This is a very simple implant that is placed between the spinous processes of the involved lumbar vertebra (see Fig. 14.6). Typically, the stenosis is only critical at one level—most often L3/4—and so only one spacer needs to be placed. Because it goes between the spinous processes, it is just a few centimeters below the skin and so a full depth spinal surgery can be avoided. The X-stop (from Medtronic) was the first of these devices (FDA approved in 2005) but other manufacturers now offer more complex variants that fit the interspinous spaces more precisely, have some flexibility, or are adjustable when they are placed so they can better fit individual variations in anatomy.

Foraminotomy: Opening the Canals

The passage that a nerve takes as it leaves the spinal canal and heads out into the body is through an opening called the *foramen,* which simply means "passage" or "tunnel." The foramen is formed by the pedicles of the vertebrae above and below it, the disk in front of it, and the joints behind it. The most common reason that a foramen gets narrowed is because the surfaces of the bony joint, or facets, have started to grow. This takes place in a fashion similar to what you may sometimes see in an older person with arthritis who has very large knuckles. Similarly, the small joints of the spine will expand. Unfortunately, their expansion often leads

Figure 14.6 Interspinous spacers for lumbar stenosis. Patients with lumbar stenosis may get relief from their claudication when they bend forward—but implants can achieve this effect by expanding the space between successive spinous processes, allowing the patient to get relief while standing straight. A—Stenofix implant from Synthes is a newer dynamic type interspinous expander that retains flexibility between the two vertebrae. It can also take pressure off the facet joints and help hold the foramen open more widely. It is approved for one or two spinal levels. B—The X-stop from Medtronic was the first type of interspinous spacer and has been used widely; it holds the vertebral pair in a fixed position. Studies of the success of the X-stop have shown improvement in 50 to 60 percent of patients. Image B reproduced with permission of Medtronic, Inc.

them to grow into the foramen and steal space from the nerve that should be passing freely through the opening.

In the cervical spine, there is also an area at the corner of the vertebral body end plate, next to the disk, that can form bone spurs, or osteophytes, that grow into the foramen. This is an area where the cervical vertebrae have something like a joint in the space between them, which is dominated by the disk. This vertebral body joint area in the neck is called the *unco-vertebral* joint.

Lumbar Foraminotomy

When overgrowth of the facet joints and their associated ligaments causes a pinched nerve in the lumbar spine, the treatment is a *foraminotomy*. This means cutting or reexpansion of the nerve canal. A lumbar foraminotomy is accomplished by making an approach from directly behind the spine, from the back, very similar to the approach for a microdiscectomy. It involves carrying out small laminotomies, or cutting openings in the lamina, to get inside, along the path of the nerve root. Then the nerve root is followed out along the narrowed tunnel, biting away bone from the surfaces behind and around it. This generally means trimming away excess bone growth on the undersurface of the facet joints. There are special devices that are curved so that they can reach out into the canal to try to get both the inside, or near, portions of the canal and the exterior, or far portions.

A pinch of a nerve root in the proximal or near part of the foraminal canal used to be most commonly diagnosed by an imaging study called the X-ray *myelogram*, which shows the root sleeves as they pass into the foramen. At present, one of the best ways to evaluate both proximal and distal (both near and far) compression in the foramen is an MR neurography study of the lumbar region (see Fig. 10.3), although narrowing or stenosis of the foramen can also be assessed from standard MRI scans and certainly from CT scans as well.

If a foraminotomy is excessive, it can compromise the stability of the spine by taking away too much of the joint. This will lead to increased back pain. However, lumbar foraminotomy is a very common operation and is very reliable when carried out carefully and thoroughly. Foraminotomies need to be considered any time that any decompression of the spinal canal is carried out. In the case of any laminectomy for central spinal canal stenosis, foraminotomies may be needed as well.

Monitored Foraminotomy

The general logic of spinal surgery is to cut through skin and soft tissues, then use various drills and choppers to clear away bone to get near the involved nerves. The Baxano foraminotomy device is a very novel change in the paradigm and may be the first step in a wider revolution of spinal surgery. The surgery starts out in conventional fashion, but instead of blindly cutting at the bone of the foramen, the surgeon places a guide into the entry of the foramen and is able to use electronics built into the instrument to check the position of the nerve as the guide is eased through the tight foramen.

A wire is then passed that is then popped through to the skin surface, and the wire allows the surgeon to pull a flat flexible rasp into the foramen. Then, while still monitoring and protecting the nerve, the surgeon can use the rasp to file away the surface of the entire foramen—from the previously accessible inner or proximal portion all the way out to the distal outer portion, which has generally been completely inaccessible from a traditional approach from inside the spine. Not only does it do a far better job than the older method, but also it represents a complete rethinking of the task, takes advantage of modern technology to turn simple instruments into smart probes, and makes the entire process far less invasive and risky.

Microscopic Cervical Foraminotomy

A foraminotomy in the cervical spine is a somewhat different operation. It is often a choice when there is a pinched nerve canal in the neck, and the surgeon and the patient hope to avoid the need to actually carry out a fusion. A cervical foraminotomy can be performed through a very small incision with microscope magnification, approaching from the back of the neck. It involves making an opening from directly behind the nerve canal just big enough to allow a very small Kerrison punch to enter. The Kerrison punch is used to reach down inside the canal and open up the space along the nerve. A posterior cervical foraminotomy is a very small operation that can often solve a difficult problem, without the more extensive disk replacement surgery needed when the foraminotomy is carried out from the front (see Fig. 14.7).

Facetectomy: Trimming Overgrown Joints

Similar to the foraminotomy, a *facetectomy* involves trimming the edges of the overgrown joints as they expand medially into the spinal canal—a situation that can cause entrapment of the nerve roots along the lateral edge of spinal canal, or *lateral recess stenosis*. The facetectomy takes care of the medial

Figure 14.7 Posterior cervical foraminotomy. If the problem in the cervical spine affects only the exiting nerve root, then a very small surgery can be done to unroof the canal through which the spinal nerve exits, the neural foramen. Image published with permission of Joe Bloch.

overgrowth of the joint into the central spinal canal, and the foraminotomy takes care of the anterior overgrowth into the foraminal nerve canal. The two are often done together, and once again, pose the risk of destabilizing the spine and leading to back pain if too much bone is removed in the course of the procedure.

Vertebrectomy: Removing the Front

A much more extensive type of decompression surgery for the spinal canal is the *vertebrectomy*, which actually involves removing most or all of the body of the vertebra. This is the large, weight-bearing, front part of the vertebra (see Fig. 14.8). This is more often done in the neck when multiple levels in the cervical spine require discectomy and removal. It is also done at any location in the spine in situations of tumor invasion, infection, or fracture when the vertebral body, or the tissue replacing it, has started to press on the spinal canal from the front.

Replacing the Supporting Column

When vertebral bodies are removed, it is essential to replace them with something that can provide vertical structural support. This usually involves placement of some kind of graft in the spine, such as a piece of leg bone (the *tibia* or *fibula*) that can provide adequate vertical strength. Grafts such as these are *allografts*, taken from a cadaver (*allo* means "other"). Usually, bone obtained in this way is extensively and harshly treated to dissolve away everything except the minerals that make up the bone and some of the toughest structural protein fibers. For this reason, the rejection problems that affect organ transplantation don't occur.

A vertebral body can also be replaced with some hipbone from the patient, called an *autograft*. In most situations, the amount of hipbone that would have to be removed to fill in the opening from a thoracic or lumbar vertebrectomy discourages the surgeon from using the patient's own hipbone to fill the space. In the neck, however, it is often reasonable to replace a single vertebra with hipbone from the patient, although it is very common to use an allograft or a synthetic to replace a full vertebral level there. A vertebrectomy can also be replaced by certain types of titanium cages or meshes that can be used to hold bone-generating materials. In this situation the intention is to provide the support and materials to help the body grow its own bone strut rather than placing actual bone in the space.

Vertebrectomy Requiring Thoracotomy

Vertebrectomy in the cervical spine can be carried out through the type of small, minimally invasive anterior approach to the neck that's used for a cervical disk

Figure 14.8 Vertebrectomy. When significant problems affect much of the vertebral body, a vertebrectomy—removal of the vertebral body—may be required. Image published with permission of Joe Bloch.

operation. However, vertebrectomy in the thoracic region generally requires opening the chest, a procedure called a *thoracotomy*. It is often carried out by a vascular or thoracic surgeon working with the spinal surgeon. An incision is made between a pair of ribs and the surgeon actually spreads the ribs apart; sometimes it is necessary to remove one of the ribs to provide adequate access to the spine.

Thoracotomies for approach to the thoracic region of the spine are carried out in some cases for treatment of thoracic disk herniations that cannot be repaired through less invasive surgeries. They are also always required in the case of a major fracture in the thoracic spine or a major problem with tumor invasion or infection destroying a vertebra. After a thoracotomy, it is often necessary to place a drainage tube, called a *thoracostomy tube* or a *chest tube*, in the chest space. This tube sits in the space between the lung and the chest wall and uses suction to drain out any fluids and extra air until the normal shape and function of the lung can be restored through natural healing. Chest tubes can either be large-diameter tubes as big as half an inch across or very small tubes when less drainage is needed. Among the various approaches to the spine, the thoracotomy may be reasonably considered as the most maximally invasive.

Kyphoplasty: Reinflating a Vertebra

One of the newer types of vertebral operations is a method for expanding a partially collapsed vertebra without the need for open surgery. Vertebrae sometimes collapse as a consequence of osteoporosis, or loss of calcium and structural strength in bone. The idea of *kyphoplasty* is to work through the skin to insert a catheter through a small incision in the back. The catheter travels down a path cut in the pedicle of the vertebra, into the collapsed vertebral body. A balloon then is expanded to push the vertebra back into its normal expanded shape, and the balloon is filled with a type of super-glue. This often makes it possible to restore the normal shape of the spine and to treat the pain of a collapsed vertebra without an open surgery (see Fig. 14.9). In other older methods there was no balloon and the glue could spread directly in the bone. This posed a risk of the glue

Figure 14.9 Kyphoplasty. The collapse of a thoracic vertebra due to osteoporosis can be treated without open surgery. The Kyphx Xpander system shown here involves a balloon passed inside a needle through the skin. Once the balloon is inflated, it can be filled with a glue that supports the vertebra once it hardens. Illustrations reproduced with permission of Kyphon/Johnson & Johnson.

backing up into the spinal canal to compress the spinal cord, but the Kyphoplasty balloon system solved this problem.

One further important advance in this area is the use of a stent system. A stent is an expandable metal cage. These are important in expanding constrictions in the arteries during angioplasties in the coronary and carotid arteries and are used in various other places in the body. The main effect of using a stent in a vertebral body is to help spread the stress of pushing the bone back into place.

One of the most remarkable stories in modern medical regulation unfolded around the vertebroplasty procedure. As this procedure was gaining support among surgeons, a variety of surgical device companies were interested in providing products and methods. In a very ill-starred and unfortunate series of events, a company called Norian tried to re-task the bone cement system it developed for broken arms and legs in order to provide vertebroplasty cement (Norian XR) for the spine. For reasons that were not fully understood until Jens Chapman and colleagues at the University of Washington made a stunning report at the Orthopedic Research Society meeting in 2004 (based on animal studies), Norian XR produced an unexpected effect when used in the spine—a high risk of death from blood clots in the heart and lung (pulmonary embolus).

By the time the report was presented at the meeting, Norian and its larger partner (Synthes) were discovering that several patients died during surgery because of the clots. Pulmonary emboli can happen during any operation, but the report showed that calcium in the glue was causing a strikingly rapid and extensive clot formation process. This was not evident in the limbs because orthopedic surgeons typically used tourniquets that stopped blood flow when operating on arms and legs—in the spine, of course, there is no tourniquet or stopped blood flow.

Because this process of calcium extrusion was not previously known or anticipated, executives at Norian did not believe that the glue could be harmful when they started trials for spinal use in 2002. Surgeons—including surgeons at Veterans Administration hospitals—were trained to use Norian XR glue in the spine for vertebroplasty, thus leading to deaths in the VA hospitals. However, the FDA had not approved the use of the glue for the spine and the decision to start the spinal use trials (although made without knowledge of the lethal risk) was not in compliance with FDA regulations. In 2009, executives at Synthes admitted responsibility for misdemeanors. In November 2011, in a remarkable first—senior executives at Synthes who had little knowledge or involvement in the work at their Norian subsidiary—were sent to prison for their criminal corporate responsibility for the debacle. Synthes is now being purchased by Johnson and Johnson.

Techniques for Removing Tumors

Tumors that spread into the spine can often be removed by using some of the techniques already described in this chapter. When a tumor is affecting the inside of the spinal canal, the surgical approach is generally dictated by the specific position of the tumor and its location relative to the spinal cord dura (see Fig. 14.10).

First, there is the issue of whether the tumor is in front of the spinal cord dura, behind it, on one side or the other, or surrounding it like a ring. Very commonly, a laminectomy will provide access for removal of any tumors that are posterior to the dural canal. Unfortunately, *metastatic* tumors that spread to the spine from other tissues such as kidney, lung, or breast have a tendency to grow inside the

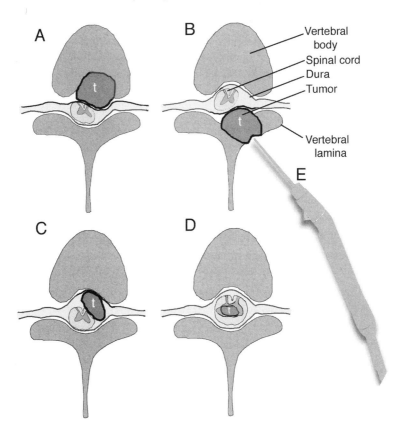

Figure 14.10 Tumor locations relative to the spinal cord. (A) The tumor (t) is outside the dura membranes (epidural) but is anterior to the spinal cord in the vertebral bone—a common location for a metastasis from breast, prostate, or lung cancer. This tumor will need surgery from the front, through the abdomen or chest. (B) Posterior epidural tumor—this can be removed from the back. An ultrasonic aspirator (E) can gently brush away the tumor without adding any pressure to the spinal cord. (C) Some tumors occur inside the dura membranes but outside the spinal cord itself—this is typical of a benign meningioma. The dura must be repaired or replaced when it is removed. (D) A tumor inside the spinal cord itself is the most difficult to remove. Aspirator outline from illustration reproduced with permission of Valleylab and Tyco Healthcare Group, LP.

vertebral body with its rich blood supply. When one of these starts to collapse a vertebra or to push on the spinal cord, an anterior approach is almost always required. If the tumor is in the thoracic region, this often means a thoracotomy, or if it is in the lumbar spine, an opening of the abdomen or flank. Metastatic tumors only very rarely occur inside the spinal dura or inside the neural tissue of the spinal cord itself.

Prior to surgery on a tumor near the spine, the surgeon tries to establish whether the tumor has a high density of blood vessels and a large amount of blood flow. If so, bleeding may limit the success of the operation, and the resulting decrease in visibility may reduce the safety of the procedure. In some cases, a tumor with excessive blood flow can be treated in advance with a technique called *embolization*. To do this, an interventional radiologist threads a small catheter into the femoral artery in the thigh and directs it gradually into the blood vessels that supply the tumor. If the blood supply to the tumor proves to be distinct from the blood supply to the spinal cord, it may then be possible essentially to pump glue into the blood vessels that feed the tumor. Later when the surgery is done, the surgeon will be able to remove the dry, nonbleeding tumor with far greater safety than without the embolization.

Once the surgeon has access to the tumor, it can be removed either mechanically, with cutting instruments, or, in some cases, with a high-powered ultrasonic aspiration device, so that the tumor can be gently removed without pulling or pushing on sensitive spinal dura or nerves nearby. These devices work with a rapidly vibrating metal tip that delivers its disruptive energy in a very small area. The tumor is washed away and sucked up into the device as it is touched by the aspirator's wand. Lasers also can play a role in evaporating tumor tissue without mechanical disturbance of neighboring neural tissue, but heat from the lased tissues, visual obstruction from laser smoke, and the risk of overpenetration by the laser beam place limits on the usefulness of lasers for this task.

The other important factor is whether the tumor is inside or outside the spinal dura. Some types of tumor that affect the spine actually grow inside the dura membranes near the nerves. When a tumor is inside the dura, the approach is usually done from the back because working inside the dura requires delicate microsurgical techniques and often requires more physical space than is available to the surgeon when approaching from the front.

Successful Tumor Treatment in the Spine

Surgery to treat the various tumors that can attack the spine is a bright spot in the whole array of cancer treatment. Unlike radiation or chemotherapy, which may be debilitating over months, the surgery is usually not very difficult for the patient to recover from. When the operation is done, the patient can move on with life. It is very often possible for the spine surgeon to remove the tumor completely, restore and protect the nerves and spinal cord, and build a solid and effective replacement for any tissues that had been destroyed by the tumor. A cancer patient who arrives at the hospital in severe pain and barely able to walk can leave with a routine surgical recovery and a fully functional spine. This field is one of the great triumphs of surgical technology.

It is still the job of the various antitumor drugs and treatments to try to stop the tumor from reoccurring. Severe injury to the spinal cord from collapse of a vertebra or growth of a tumor actually within the neural tissue of the spinal cord or nerves can prove impossible to overcome. However, successful repair of the tumor-damaged spine is now the routine.

A View of Spinal Surgery

The advance of technology has had a huge impact on the basic elements of spinal surgery during the past 50 years. The basic job of taking pressure away from the nerves and spinal cord has changed little during this time, but the safety, efficiency, and gentleness on the body as a whole have improved tremendously.

When a nerve or the spinal cord is being compressed so that the individual is suffering pain, numbness, or weakness, there are fewer and fewer reasons not to proceed with a corrective operation. This is because the accuracy of diagnosis, the development of highly specialized equipment, and the very high levels of training of today's spinal surgeons have contributed to a transformation out of the realm of heroic high-risk care into a matter of safe and routine treatment. Due to some of the methods and technologies discussed in the chapters of this book, many surgeries that required two weeks of hospitalization 30 years ago can now be done on an outpatient basis with return to work in just a few days.

15

Surgery Inside the Spinal Dural Lining

The vast majority of spinal surgery takes place without opening the *dura membranes* around the nerves and spinal cord. However, in a number of situations the spinal surgeon, particularly the neurosurgeon, may need to go inside the dura to treat *intradural* problems that involve the membranes and the fluid inside them.

For the most part, the dura can be opened and closed and reliably sealed. It is only in rare situations, either because a leak is not anticipated or because there is some small fault in the sealing, that leakage of spinal fluid becomes a problem. When it does occur, the dura can often simply be sealed with additional sutures, an intentionally formed clot, or a synthetic sealant. Sometimes a drain has to be placed; sometimes a new surgery is required to seal the leakage.

Inadvertent Durotomy: Handling Tears and Leaks

The most common reason for surgery involving the dura membranes is an accidental tear or inadvertent opening of the dura that allows the leakage of spinal fluid. *Cerebrospinal fluid* (CSF) is a crystal-clear liquid strained out of the bloodstream by the brain. Its purpose is to bathe and to float the brain and spinal cord and to carry nutrients into the brain without allowing direct blood flow throughout the sensitive tissues of the *central nervous system*. The brain produces about a cupful of CSF every day, in a high-pressure filtration system inside its ventricles, the fluid spaces of the brain. As the new fluid is produced, it gradually flows out around the base of the brain and down the spinal canal, inside the dura and around the cord. From the canal, the CSF is squeezed through more filters, like microscopic one-way valves, back into the bloodstream in a steady flow.

When Cerebrospinal Fluid Escapes

A variety of neurosurgical problems have to do with blockage of the normal flow of spinal fluid, but these don't generally concern the spine surgeon. However, if the dura membrane is torn or cut open, that cupful of fluid that is produced every day will flow out through the tear or cut rather than forcing its way through the microscopic valves back into the bloodstream as it should.

After a fresh spine surgery that inadvertently punctures the dura, CSF may make its way up through the different layers of the closure and out through the skin. Once a continuous drainage of fluid occurs, the tear or opening in the dura membranes is relatively unlikely to close by itself, and as long as fluid is flowing out, bacteria can follow the draining fluid back into the spine. In addition, if the escaping flow is too great, the normal pressure of the CSF throughout the central nervous system can be reduced, which can lead to headaches.

Sometimes the dura just can't be closed, as in some of the congenital malformations. In such situations, CSF is diverted from the surgical wound by putting a small tube into the spinal canal at a different location, to drain the fluid through a sealed system into an external drainage bag. In this way, the pressure of the spinal fluid flow on the wound is reduced and the area of surgery is allowed to heal. Once the healing is complete, the tube is withdrawn and the tube's course is carefully sealed. In this way, a *lumbar drain*, as it is called in the low back, can facilitate the closure of a difficult spinal leak.

Dural Repair with Sutures and Membranes: Patching Things Up

When a tear of the dura is seen at the time of surgery, it is usually possible for the surgeon to put some small, fine sutures in the membranes to seal the resulting leak. But sometimes the leak is inaccessible, difficult to locate, or intermittent; or it may not be evident at the time of surgery, demonstrating itself only when the patient stands or exerts himself or herself after surgery. Occasionally, the dura becomes extensively adherent or scarred after a surgery. If a second surgery is later needed in the same areas, the new operation may cause an unavoidable large opening in the dura that can't be simply sewn closed. When these situations occur, there are a variety of dural substitutes that are used to patch, replace, or re-create the membranes and seal up the spinal fluid inside.

Bovine dura from cows is a safe and effective *xenograft*—a graft from another species. However, dural substitutes that can be manufactured from synthetics are increasingly important. Another natural source is used in intradural surgery, in this case to relieve compression at the first cervical vertebra and the base of the skull for foramen magnum syndrome and Arnold-Chiari type I malformation (explained in chapter 8): A sheet of periosteum, the lining of the bone, can be taken from the base of the skull and transplanted into a dural opening, so the patient's own body has produced the autograft tissue for the dural patch.

Synthetic membranes, some made of Gore-Tex, have the advantage of being available in whatever size is needed, but because they are not living tissue, they may not provide an adequate framework for natural dural cells to regrow and provide a tight seal. Also, when repairing a large opening in the spinal cord, the surgeon always has to worry about the nerves inside becoming stuck to the dura, so sometimes very smooth Gore-Tex sheeting is placed on the inside, and then another dural substitute is used on the outside. A new, totally synthetic material called Duragen, for instance, can cover the opening and allow dural cells to grow rapidly across it, forming a new membrane.

Sealing the Dura with Blood and Glue

Some spine patients undergo a diagnostic myelogram to examine the membranes of the spinal cord on an X-ray or CT scan, which involves injecting marker dye through a needle into fluid in the spinal canal. If CSF then leaks out of the injection hole, the patient may experience a headache. Such a leak may have to be treated by injecting blood over the puncture and using the resulting blood clot to seal it; very rarely, surgery is needed to stop the fluid from leaking.

One of the most widely used means of sealing and double-sealing any leakage of spinal fluid is to apply what is called a *tissue glue*. For many years the substance used was very similar to the components that come out of your bloodstream to make a clot or a scab. The *clotting factors* were purified from blood, and then as they were poured on the site of the leak they were mixed with *activating factors,* and a kind of clot was formed.

When tissue glue is used, it is important to consider its similarity to a blood transfusion, in that the source of the material is typically from multiple human donors; but this type of prepared blood product is very carefully screened. Tissue glue formerly was the only choice when it was necessary to seal a leak of this kind, because in the past there were really are no good synthetic alternatives. Another reason that tissue glue was so attractive relative to available synthetic patches was that it was dissolved by the body after a few weeks' time, once the body had a chance to reseal the dura on its own.

In 2009, however, the FDA approved an excellent substitute for human tissue glue called Duraseal (from Covidien). This is an adherent, two-component *hydrogel glue* that polymerizes when the components mix at the site of the leak as they squirt out of the two closely placed nozzles of a double barreled syringe. It has performance characteristics similar to human donor tissue glue, but it makes a better seal because it is more adherent and does not mix and dissolve in flowing CSF to the same extent that affected the use of tissue glue. Like tissue glue, Duraseal gets absorbed over a few weeks. This completely avoids the infection risk that inevitably accompanied the use of human-pooled donor glues.

Formal Durotomy: A Grand Opening

When the surgeon needs to get inside the dura membranes, a laminectomy is carried out to remove the bony arch at the back of the spinal canal, and a long incision is made in the middle of the dura from top to bottom. This incision is made very carefully so as not to damage the easily injured nerves inside the membranes. The sides of the dura are held open, the arachnoid, or innermost sealing membrane is opened, and the surgeon, using an operating microscope, has direct access to the nerves and spinal cord within (see Fig. 15.1).

Functional Surgery: Fine-Tuning for Cerebral Palsy Treatment

One of the most delicate and complex types of intradural surgery is a treatment for cases of *cerebral palsy* in which a child has a very severe *spasticity* or increased tone in the legs, thus making it difficult both to walk and to operate the rigid muscles. Cerebral palsy comes about during birth, and the effects are seen with growth. The mechanics of the condition involve the normal reflexes, such as your leg swinging when your doctor taps on your knee. In cerebral

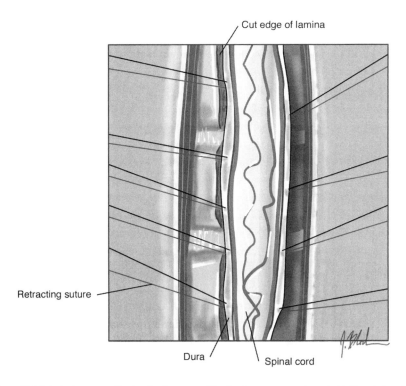

Figure 15.1 Intradural exposure. The dura has been opened to allow for surgery on a tumor inside the spinal cord. Small threads hold the edges of the dura open. After the surgery, the dura is closed to achieve a watertight seal to prevent leakage of cerebrospinal fluid. Image published with permission of Joe Bloch.

palsy, the tone of that circuitry is greatly increased, so that all of the muscles are working hard against each other all the time, making the leg, for instance, very stiff and rigid.

It turns out that by cutting certain fractions of the small nerve rootlets involved in the reflex circuitry, the overall muscle tone can be relaxed so that the intentional control signals coming down from the brain can be heard against the "background noise" of the abnormal nerve activity. This elaborate surgery involves mapping and monitoring many different parameters of sensory and muscle function during the operation, to identify and cut some of these small, sensory nerve fibers.

Spine Surgery to Interrupt Pain Signals

Another type of unusual intradural surgery is a treatment for patients with severe cancer pain: an operation on the spinal cord itself that is intended to block, burn, or interrupt some of the pain circuitry inside the cord. This involves opening the dura, getting a view of the spinal cord, sometimes mapping its surface, and placing very fine needles into specific locations within the cord that normally conduct pain sensation. Radiofrequency or another type of signal is then used to heat the tips of the needles purposely to damage and disrupt the normal pain-perception circuits. Obviously, this kind of pain treatment must be considered only when all other measures have been exhausted because of the high risk of injury to surrounding normal areas of the spinal cord.

Other, more intensive operations inside the spinal cord may be tried to interrupt pain signals; however, these are undertaken as last-resort measures, because it is very easy for this kind of treatment to disrupt normal movement and sensation. Even when the procedure is successful, the spinal cord in this situation may, remarkably and unfortunately, regrow the pain circuitry, so after a number of months the pain may actually recur. This is one of the few cases where recovery of the spinal cord's normal function after injury is not helpful for the patient. That is why these last-ditch measures are usually reserved for people who have terminal cancer and overwhelming pain problems that can't be successfully treated in any other way.

Tumor Excision: Lumps in the Cord

Another reason for operating inside the dura is to treat tumors that occur in the spinal cord. Some of these tumors are actually attached to the membranes, such as a *meningioma* growing out of the *meninges* (another technical term for membranes like the dura). The dura have to be opened to remove a meningioma inside them, and a section of the dura might even have to be replaced (see Fig. 14.10).

Adherent tumors that grow out of the edges of nerves can sometimes be peeled off the nerve, but tumors that occur within the spinal cord itself are more difficult to remove. Some of these tumors have very well-defined borders that separate them from the surrounding tissue; in that case, with a very meticulous technique, the surgeon can gradually collapse and then remove the tumor by drawing it out from the surrounding spinal cord without injuring the cord tissue.

Some tumors actually do occur inside the tissue of the spinal cord. Most commonly, these are neural-type tumors that arise from some of the cellular components that make up the tissue of the spinal cord. Surgery inside the dura and inside the spinal cord is a very delicate matter. It is undertaken under microscopic magnification and with frequent reliance on electrical stimulation to help to distinguish tumor from spinal cord tissue. The likelihood of success in removing a tumor of this type depends on the exact tissue type of the tumor and whether or not it has perceptible edges separating it from the surrounding spinal cord neural tissue. Often the exact type of the tumor and hence the likelihood of success cannot be determined until the surgery is well under way and a sample is obtained from inside the tumor.

It is often preferable to use radiation treatments for the difficult problem of a tumor inside the spinal cord; however, risks are certainly involved with radiation as well, because spinal cord tissue itself is very sensitive to radiation. Any radiation beam that passes through the spinal cord may cause significant damage to the cord in the course of trying to treat the tumor. For this reason, direct surgical removal of spinal cord tumors is sometimes still necessary.

Closing Time

Whatever problem led the surgeon to operate on the dura membranes, once these special, deep layers are taken care of through dural replacement, watertight suture, tissue glue, or any other implant, -the levels above, such as the major fascia, must be very tightly closed. Sometimes a nonabsorbable suture is used, because absorbable sutures that are placed in the fascia will break down after two to four weeks, and the skin is usually closed with an extra-tight sealing technique. Glue may be used on the skin surface. Drains that might normally be used to allow any extra blood to escape from a surgical wound can't be used, because these tend to promote the flow and escape of spinal fluid. Instead of encouraging you to get up and out of bed the day after surgery, you may be asked to remain lying flat for two or more days.

When spinal surgery was in its infancy at the beginning of the twentieth century, the dura seemed to be a sort of insurmountable barrier that the surgeon must not cross. Openings of the dura still present a challenge and require special attention from the surgeon; however, this is yet another area where advances in technology have reduced a major obstacle, thus extending the range of conditions that can be safely treated. At the same time, the new technologies for sealing and rebuilding the dura have relieved most of the concerns that used to surround the potential for leakage of spinal fluid during spinal surgery.

16

Spine Carpentry: History and Principles of Rebuilding the Broken Spine

The beginnings of spine carpentry are closely linked to the discovery of X-rays in the 1890s, and the spine surgeon's tool kit has gradually developed over the years since then. Before that time, surgeons did not know exactly what had gone wrong in the patient's spine or exactly what they needed to fix. Once the basic concept of bone fusion was understood, the advent of X-ray imaging set the stage for the development of spine fusion surgery. When faced with a clear picture of a fractured or collapsed bone, the human imagination is immediately driven to contemplate what can be done to repair what is broken.

Surgeons can now expect to correct safely virtually any mechanical problem anywhere in the spine. Ongoing advances from the fields of computer technology, mechanical engineering, and genetic engineering should make surgical success rates even higher and spine surgeries even safer and shorter. The last remaining frontier for spine surgery is restorative operations that can return normal function to the damaged spine and spinal cord.

Traction and Manual Reduction: Restoring Spinal Alignment

One of the most spectacular moments in my work with the spine came late one summer night in a busy emergency room in Seattle when I was the neurosurgeon on call. A man had fractured his neck in a car crash a few blocks from the hospital, where paramedics found him unable to move and struggling to breathe, with his blood pressure falling. At the ER, his neck X-ray showed a classic spinal nightmare: a fracture in the upper cervical spine, with "jumped facets" (abnormally locked and overlapping joints that prevent the spine from slipping back into alignment) clearly crushing the spinal cord. A high-dose steroid infusion was started, but there is no medication that offers more than the slightest promise of improvement from this devastating situation.

Watching the pale fluorescent video screen of a real-time cine–X-ray for guidance, and using the assistance of spinal traction tongs placed in his skull, I was able to unlock the facets, first left and then right, to pull the man's fractured and displaced cervical spine back into alignment. Moments later he began to move his legs, the blood pressure started to climb back toward normal, and he took his first deep breath since the moment of the accident.

The moment before, he was an anguished new quadriplegic; a moment later, he was once again able to move his arms and legs. It's more common in these circumstances just to get a slightly improved sense of touch in the legs at first, and then to see more complete improvement only gradually over days and weeks, so the events that night were particularly stunning and memorable for everyone in the ER. Sometimes in spinal care, the seemingly impossible miracle can happen.

Pins and Weights

The fastest way to get the pressure of a fractured, malaligned vertebra off of the spinal cord is to pull on the patient's head. With enough pulling, or *traction*, the bones tend to slip back into their correct position. To accomplish anything useful, though, a great deal of force has to be applied, and in a very precisely controlled fashion. The best way to get this done is to screw pins into the patient's skull, deep enough so that they won't pull out, but of course not so deep as to puncture the surface of the brain inside.

Once the traction pins are properly placed, the patient's feet can be strapped to one end of the stretcher and weights can be used to pull on the skull with up to sixty or seventy pounds of force if needed. The weights are put on slowly, one by one, gradually building up the force. After each weight is added, a new X-ray is taken to see whether the bones are moving into correct alignment and to be sure that nothing in the spine is getting stretched too far.

Unlocking a Fracture

Sometimes, though, the traction approach just doesn't work. Parts of the fracture may form a kind of "lock" that won't pull apart no matter how much straight tension is put on them. When that happens, the next step is either emergency surgery or what amounts to using a few twists and bends on the patient's neck to get the bones unlocked. This sort of technique is described by the somewhat antiseptic medical term of *manual reduction*.

The surgery option is comparatively safe and controllable, but even emergency surgery takes time. In the most streamlined of trauma centers, it can take two to three hours from making the decision to operate until the moment when the pressure is taken off the spinal cord. When the spinal cord is under severe pressure, three hours can very literally be the same as forever; by the time the pressure is removed, it may be too late to save the spinal cord. When the pressure on the cord doesn't appear to be too severe and there isn't any paralysis,

Figure 16.1 Traction for cervical fracture reduction. Forty pounds of weights are hanging from a rope that runs over a pulley and then connects to traction tongs attached to the skull. The X-ray fluoroscopy machine provides a real-time view showing the effectiveness of the weights for pulling a fractured and collapsed spine back into alignment. This type of treatment is done urgently in the emergency room for some types of neck fractures.

there's time to prepare for surgery. Arrangements are made to assemble nurses, technicians, and anesthesiologists; intravenous lines are put in and a fiber-optic video system is used to slip a breathing tube down the patient's throat; the skin is painted with iodine; and surgical drapes are positioned. Then, once everything is ready, the incision is made, and after careful dissection down to the spinal fracture, the locked bone is drilled away to allow the spine to slip back into alignment. But when the cord dictates that there's no time for all that, the only option is the bending and twisting of manual reduction.

The key to success in manual reduction is to watch the bones move while the reduction is performed. Static X-rays taken after the fact are worse than useless for getting this particular job done; fortunately, there is an imaging system called *fluoroscopy* that provides X-ray views in real-time motion. The apparatus is mounted on a device called a *"C-arm"* that can be wheeled into place in the emergency room. The C-arm is positioned so that the X-ray source on one end of the "C" transmits from one side of the patient's neck to the fluoroscopic detector on the other end, on the opposite side of the neck. The whole system is hooked up to a video screen (see Fig. 16.1). Once the equipment is in place and everyone is wearing lead gowns, the fluoroscopic system is switched on. Then the surgeon very slowly and deliberately pulls, bends, and twists the patient's neck while watching the bones move on the screen. Usually, with all the weights already pulling on the traction system, it takes only a small, precise movement to undo the bone lock and get the spine back into alignment.

Fixation and Fusion: Restoring Spinal Strength

The problem after manually correcting a severe fracture is what to do next. How are the fractured bones of the spine kept from slipping back out of alignment and causing more damage? Usually, once the fracture has been unlocked and pulled straight, a traction system is used to keep the spine in alignment. However, you can't stay in traction very long: While you're lying flat with your feet strapped to the end of the bed, bed sores start to develop, your lungs get in trouble, and blood clots start forming in your veins. In fact, as recently as the mid-1970s, 95 percent of people in this situation went on to die from the injury.

The answer to this problem has been the development of what can be called "spine carpentry": the art and science of using screws, bolts, cables, rods, metal plates, clamps, and other hardware to fix the broken spine. It is now extremely rare for anyone to die from a vertebral fracture. Once a spine fracture is slipped into alignment, the patient can go to the operating room for spinal reconstruction and be out of bed and starting physical therapy the following morning. There is still a long way to go in repair of the spinal cord itself, but the bones around it are now fully repairable.

Tools, Implants, and Hardware for Bone Repair

The operating room for a major spine surgery is filled with tables covered by many hundreds of pieces of hardware, as well as drills, wire cutters, power saws, hammers, reamers, and gouges; virtually everything used to repair furniture or build a house has its equivalent in spine carpentry. An assortment of titanium alloy and space-age carbon-fiber implants, as well as an advanced array of three-dimensional, computer-guided, and robotic devices, are also available to the spine surgeon. With all of these tools in hand, there is virtually no mechanical problem or structural failure at any location in the spine that cannot be accurately repaired.

Bone is not entirely like wood, so some things that work for wood carpentry don't work out for bones. The first important difference is that bone is not solid. Most bones have a hard outer shell called a cortex. Then, beginning just a few millimeters below the surface, the bone is made of soft marrow percolating between tiny, fragile spikes woven into a kind of honeycomb. In bones that carry the most stresses, such as the leg bones, the cortex can be nearly half an inch thick, but in most parts of the vertebral column, the cortex is much, much thinner. A few decades ago, when spine surgeons really did not know how to proceed, screws didn't seem to be the right thing to use in the spine; a screw could hold in the cortex, but then it couldn't get any purchase once it passed a few millimeters into the softer bone.

Fortunately, bones do participate in repairing themselves. The problem is how to hold them in place safely while the healing is under way, and that's where all the hardware comes in. For a crack in a bone in the arm, it's usually enough simply to put a cast on the outside. For a fracture in the neck, however, it's essentially impossible to immobilize the bones completely from the outside by using braces or collars.

Fusion in the Spine: We Have More Joints Than We Need

The objective in spine carpentry is almost always to get pieces of bone to grow together into one solid piece. Obviously, this is true anywhere in the body when the objective is to get new bone to grow across a fracture. In spine surgery, however, it is also often useful to fuse bones together that used to be separate.

To make two separate bones fuse, you scrape off the natural, protective coating of the bone on the surfaces that you wish to fuse, position the surfaces against each other, and hold the bones in that position for a month or two. If the two bones don't quite touch each other at the start, you can place some chips or pieces of bone taken from elsewhere into the gap. A surgeon can borrow bone from a few places in the body, mostly along the edges of the pelvis. Alternatively, donor cadaver bone can be used with relatively little risk of rejection.

Fusing two bones together is rarely done in other parts of the body, but fusions of the spine are now performed for hundreds of thousands of patients every year. The use of fusion in the spine is so widespread because it is not absolutely essential to have all of the vertebrae moving freely. For example, when two of the seven separate vertebrae in your cervical spine are fused together into one bigger bone, you really can't tell the difference in neck mobility; fuse three, and you may have a little stiffness; but only after four cervical vertebrae are fused will the rigidity get very noticeable. The situation in the lumbar region is similar to the neck in that one or two fusions don't have much impact on your mobility. In the chest, all twelve vertebrae could be fused together and you really wouldn't notice much more stiffness than is usual for the thoracic region.

If you consider that the contacts between each pair of vertebral bones include three joints, and then add up all the joints in the entire spine, you get about seventy spine joints. That's a greater number than all the rest of the joints in the body-arms, legs, hands, feet, and jaw. Having all of these vertebral joints has more to do with the history of the human body plan and the evolution of the spine than it does with any great need to move every one of these joints.

It's strange to think that you could probably fuse fifty different spinal joints and never notice an effect on your mobility.

Perhaps because the negative impact of fusing two bones in the spine is so limited, artificial joints for the spine have only come into use very recently. When a knee or hip joint is damaged, putting in an artificial replacement makes far more sense than fusing the joint so that you can't move it anymore. The risks and difficulties of surgically replacing a joint in the spine, however, have far outweighed the life impact of a fusion, so fusion is still the most common approach to the problem of a spine fracture.

Wrapping with Wires

The basic concept of bone fusion is simple, but usually the main difficulty in getting two spinal bones to fuse is the task of holding those bones in place for a few months. The first approach to this issue, proposed in the 1890s, involved wrapping stiff metal wires around convenient parts of the two bones to be fused, then twisting the wires to tighten up the whole assembly. This *fixation* approach to holding bones together is still very regularly taken in spine surgery. The use of wires in the spine, however, is not risk-free. Sometimes the wires have to be looped around parts of the vertebrae in such a way that they can put pressure on nerves, thereby occasionally causing the catastrophe of a paralysis from spine surgery. This problem has helped motivate the drive to find various other means of fixation in the spine.

Bone-Carving Techniques

One surgeon who tried to find a way to treat spinal instability without the use of wires is Ralph Cloward, a man who is without doubt the greatest "spinal carpenter" of them all. With all of our new technology, there may never again be a need for such a fine craftsman, but his work still has a heavy influence on many procedures in modern spinal surgery. Cloward's operating concept is reminiscent of the "mortise-and-tenon" approach to carpentry, the way that master carpenters are able to build a piece of furniture, or even an entire house, without the use of a single nail or screw. Success depends on a nearly perfect understanding of mechanical stresses and on unerring accuracy in wood carving to make the piece with the slot and the piece with the corresponding projection hold together as strongly as any two pieces of wood fastened together by screws.

In the late 1950s, Cloward showed how a mortise-and-tenon approach could be used for fusions of the cervical spine. In his technique, a cylindrical saw is used to cut a dowel of bone out of the hip and a matched drill is used to cut through the two neck vertebrae to be fused. The disk material between the two vertebrae is removed from the front and the carefully shaped hipbone graft is wedged in to fill the disk space. After it is tapped into place, the graft then fuses with the vertebrae above and below it. Similar techniques use classical "tongue-and-groove" carpentry, in which the graft is shaped with ridges that fit into grooves on the surfaces of the two bones to be fused, so that the graft holds the whole assembly together. Both approaches can make wires and screws unnecessary. However, getting good results requires a high level of craftsmanship, and these techniques can be foiled when the patient's spinal anatomy isn't quite normal, the bone is a little too soft, or the fracture is a bit too complex.

Rods and Hooks to Straighten the Spine

During the 1950s, spinal surgeons faced a new and growing problem posed by children who had survived polio infections. In many cases, the effects of the paralysis led to an abnormal curvature of the spine, or scoliosis, which progressed slowly into a painful and disabling problem long after the polio itself was gone. Faced with this problem, orthopedic surgeon Paul Harrington conceived of a method to force a patient's back into a straight line that was a true breakthrough in surgical thinking: He devised an implantable rod-and-hook system capable of applying tremendous force to the spine. In retrospect, the *Harrington rod* is very crude, but it transformed the field because it could do something that spine surgeons had never imagined possible.

The Harrington Rod: Success and Failure

Harrington's system was a way of putting traction on a bent, fractured, or collapsed spine with a device that could pull the spine back into its normal alignment and length and be buried permanently below the skin. His idea also differed from much of what had gone before because an extended length of the spine, including curvatures stretching across more than a dozen vertebrae, could now be treated with a single device. Since the advent of the first Harrington rod, there has been a relentless series of technological advances and refinements, and many modern devices for this purpose bear little resemblance to the original. Nonetheless, they all share the underlying concept of using a mechanical implant to take hold of the spine and reshape it (see Fig. 16.2).

Essentially, the Harrington system involves a rod with a solid hook on one end and a second hook on the other end that rides on a kind of ratchet. The solid hook is placed on a vertebra at the lower end of the curved spine and the second hook is used to catch hold of a vertebra at the top end of the curvature. Next, the surgeon pushes the top hook upward, snapping along the ratchets of the upper part of the rod, and straightening the spine further with every click of the ratchet. Once a good position of alignment is reached, the surgical incision is closed over the rod. With this operation, a child with scoliosis could rapidly regain a straight spine. Harrington rods were used in more and more situations over the following

Figure 16.2 Correction of spinal deformity. Long rod systems involving pedicle screws (see Fig.16.3) and hooks can be used to correct scoliosis (see Fig.8.1) and other major deformities of the spine. Monarch System illustration reproduced with permission of Depuy Spine Inc., Johnson & Johnson.

decade and sometimes made it possible to correct severe spinal fractures as well. But useful as they were, Harrington rod surgeries were often plagued by failure.

As years passed, more and more of the implanted rods fractured and the hooks pulled out, causing corrections of curved spines suddenly to fail. The initial response to these failures was to modify the basic design by adding more hooks to redistribute the stress and putting in wires along with the hooks. Every hook placement and every wire pass, however, increased the rate of nerve injury during surgery. To improve the situation, efforts were made in the mid-1970s toward a totally different approach: operating through the chest and abdomen and placing screws into the vertebral bodies to support rods. The first designs of this type, unfortunately, were plagued by screw breakage and vertebral fracturing because the biomechanics of proper screw placement in the spine were not fully understood. Some broken screws even caused sudden death through massive internal bleeding when the sharp metal edges sliced open the aorta. It should be kept in mind, however, that without these devices, many patients were left to face progressive paralysis and certain death.

The Luque System: Wires and Rectangles

Fortunately, by the early 1980s, two new types of spinal correction devices were introduced that soon replaced most uses of Harrington rods. The first device, the *Luque system*, was nothing more than a plain metal rod tied to the vertebrae with wires. This carried all the risks inherent in passing wires near the nerves but did not have the corrective power of the Harrington system. It was an improvement, in a way, because its advocates understood that correcting the spinal anatomy had to involve preparing for fusion. Once the spine was placed into rough alignment and prepared for fusion, the Luque rod was then secured to hold the spine in position while fusion took place. The spine was expected to achieve bony fusion before any fracturing of rods or pull-out of wires would take place, and it was thought that the rods and wires would eventually face very little stress.

The Luque system had nearly as many complications as the Harrington rod, but it gained favor through a strange twist of U.S. regulatory law around the time of its introduction, when the U.S. Food and Drug Administration (FDA) began applying new rules to implanted surgical devices. In evaluating the Luque system, the FDA's only concern was that the wires and rods were physically no different from simple rods and wires that had already been used for decades for other surgical purposes. The Luque rod system was therefore "grandfathered in" as acceptable, even though it posed a high risk of patient injury from placement of the wires.

Screws to Use in the Spine

The second development to succeed the Harrington rod, called the *pedicle screw*, was a tremendous advance and avoided nearly all of the complications of the Harrington and Luque systems. The pedicle screw is still the mainstay of spinal reconstructive surgery. About ten years after its introduction, however, the pedicle screw became the subject of one of the largest and most destructive legal conflagrations in medical history.

The Arrival of the Pedicle Screw

By the early 1980s, orthopedic surgeons had been using screws to repair bone fractures for a hundred years, and some of these had been used with miserable effect in the spine since the 1950s. Arthur Steffee, an orthopedic surgeon from Ohio, designed a slightly modified screw that was optimized to work efficiently in the spine. The key to the design of the Steffee screw was a method of placing it into one of the strongest parts of the vertebra, the pedicle, where it could function reliably without fracturing (see Fig. 16.3).

Unlike previous devices, these screws avoided the risk of injuring the nerves or spinal cord by staying completely within the vertebral bone. Pedicle screws provided good control of vertebral position for treating a wide variety of problems, from curvature of the spine to fractures, and they also connected to a redesigned rod-and-hook system, becoming a part of new implants that did all the work of the old Harrington rods. The pedicle screw was rapidly accepted by thousands of spine surgeons because it represented a tremendous advance in safety and flexibility and solved worries and frustrations that many surgeons had faced for decades. Within a few years, pedicle screws were being used with great success in a great many of spine operations. Many of the feared complications of spine fixation in the 1960s and 1970s essentially disappeared.

The screws' safety and ease of use led to their application to more routine spine problems, such as pain from arthritic joints. Instead of reserving spinal fixation for dramatic cases of collapse and impending paralysis, surgeons began using fixation and fusion to treat many previously untreatable types of back pain problems. Back pain, as described in detail in chapter 7, can be due to many different causes, and of the tens of millions of cases of severe back pain in the United States each year, less than 2 percent are treatable by surgery. Nonetheless, with the pedicle screw, it now became possible to help hundreds of thousands of patients who in the past were left disabled and in pain with no hope of treatment.

Controversy and Litigation

By 1990, over 300,000 operations had been performed with pedicle screws. The failure and complication rate remained extremely low; however, even with a 90 percent success rate, that would leave 30,000 patients in pain and suffering after the surgery. If one-half of 1 percent actually suffered neurologic injury through incorrect placement of a screw, that could be more than 1000 patients with a numb, weak leg as result of misplaced pedicle screws.

Up until 1993, most patients understood that failure to correct back pain was a well-known risk of spine surgery, and such a failure virtually never led to litigation. If a screw was misplaced in the operation, causing a nerve injury, the individual surgeon faced a malpractice suit, as it seemed obvious that the blame lay with the surgeon and not with the screw itself. Then, on December 17, 1993, the

Figure 16.3 Pedicle screws. Many major lumbar spine operations require the use of pedicle screws. The pedicle linking the vertebral body to the lamina has some of the densest bone in the spine. Once screws have been placed in the pedicles of the involved vertebrae, the screws can be positioned along rods and tightened to lock the vertebrae into a fixed position. This is often done as part of a spinal fusion surgery. In this illustration, the space between L5 and S1 is being reopened. Moss Miami System illustration reproduced with permission of Depuy Spine Inc., Johnson & Johnson.

ABC news show *20/20* ran an incendiary segment in which the director of the FDA, Richard Kessler, expressed frustration with pedicle screws.

Although approval of the Luque system had been grandfathered in under earlier approval of wires for other spine devices, the FDA had decided that pedicle screws should be declared "experimental" because they differed in shape (being longer and heavier) from other orthopedic screws—even though, by this time, pedicle screws had been placed in far more spine patients than any other device. The FDA had large-scale studies under way to evaluate the safety of the screws, but these were not yet completed when the show aired. Surgeons, meanwhile, had become accustomed to the screws and had no safe alternative to their use. The FDA has no actual jurisdiction over surgical practice; technically, the FDA can comment only on advertising claims by manufacturers. Nonetheless, on *20/20*, Kessler seemingly expressed that he expected surgeons to stop using pedicle screws.

The TV show prompted a vigorous legal response. Within weeks of the broadcast, thousands of lawsuits were launched, claiming billions of dollars in damages to a huge class of plaintiffs. Lawsuits were directed in a blanket fashion at every surgeon in the United States who had ever placed a pedicle screw. In July of 1994, the FDA completed its study and made an initial recommendation in favor of pedicle screws, but by then, the litigation was already launched.

Resolution and Results

In the 1980s, Steffee had founded a company called Acromed to sell his pedicle screws. Along with other spinal implant manufacturers such as Danek, Acromed fought the pedicle screw litigation in court. However, Acromed made a fatal choice: it decided to pay a settlement of a $100 million even though Steffee believed that the lawsuits were meritless.

Months after the Acromed settlement, the FDA ruled favorably on pedicle screws, and the litigation evaporated, after five years of Sturm und Drang. Faced with overwhelming evidence of the screws' safety and medical benefits, both the FDA and the courts put an end to the whole mess. The FDA took seventeen years to finish its analysis of pedicle screws, and the whole experience was vastly unproductive for all involved. Newer surgical devices are generally evaluated and approved in a far more efficient and constructive manner.

Thoracic Spine Fixation with Rods and Plates

In the days before shoulder belts were in general use and long before the arrival of the airbag, "seat belt fractures" were a bane of the spine surgeon. If you're wearing only a lap belt, a car accident can bend you violently over the belt, which can lead to one of the low thoracic or upper lumbar vertebrae being crushed. With all the pressure from the vertebrae above and below it, the vertebra in the middle, behind the lap belt, literally bursts; and because of the back's forward-bending flexion in that moment, the posterior part of the vertebral body blows out backward into the spinal cord, causing paralysis of the legs.

During most of the 1970s, there was no good way to repair the seat-belt fracture. Harrington rods were tried but usually yielded fairly poor results. Then in the early1980s, with the introduction of pedicle screws and more advanced rod systems, surgeries were attempted from the posterior to make the broken spine straight again. Unfortunately, this often left the bone fragments in the spinal canal. The surgeon could also perform a double operation: in front to pull the fragments out of the cord, and in back to stabilize. It turned out, however, that despite this huge operation, the work in front so destabilized the spine that the rod in back often wouldn't hold.

The first really successful device for treating this type of fracture was subsequently introduced by orthopedist Kiyoshi Kaneda. This involves an adjustable frame with two screw holes at one end and two at the other. The top of the device could be screwed into the vertebra above the fracture and the second two screws placed into the vertebra below the fracture. The surgeon could then adjust the size and compression across the space where the fractured vertebra had been removed and into which some sort of graft material had been placed. A surgeon could now approach the spinal column through the chest or abdomen, pull out the fragments, replace the broken vertebra, and install the Kaneda device for support. No additional posterior surgery is needed for more stabilization, and the Kaneda device helps to assure that the graft is held in place. A variety of similar systems is now available (see Fig. 18.3).

In some cases, it's actually possible to implant a Kaneda-type device endoscopically, without actually doing a full-scale operation. For an endoscopic operation, rather than making a big incision, the surgeon makes a small slit in the skin through which a tiny fiber-optic light and video camera can be slipped into the chest. Another two or three small openings are made to allow specially designed surgical instruments to be passed in as well, and the surgeon watches the procedure on a video screen while working inside the closed chest wall. Endoscopic placement of a *Z-plate* to repair a thoracic vertebral fracture is a dramatic improvement over the extensive front-and-back surgeries from just ten years ago. These differ from the Kaneda device in that they have no moving parts and so are simpler to use. The surgeon selects a plate of approximately the correct size and can use the slotted screw holes on the plate to do any final adjustment needed.

Screws and Plates to Master the Cervical Spine Fracture

A good example of a problem for which the Cloward mortise-and-tenon procedure won't work is the type of totally unstable neck fracture suffered by the patient at the beginning of this chapter. To put the pieces of this fracture back together, an incision is made at the front of the neck and the surgeon dissects down past the *jugular vein, carotid artery,* and *trachea* (windpipe) to reach the front of the spine. The crushed vertebral body is removed and replaced with a bone graft, and then a screw-and-plate system is needed to hold the whole thing together.

A screw-and-plate system for the front of the spine in the neck has to lie very smooth and flat; the *esophagus* runs directly over the plate, so if the hardware's profile is too high, then the patient will have never-ending problems with swallowing. Also, the screws holding the plates in place lie under the esophagus, trachea, *larynx* (voice box), and carotid artery, and entertaining the possibility of a loose or broken screw in these locations is out of the question. These screws are designed with locking systems to prevent "back-out" of the screws. The first generation of metal plates for the front of the cervical vertebrae often proved to be too weak and had a risk of fracturing, but newer plates of advanced alloys have all the necessary strength against repeated bending without having to be thicker.

To treat a totally disrupted cervical spine, however, the anterior plate has to be supplemented with some sort of fixation in the back of the neck, because without the additional fixation, the anterior plate will bend like a parallelogram and the whole construct will collapse, with disastrous consequences. Putting rods and screws into the back of the neck is among the most difficult types of hardware placement in the spine. Each screw has to thread through a narrow zone of bone in a cervical vertebra to avoid injuring the neck's nerves and arteries; this is such a treacherous operation that many surgeons insist on using a high-tech, computer-image guidance system to do it. Once put together, a plate or rod at the back of the spine provides very good stability (see Fig. 16.4).

Even these screw-and-rod systems can be too weak, however, when the patient's cortical bone is too soft to hold screws, and there are certain patients whose cervical spines are very difficult to repair successfully. In some situations the screw and rod is additionally supplemented by a bone strut and cable system that lashes together the spinous processes as well.

Cages and Interbody Implants for Lumbar Spine Fusion

The concept of implanting a cage-like spacer between lumbar vertebrae came from George Bagby, an orthopedist and veterinarian who first used them to treat cervical disk problems in race horses. His original device was a cylinder

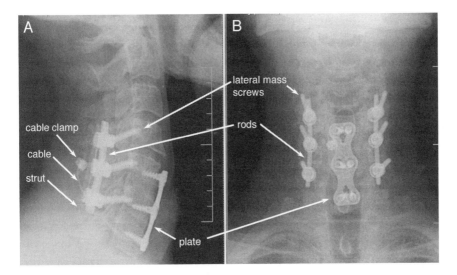

Figure 16.4 Instrumented cervical spine fracture. These X-rays in lateral (A) and anterior-posterior (B) view show a major spinal repair involving four types of spinal reconstruction technology. Several of the vertebral disks have been replaced with bone graft material. A plate and screws have been used to lock the vertebral bodies of C5, C6, and C7 tightly against the graft. From a posterior approach, lateral mass screws at C4, C5, and C6 are linked together to prevent rotation and lateral bending. A thin titanium cable and cable clamp have also been used to lash a strut of bone onto the spinous processes of C4 to C7 to resist flexion forward.

or cage filled with bone chips and implanted in the disk space. Natural tension and weight between the vertebrae held the implant in place until new bone grew through it. Bagby's idea was further developed into threaded titanium cages by the neurosurgeon Charles Ray and by the orthopedist Stephen Kuslich, among others; such devices include the BAK cage or Interbody Fusion System and the Ray Threaded Fusion Cage. A similar device made of cadaver bone was introduced by the Danek Corporation, and many different generations of improved cages and threaded dowels have followed.

These *interbody implants* have greatly simplified the work of lumbar fusion, but in many cases pedicle screws must be used along with the implant to get a good result. Even together, however, the screws and implants have not yet made lumbar spine fusion a completely reliable operation (see Fig. 16.5).

Fusion rates with these systems are good, in fact, and the rate of complications is low, but correctly identifying which back-pain patients can be helped by lumbar fusion is still a problem. Also, despite their improving ease of use, there are still many cases in which the implants are not placed in the optimal position; even in the best of hands, accurate placement of interbody implants and pedicle screws still poses challenges. As the years progress since the introduction of these devices, reassessments of their success in producing fusion continue.

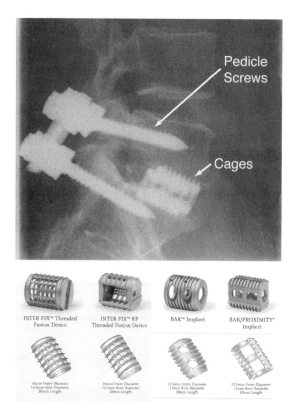

Figure 16.5 Lumbar fusion cages. These titanium cages may be placed in the disk space to provide support and to limit movement. The x-ray shows a patient in whom pedicle screws (see Fig. 16.3) have also been placed. The cages are typically filled with bone graft material and bone growth-promoting proteins. Cage comparison Illustration reproduced with permission of Medtronic, Inc.

Perhaps because of the presence of the interbody implants, fusion often takes as long as several years.

Updated Tools to Extend and Optimize the Process

Aside from the major changes in the fixation methods and devices, the advance of the safety and efficacy of fusions is dependent on the improvement of the tools used to place the screws and interbody implants. Several advances have made it possible to place the fixation screws and devices through a series of small minimally invasive incisions instead of the very large openings used in the past. This helps reduce blood loss, postoperative pain, and the tissue disruption that makes recovery difficult. Examples of advances include a channeled device that allows a guide probe to be introduced into the disk space, the surgeon can then pass a disk chopping/removal device through the guide, knowing that the guide will lead the device into the disk space where a comprehensive disk removal and preparation of the disk space can be carried out without requiring the surgeon to have the disk space in view.

Tubes for the placement of pedicle screws have been particularly important for very large complex fusions that are done for problems such as scoliosis where ten or fifteen spinal levels may require fusion. The tube is passed through a small incision in the skin and then docked on the bone at the appropriate entry point. The surgeon can then drill and place the screws without any more exposure than is required to place the tube. In this fashion, the thirty screws that may be required are put in place through multiple tubes (see Fig. 16.6). The ends of the screws are connected to extenders and these can be used to correct the spine curvature of the scoliosis once all the screws are in place. Then, once the spine is properly aligned, a flexible rod system can be passed under the skin from screw to screw so that the whole large complex construct can be assembled on a relatively minimally invasive basis (at least much less invasive than the traditional extended length scoliosis correction).

Figure 16.6 Phoenix Orthofix fusion system for minimal access. Use of tube connectors on pedicle screws makes it possible to maintain access to the screw head from outside the skin surface. The tube and screw can be placed through a small opening without extensive disruption of tissues. The rod can be passed through a small opening in the skin and advanced along a line passing across the screw heads. Various wrenches and screwdrivers can be applied through the tubes to assemble and secure the instrumentation construct. Image reproduced with permission of Orthofix.

Additional aids to working in small spaces are additions to the small retractor blades that are used. By building fiberoptic lighting, irrigation, and suction into the retractor blades, the tools to do each of these functions are no longer needed, and the space for the tools are no longer needed. All that work is done by the thin retractor blades so that the only space needed is the exact exposure to enter the disk or to drive the screw.

Entirely novel approach systems have also been developed in ways that can truly transform the process of completing a fusion. The most important of these in 2012 is the NuVasive XLIF (XLIF = extreme lateral interbody fusion) system. In the past, surgeons had approached the spine from the front by going through the abdomen (moving aside intestines, aorta, and vena cava) or from the back, delicately working around the spinal nerves and dural sack. NuVasive provided an entire system of retractors, implants, access devices, and electronic nerve detection devices that allowed for access from the side. There is still risk of traction to the spinal nerves at the sides of the vertebrae, but this approach and similar systems from other manufacturers has resulted in a far less invasive surgery for many patients needing lumbar fusions (see Figs. 19.1, 19.2, and 19.3).

Advanced Technology for Spinal Repair

Currently improved reconstructive spine surgeries are beginning to include the use of artificial replacement disks similar in concept to the artificial hips and artificial knees that have been in successful use for many years. *Facet arthroplasty—* surgery to replace or repair the posterior facet portions of the vertebrae—has lagged behind the development of disk replacements. However, early results with disk replacement suggest that replacement of both the disk and the facet joints will be required in many cases.

Carbon-Fiber Implants: New Material and New Structures

In 1996, a new entry in the spine carpenter's tool kit arrived: the carbon-fiber implant, and it came from Dr. Steffee. Out of Steffee's frustration with the pedicle screw battle grew his interest in introducing carbon-fiber implants to replace the use of steel and titanium in the spine. These new-generation materials provide certain advantages over metals: they don't interfere with MRI or CT scanning, and they transmit the forces needed to promote the growth of new bone for fusion.

At that time, all of the manufacturers of carbon-fiber materials, however, were in the military aircraft business, and they feared being bankrupted if there ever were product-liability litigation against any carbon-fiber implant. Product-liability litigation is intended to keep bad products off the market, and the attorneys involved should feel that it will help to motivate the development and improvement of new products. But the tactics sometimes become so aggressive that innovation itself is the target. Fortunately, commitment to what is best for patients in the difficult and challenging field of spine surgery once again overcame fear of the entrepreneurial litigation strategies of the product liability attorneys.

The first carbon-fiber spine implant was a spacer intended to hold adjacent lumbar vertebrae apart while new bone fused between them. Since 1996, a series of carbon-fiber devices designed as spacers and supports for lumbar fusion have been approved by the FDA (see Fig. 16.7). At present, carbon fiber is just one of a variety of advanced materials being explored for use in spinal surgery (see chapter 21).

Computer Guidance for Placing Screws

Computer image-guidance systems for placing screws in the human spine are among the most advanced pieces of technology ever developed and are often used to supplement the old "freehand" techniques. These systems are still new, awkward, expensive, and time-consuming, so computer guidance is currently used only for the most difficult and high-risk operations.

Various techniques for fusing C1 to C2—at the very top of the spine—have been developed over the years. The oldest of these involve wires and cables and carefully carved bone struts. These procedures had low success rates and required the patient to spend months wearing an elaborate "halo" brace attached to four screws sticking into the skull. A new type of surgery using carefully placed *transarticular screws* greatly improved the success rate and made the halo brace unnecessary.

Placing screws in some areas of the cervical vertebrae requires a very high degree of accuracy to achieve good, safe positioning. The simultaneous development of computer image guidance for the screw placements has helped to make the whole advance feasible.

So how do these guidance systems work? The first step is for the computer to form a detailed three-dimensional image of the patient's cervical vertebrae from a very high-resolution, X-ray CT scan of the neck. The computer reads the scanner output and, in its memory, re-creates a volume image of each vertebra, which can be rotated in any direction in the cyberspace of the computer (see Fig. 16.8).

The next step is for the computer to "learn" exactly where the patient's real vertebrae are in the operating room, a feat that is accomplished in different ways in competing systems. Once the muscle is cleared away from the surface of the bones designated for surgery, the computer's location process can begin. Usually, a three-lens camera array is set up in the operating room and the

TANTALUM MARKER BEADS
Allow radiographic location and orientation of the implant.

SURFACE TEETH
Increased stability, minimizing risk of retropulsion.

HORIZONTAL STRUTS
Optimal strength and surface area to maintain disc height.

OPEN DESIGN
Maximizes bone graft-to-endplate surface contact. Provides ample room for vascularization and bone healing.

INSERTION HOLE
Secure attachment to Cage Inserter.

Figure 16.7 Carbon-fiber fusion cages. Carbon-fiber cages have an elasticity similar to bone. Unlike metal fusion cages (see Fig. 16.5), they do not degrade the accuracy of CAT scans and MRIs obtained after surgery. Illustration reproduced with permission of Depuy Spine Inc., Johnson & Johnson.

Figure 16.8 Computed-image guidance. This CBYON guidance computer is being used to plot a course for placement of a cervical lateral mass screw. The three-dimensional reconstruction capabilities of the system allow the surgeon to identify and follow a safe course through the bone of the vertebra.

surgeon attaches a device to one of the patient's vertebrae to provide a frame of reference for the computer. The device has three LEDs (light-emitting diodes), each flashing at a particular frequency that the computer can identify. From the lenses and LEDs, the computer "knows" exactly where the frame-of-reference device is.

The surgeon then "teaches" the computer where each target vertebra is relative to the frame-of-reference device by using a probe with its own LED trio. The probe is touched to a number of points on the surface of a vertebra, and at each point of contact, the surgeon steps on a pedal to instruct the computer to remember where that point is in space. After five or six points are mapped, the computer compares their positions with its data about the shape of the vertebra from the patient's CT scan, fitting the map of surface points to the image in its memory. It then informs the surgeon that it knows the exact location of the vertebra in the room and its exact orientation in space.

The surgeon checks to see whether the computer has gotten it right, down to the millimeter, by touching the probe to various points on the surface of the vertebra as the computer watches through its three camera lenses. An image of the vertebra appears on the computer screen, and for any vertebral feature now touched with the probe, the computer will display an image of the probe at that spot on the image of the vertebra. It also shows the exact angle at which the surgeon is holding the probe. There has also been early development of methods of "injecting" nerve images into the computer simulated view and guidance frame to further improve the usefulness of guided systems.

If everything checks out, the surgeon moves on to the next steps, using specially made instruments, each with their own set of LEDs attached to the handle. The tip of the instrument is touched to a marking pad and a press of the foot-pedal tells the computer to learn where the tip is from the LEDs on the handle. Now when the instrument is brought into contact with the vertebra, the computer screen displays a real-time, moving image of the instrument touching the image of the vertebra. Through this process, the computer can use the links between patient, image, and instrument to guide the surgeon through the inside of tissues he or she cannot see directly.

For the most part, a surgeon still can't rely solely on a computer image-guidance system. There's always an increased risk in proceeding freehand, however. Currently, surgeons working freehand or with computer guidance do a better job at placing screws than the new surgical robots, but in another ten years, the computers and robots may be better and more reliable than the surgeons working freehand.

Surgery in a Scanner

The present frontier of image-guided surgery for correcting spinal disorders offers the potential for carrying out the operation inside a specially designed, open MRI scanner. This working environment allows the surgeon to have a nearly perfect view of where an implant is being placed and how the vertebrae are positioned around it. Putting metal implants in a patient within an open MRI scanner is not entirely feasible because the image is degraded by the metal at exactly the site the surgeon needs to see; in the future, however, this should be possible with nonmetallic implants.

The advantage of real-time MRI over the previously described computer image-guidance system is that the computer systems are limited to working from an image of the spine obtained before surgery that cannot account for any changes that might occur during the operation. Also, the computer's frame of reference identifies where one vertebra is, but during surgery it's often necessary to track the independent motions of two or three vertebrae simultaneously (see Fig. 16.9).

Figure 16.9 Open MR surgery. The surgeon can use the scanner during surgery to locate the target problem precisely and to monitor the effectiveness or completeness of surgery as it is done. Photograph of Concerto Interventional MR system reproduced with permission of Siemens AG.

Another great advantage of open MRI-guided surgery is that it can be performed through very small surgical incisions. Image-guidance systems require an extensive exposure of the spine—a large incision—so that the computer can accurately learn the position of the vertebra. In open MRI-guided surgery, however, the surgeon sees the interior of the tissues in real time on a flat screen, thus the incision needs to be only large enough to get the surgical instruments into place.

Surgery inside large closed scanners is being investigated—but this requires very complex MRI compatible robots. Systems of this type are under development for brain surgery by companies such as IMRIS, but it is not clear whether this will ever make more sense than surgeon and X-ray/CT guidance for spinal work.

The Future of Spinal Carpentry

In the 1950s, when spinal reconstruction was first becoming possible, surgeons relied on a tool kit and strategies very close to the ones used by a carpenter doing woodwork. Five decades later, spinal surgery resembles almost nothing else in human experience: three-dimensional computer tracking systems, real-time moving images in MRI, unique advanced materials, and biotech proteins. Fortunately, this field has continued to draw the best and the brightest of surgeons and engineers fascinated by the problem of rebuilding the damaged human spine with the utmost of safety and the minimum of risk and discomfort to the patient. There are already huge improvements from this progress that greatly benefit the patient faced today with the need for any scale of spinal repair and reconstruction.

17

Fixing the Cervical Spine: Surgical Approaches for the Neck

A number of problems in the cervical spine can require surgery, from degenerative conditions to fractures and tumors. Three types of "end-point problems" in particular, often require neck surgery.

The first is a mechanical pain when the neck turns or moves. The pain may be caused when cervical vertebrae rub directly against each other, when a disk is disrupted, or from an impaired facet joint posteriorly. The second type of end-point problem also produces pain and possibly numbness or weakness, but the symptoms extend to the arms, hands, and fingers rather than being felt only as a pain at the midline of the neck. This results from pinches of the nerves that travel out through the cervical spine's foramina (nerve canals) that happen when the canals are narrowed by abnormally overgrown bone, as in *arthritis* or *arthropathy*, or are impinged on by disk herniation. Third, and always of great concern when it occurs in the neck, is any pressure on the spinal cord itself. Cord compression can be manifested as impaired balance, by altered bowel or bladder function, or as numbness extending all the way down to the legs. Any significant pressure on the spinal cord can also subsequently lead to even more serious problems, such as the complete inability to walk.

If disk or vertebral problems in your neck have reached the point where surgery may be needed, it is likely that your surgeon has talked to you about a disk removal, an implant, or a fusion. Obviously, in an arena as exacting and technical as spinal surgery in the neck, you are going to rely on advice from your surgeon. However, if you've had a second opinion, you may have competing recommendations. Moreover, the surgeon may have asked your opinion about other choices that need to be made. Hopefully, the information that follows can help you in making informed choices.

The Anterior Cervical Approach

Whatever problem requires cervical spine surgery, the solution is most often the anterior approach (from the front) because of the situation of the nerves and spinal cord in the neck. In the lumbar region of the spine, for example, the spinal canal contains only the tail ends of some small nerves floating in cerebrospinal fluid, and these can be pulled out of the way or retracted for the surgeon to reach through to the disks from the back. In the cervical spine, however, the canal is filled with the spinal cord, and it is not safe for the surgeon to retract the cord to get around to the disks in front of it. Therefore, when at all possible, it is better to come from the front of the neck to deal with a damaged disk and to leave the spinal cord alone.

It is also the case that an anterior approach in the neck is easily done for the surgeon and usually has a rapid recovery time for the patient, while anterior surgery for the lumbar region involves opening the abdomen and moving major internal organs and blood vessels—generally requiring a second specialist such as a vascular surgeon. This is another reason why cervical surgeries are more commonly done from the front than surgeries in other parts of the spine.

For the most part, recovery from an anterior cervical surgery is not very painful and is relatively easy. Any surgery obviously has its risks, and certainly a surgery in the neck carries the very tiny chance of an injury to the spinal cord that could cause significant symptoms affecting the arms and legs, but an anterior cervical approach is very commonly done and is, in general, very safe.

One of the main risks, however, is temporary hoarseness, because the nerve to the vocal cords passes by the course that the surgeon takes from the front of the neck to the spine. Because of this possibility, people who rely on their voice for their work, such as singers, attorneys, teachers, and a variety of other professionals, may want the surgeon to carefully consider any alternatives to the anterior approach.

Discectomy and Foraminotomy: Clearing a Space

For an anterior cervical approach, a horizontal incision is made in a skinfold on either the right or the left side of the neck. The incision is usually between three and five centimeters in length (although some are longer). It starts in the midline between right and left side and is usually just below the Adam's apple. The surgeon uses gentle techniques to dissect bluntly down through the tissues of the neck. Protective retractors push the esophagus and trachea away from the surgeon and pull the carotid artery toward the surgeon, providing protected access to the front of the spinal column (see Fig. 17.1).

At this point, an X-ray is always taken to help the surgeon to be sure to identify the correct spinal level for the operation. Once the X-ray confirms the

Figure 17.1 Exposure and approach for anterior cervical discectomy. The retractor blades hold the esophagus, trachea, jugular veins, and carotid arteries (A) (top). With the retractor system in place, the surgeon has a clear straight safe view into the disk spaces between the vertebrae (B) (bottom). Illustration reproduced with permission of Medtronic, Inc.

correct level, the operating microscope is generally brought into place to provide its superior magnification and illumination for the delicate task of removing the disk.

In general, because degenerating disks lose their height, the surgeon also needs to stretch the neck in some way while working. This can be accomplished in a number of ways. One is to attach a sort of halter to the patient's head and tie this to some weights. However, by spreading only the disk space itself, the disk can generally be opened more rapidly and safely. The disk space can be opened up using a hinged spreading tool inserted into the disk. Another alternative is to screw some pins into the vertebrae above and below the disk and to use a ratchet device to push the pins apart. In any case, one of these strategies is needed to get a good safe view into the deepest part of the disk space.

At this point, the surgery generally requires the use of a high-speed drill to gently dust away any bony osteophytes or bone spurs. The same gentle technique is also directed out toward the sides of the disk space to open a path into the cervical foramen, or nerve canal. At various moments, a very small curette is used to develop tissue planes, to feel under the edge of the vertebra, and to explore and enlarge the entry into the foramen. The curette, punches, and even the drill are then used to complete the foraminotomy. The surgeon checks the completeness of the foraminotomy by passing a small probe out through the foramen along the exiting nerve root. If the space is still tight, there is more work to do.

In most anterior cervical discectomies, the final step of decompression is to lift and cut the posterior longitudinal ligament. This is the ligament that separates the disk from the dura. If any disk fragments have herniated through the ligament, they can't be removed unless the ligament is opened.

One last step after decompression is to prepare the vertebral surfaces. Since some sort of fusion of the surfaces is almost always desired, the surgeon prepares them by scraping away any cartilage that lines the disk space and by drilling and scraping to remove periosteum as well. Once the preparation is completed, the disk space can be measured in all its dimensions to determine the optimal size of any implant to replace the disk.

One option is simply to scrape the exposed end plates of the two surrounding vertebrae and to let the vertebrae settle onto each other. Although this is generally the most painful option in the short term, these vertebrae will very often go on to fuse together well. The problem with this procedure, however, is that in as many as 10 to 20 percent of cases, fusion never takes place and the patient has worse neck pain than before; therefore, it is generally felt that a simple fusion is not optimal. Usually, the space left by removing a disk is filled with some sort of implant.

Implants and Fusion: Filling the Space

The first advantage of a bone graft implant is the immediate immobilization of the vertebrae above and below it. If your original problem was neck pain from abnormal vertebral movement, this stops that movement and relieves the pain. Then, once fusion with the implant occurs, the process of arthritis(the abnormal formation of new bone by the pressures of abnormal movement) should stop at that level in the cervical spine because all the movement at that level is stopped.

The implant helps to preserve the normal curvature of the neck and also holds the vertebrae widely separated. This protects the size of the opening made in the foraminotomy done during surgery. The implant also ensures that the vertebral bodies do not collapse together and once again start pinching an exiting nerve.

Sometimes surgery is necessary at more than one level in the cervical spine, as two or three disks may herniate, and the same anterior cervical procedures can be carried out for a second and even a third level all at once. Having a single fusion of two vertebrae really doesn't noticeably affect your neck mobility; having two fusions to hold together three vertebrae, however, has perceptible effects; and if you have three levels done, the result is even more noticeable. Some professionals, such as dental hygienists or cinematographers, can't continue to do their jobs after a three-level fusion. Nonetheless, the surgery, if required, is certainly technically feasible.

One important concern with cervical fusion is whether things will proceed as intended after the operation. Sometimes even though the correct graft is in place, the vertebrae above and below the graft fail to fuse with it into a nice, solid piece. When that happens, a false joint or *pseudoarthrosis* forms, which can be very painful and requires additional surgery. A variety of surgical modifications are used to reduce the chances of failed fusion, but even taking all these measures, it still isn't possible to bring the chances down to zero.

Autografts, Allografts, and Alternatives

There is a wide set of choices as to what can be placed in an empty disk space, such as a piece of bone, other natural materials such as coral, or completely synthetic calcium-based or even plastic structures. As often as a surgeon asks the patient what his preference is, another surgeon tells the patient what he or she recommends and proceeds accordingly. In either case, it is helpful for the patient to know about the options.

One of the most traditional and still widely used disk implants is a small piece of the patient's own hip bone. The piece needed is a little bit less than a half-inch wide and a little bit more than a half-inch deep. Because of the shape of the hip, this *autograft* (donor bone from the patient's own body) comes out shaped somewhat like a disk, and can be tapped securely into place in the spinal column.

Alternatively, an identically shaped piece of bone can be taken from a cadaver. The bone is specially treated so there is virtually no risk of rejection by the patient. This *allograft* (donor bone from another person) is simply a scaffold of calcium phosphate crystal and lacks the live, bone-forming cells that come with a person's own hipbone. However, because the disk space between two vertebrae in the neck is fairly small, bone cells can grow down from the vertebra above it and up from the vertebra below it to fill in the scaffold, essentially turning the dead graft into living tissue.

Although using tissue from a donor raises concerns about disease transmission, a bone allograft is considered to be very safe. When you receive a blood transfusion or a solid organ such as a liver, only so much can be done to clear the tissue of any bacteria or viruses; a bone graft, however, can be very aggressively treated to clear out any living tissue in it and still be useful. There is a small price to be paid for using donor bone in that the rate of fusion success does drop several percentage points, but there is also a significant advantage in not having an operation on your hip. Very often, the hipbone donation site is the most painful thing after your surgery and may go on to give you hip pain, leg pain, and other symptoms that greatly delay your complete recovery and may even become a long-standing, almost permanent pain problem. Therefore, taking the slightly increased risk of fusion failure with an allograft may be worthwhile.

Titanium Plates, Screws, and Cages to Resist Movement during Healing

One way to promote proper fusion is to reduce movement of the spine during the first weeks after surgery, until the new bone formation can progress and start to solidify. This is important when a single cervical level is fused and even more important when two levels are fused. The simplest way to do this is to have the patient wear a neck collar, and this is almost always prescribed. Nonetheless, no collar provides complete immobility. In theory, the more effectively a collar holds your head rigidly in space, the more intolerable it will be to wear. A far more effective method is to put a small titanium plate in front of the graft and screw it into the vertebra above and below the graft, holding them rigidly fixed while the fusion takes place (see Fig. 17.2).

For bone to grow naturally, it requires some physical stress to be applied to it, so often the plate allows for a little bit of "play" or bending, and the screws that hold it to the vertebrae have some mobility. One recent advance in cervical plates that addresses this issue is a plate with a built-in ratchet system. The plate can actually get shorter over time as the implant settles and shrinks during the fusion process. The plate cannot get longer. This addresses a problem with traditional plates that have no flexibility—if the implant shrinks at all, the plate could pull the vertebral surface away from the implant by holding it rigidly in place—thus making fusion less likely to occur.

The plate has a definite, positive effect on the rate of fusion, increasing the success rate by another 5 percent, whether you use donor bone (95 percent success with a plate) or your own hip bone (98 percent). Also, with good placement of a plate, you may be able to do away with the need for a neck collar. Many surgeons who use plates don't prescribe a cervical collar at all, while others suggest that one be worn part of the time simply to protect against the impact of a fall or a car accident during your recovery.

Figure 17.2 Cervical plates and dynamic adjustment. In older generation anterior cervical plates, the screws held the vertebral bodies in place at the configuration existing immediately at the end of surgery (A, B). However, if the implant underwent loss of height during healing, then the screws actually hold the vertebrae apart from each other and prevent successful fusion. In many newer plate designs, the construction allows for dynamic shortening after placement if the implant shrinks or partially collapses through the vertebral endplate. C—Dynatran plates from Stryker have a central open slot so the surgeon can more readily see the underlying vertebra and disk space once the plate is lowered in into position. Pins can be used to readjust the position of the vertebrae beneath the plate. D—Dynatran cervical plates also can be converted into dynamic functioning by removal of a retaining strip. The screws attach to the plate at a ring that allows the screws to reorient if the plate shortens. E—The Atlantis translational plate from Medtronic uses a central locking screw to keep the pair of screws from backing out, but still allows the screws to reorient if the plate shortens in dynamic functioning. Images A, B, C, D reproduced with permission of Orthofix. Image E with permission of Medtronic, Inc.

Most cervical spine plates are made of a medical-grade titanium alloy. The titanium is nonferrous, which means it doesn't set off a metal detector in the airport, which is helpful to know. The development of specialized screws for the plates has advanced tremendously. Small changes in relationship between the diameter and length of the screws as well as the thickness, sharpness, and angle of the threads make big differences in their efficacy and safety.

Some new types of plates are actually made of biologically *resorbable* materials. This may be attractive for patients who really aren't comfortable with the thought of having a metal plate left permanently in their neck. However, the process of resorbing the plate may involve inflammation, and these materials may not be as effective as metal when a fusion is proceeding slowly.

Other advances in the technology of cervical plates include efforts to make them thinner and narrower, or even to use a single midline screw rather than two screws at each involved vertebral level. One interesting advance that does away with the plate altogether is a "zero profile" device in which an artificial disk space implant actually has the screws built into it, so that the entire device drops in below the level of the vertebra (see Fig. 17.3). This is expected to greatly reduce the occurrence of both hoarseness and swallowing difficulties that can occur after a cervical spine anterior fusion.

However, although the mechanical effect of the plate on the front of the vertebra can affect the quality of speech and the smoothness of swallowing—it is worth noting that both of these problems can occur because of effects on the nerves that occur during the retraction of surgery or due to adhesions on the nerves that develop during the healing after surgery. In some cases, surgeries have been done to release the involved nerves (or to remove a plate) in order to restore the voice or the swallowing process.

Important questions about plates include whether they will ever become loose and whether the screws will ever come out and injure the vital structures in the neck. The risk of these events isn't completely zero. If the fusion works so that the bones become solid, then the plate never moves and the screws will remain in place. However, if the fusion fails for any reason, the many thousands of vertebral movements per day will gradually loosen the screws. As a result, they may back out into the interior of the neck, and the plate itself may even fracture. This almost always requires repeat surgery to remove the metal and redo the operation from the front.

A different type of implant is a circular, usually titanium cage, typically containing small bone chips taken from the patient or perhaps a synthetic bone-forming material. Once slid or screwed into the disk space from the front, the cage has the job of holding the vertebrae in place while the material inside grows into the spine. The main disadvantage of titanium cages is that they may, in fact, provide

Figure 17.3 Very low-profile cervical implant and fixation devices. Historically, the intervertebral implant has been considered separately from the fixation plate and screw device. Recently manufacturers have developed unitary devices that incorporate both the intervertebral implant and the fixation screws into a single device. Additionally, cervical plates have been the subject of concern when patients have swallowing problems due to the plate protruding into the esophagus as it sits on the surface of the vertebrae. A & B—The PEEK Prevail device from Medtronic uses PEEK (poly-ether-ether-ketone) plastic and a single midline screw. Images A & B reproduced with permission of Medtronic. C & D—the Zero-P (zero profile) implant from Synthes provides more extensive screw fixation, and allows for bone graft material to be placed in the center of the PEEK ring of the device. Images C & D reproduced with permission of Synthes.

too much protection so that the fusion never occurs, and once again, the whole system may loosen and the device can slide into the structures of the neck— either forward into the esophagus or backward into the spinal canal.

In the lumbar spine, the materials used to promote the fusion often include a bioengineered "bone morphogenetic protein" or BMP. This cannot be used for cervical spine surgeries. Although it may be helpful in small doses, too many patients have had intense inflammatory reactions after using BMP. This was hard to detect in the lumbar spine where it just mixes in with post-operative back pain, but in the neck it caused severe breathing and swallowing difficulties in some patients. Because of this the FDA issued a warning in July of 2008 that has effectively terminated the use of BMP in the neck.

Over the course of four years, the FDA had received 38 similar reports of life-threatening breathing difficulties developing 2 to 14 days after the use of BMP in cervical spine surgery. This probably represented less than a one-in-a-thousand risk, but the usefulness of BMP in the neck is not as great as in the lumbar region because cervical spine fusion rates without BMP are very high. So severe risk plus low utility equals no more use.

The Future of Artificial Disks: Will They Work?

Most interesting among the new approaches to filling the empty disk space, however, is the artificial disk. Just as joint replacement with artificial hips and knees has become increasingly widespread over the past fifteen years, the recent arrival of artificial disks promises to change the way much of spine surgery is done.

The big advantage of an artificial disk is that it won't place abnormal stresses on the vertebrae above or below it. This is always a problem with spinal fusion: if a segment is stiffened, then the joints above or below it experience more wear and tear and may break down and require fusion themselves. Ideally, the surgeon would like to clean out the targeted disk space, open up the nerve canals, and then hold the disk space open but still maintain some spinal mobility. If this can be accomplished, it is much less likely that the problem will progress to require more surgery five years or ten years down the line, or potentially even sooner, on the level above or below the targeted disk space.

The various artificial disks have a metal and plastic composition that allows the vertebrae to move in the way that they normally move with the natural disk in place. The surfaces of the artificial disk are designed to grab firmly onto the adjacent vertebrae, which can partially grow into it, so it will stay in its precise intended location (see Figs. 17.4 and 17.5).

The risk of implanting an artificial disk is due to the potential for this adhesion of the unit to the bone above and below to fail, which would allow the artificial disk to slip out into the neck or, even worse, backward toward the nerves and spinal cord. With proper design, however, the expectation is that the failure rate with artificial disks will be very low.

Another problem that has turned up with early experience in using these disks is that they may not be as effective as fusion for treating neck pain. This is because arthritic changes affecting the facet joints in the posterior side of the spine may actually be aggravated by the unnatural movement of the artificial disk. When neck pain from movement and instability is a primary motive for surgery, a fusion may continue to be the most effective option.

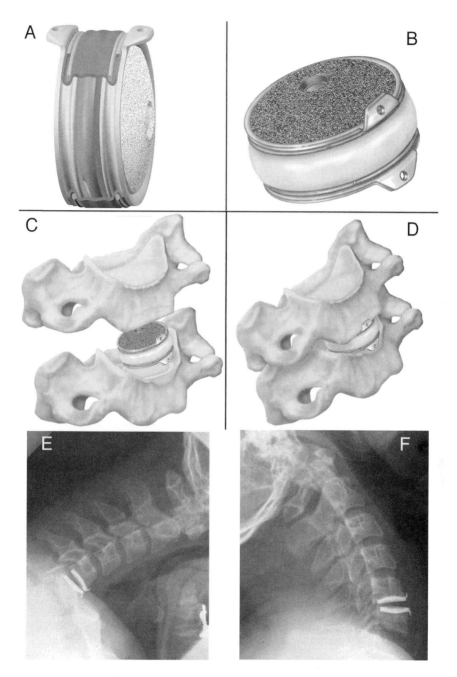

Figure 17.4 Bryan artificial cervical disk. Artificial disks preserve the mobility of the spine. Currently in the United States, artificial cervical disks are approved only for use at a single spinal level. Illustration reproduced with permission of Medtronic, Inc.

Figure 17.5 Synthes ProDisc C Nova cervical artificial disk. The surfaces of the implant include flat areas and keels coated with a sputtered titanium surfacing that allows bone to grow into the surface of the implant to better secure it. The ultra high molecular weight polyethylene (UHMWP) ball meets a cobalt-chromium-molybdenum (CoCrMo alloy) surface to provide multiple types and directions of motion. Images reproduced with permission of Synthes.

Artificial disks are a relatively new technology, with no five-year, ten-year, or fifteen-year track record in the United States. At the time of this writing, the ProDisc-C, the Bryan Disc, the Prestige Disc, and the Secure-C disc have been approved by the FDA for use in single-level disk replacements. Nonetheless, many insurance companies are still hesitant to pay for them. A certain percentage do slip and a certain percentage of implant sites fuse despite the artificial disk.

Placement of these disks at two or three levels has been offered in Europe and Asia for many years and is done "off label" (without FDA or manufacturer endorsement) by some surgeons in the US. When you are being considered for placement of an artificial disk, you have to understand that no one really knows what happens over the course of many, many years with these devices. Do they break down, do they need replacement, and what happens when they break? We just don't know the long-term results, but the potential advantages of artificial disks certainly make them a very viable option to consider.

The Posterior Cervical Approach

Although many cervical spine surgeries are carried out from the front of the neck, there are several important reasons why they sometimes can be carried out from the posterior (the back) of the neck instead. Posterior approaches are useful in repairing fractures, removing tumors, or repairing normal wear and tear. The four most common reasons for the surgeon to recommend a posterior approach are (1) fusions at the very top end of the spine, (2) decompressions of the spinal cord or fusions requiring surgery at three or more levels, (3) the need for a foraminotomy only, without any other problem to treat (see chapter 14), and (4) repair of a failed fusion.

The recovery from posterior cervical surgery usually takes a little bit longer than from surgery through the front of the neck, because much more muscle is opened up and separated from its normal attachment to the spine. However, the soreness from this usually clears up in two to four weeks. As with an anterior surgical approach, it is common to need to use a cervical collar for a while after the operation if there is a fusion involved.

Fusion and Decompression at the Very Top of the Spine

The scale of a posterior cervical surgery, in terms of the size of the incision and the recovery afterward, is not much different whether two, six, or seven levels are to be fused. Fusions are sometimes performed from the back of the neck because it is relatively straightforward to fuse three, four, five, six, or even more vertebrae, as well as fuse vertebrae in the thoracic region if needed. From the front of the neck, one or two can be easily fused, but three at the same time is difficult, and beyond that the dissection may be too extensive to be carried out easily and safely from the front.

Another advantage of the posterior approach is that it provides good access in cases when the very highest vertebrae, C1 and C2, have to be fused (see Fig. 17.6). Also, if the skull is to be fused onto the top of the spine, as is sometimes required in unusual types of arthritic degeneration, a posterior approach is the most viable. Surgery to take pressure off the spinal cord at C1 and C2 is very difficult from the front and may even require going through the mouth (*transorally*) in order to reach the problematic vertebral bone. If the surgery can be carried out from the back, however, the opening and closing are almost trivial compared with the difficulty of an anterior or transoral approach.

Figure 17.6 C1 to C2 fusion. Lateral mass screws can provide fixation between C1 and C2. Illustration reproduced with permission of the *Journal of Neurosurgery*. Reprinted from John K. Stokes, J. Patrick Johnson. Posterior atlanto-axial stabilization: new alternative to C1-2 transarticular screws. *Neurosurgical Focus* 12(1): A6, 2002.

Lateral Mass Screws: Precision Required

There are two general types of posterior cervical fusion methods. The most commonly used technique relies on screws and rods and involves placing a screw into each of the vertebrae involved and linking them together with the rod. Of all the different types of screws that surgeons place in the spine or even in the body, screws used for posterior fusion of the neck are among the most difficult to place accurately and involve the greatest risks. They certainly can be placed very safely, but the problem when working from the back is that the only place for the screw to go is through an area of the vertebra called the *lateral mass*. As it passes through a very tight space of bone, the lateral mass screw must avoid the main cervical spinal nerves as they exit the spine and also one of the major arteries, the vertebral artery, which is winding its way up to the brain.

An experienced surgeon uses known landmarks and angles to place these screws accurately and safely, but given the risks, nerves may also be monitored electronically during the course of the placement to make sure that screws aren't beginning to pinch them, and three-dimensional computer-image guidance systems are sometimes used as well (see Fig. 16.8). There is still no replacement for a skilled surgeon, because the computer-guided systems are subject to their own computer-based weaknesses and, at least as of the time of this writing, the safety of the image guidance is still not as good as the safety offered by an experienced surgeon working freehand. For a surgeon who does not often perform this operation, however, computer guidance can be a tremendous help.

Lateral mass screws have been used for fusions of vertebrae from the C3 level down to C7 for many years, beginning in the late 1970s (see Fig. 17.7). This technique has also recently been extended to include fusions up through the first and

Figure 17.7 Synthes Synapse cervical lateral mass screws. Screws placed in the pedicles of thoracic vertebrae and in the lateral masses of the cervical vertebrae can be used to provide fixation for fusion across the low neck and upper thoracic spine. Image reproduced by permission of Synthes.

second cervical vertebrae as well. The back of the skull (or *occiput*) can even be included by securing a type of plate onto the base of the skull and then attaching this plate to the rod system in the neck; however, this does place a great deal of stress on the fusion devices and is used only in very specialized circumstances.

Struts, Cables, and Claws: Designer Assembly

A second and entirely different approach to fusion in the posterior cervical spine is often a nice addition to the screw-and-rod method. Its basic principle is to take struts of donor cadaver bone—although other materials can be used—and to attach these with wires or cables to the spinous processes that stick out posteriorly from the vertebrae of the neck. This type of fusion was used with poor effect for many years as the primary method of fixation and fusion. But when lateral mass screws and spinous-process wiring are used together, they neatly cover each other's weak points. In this fashion, it is possible to achieve a very rigid assembly. This combination is also helpful when a fusion has failed anteriorly and the posterior approach is being used as a second try to achieve fusion (see Fig. 16.4).

Spinous process fusions have very good leverage for controlling natural flexion or extension of the neck, but because of their midline position, they are not very good at controlling the neck's twisting and turning. Lateral mass screws effectively limit twisting and turning but have very little leverage to control flexion and extension. Lateral mass screws are also particularly susceptible to failure when they are placed into bone that is soft due to osteoporosis, so combining the screws and a spinous process assembly is often a good choice for the surgeon when that condition is expected, whether the fusion is in the lower cervical spine or in the top two vertebrae.

Various other devices have been designed to try incorporating the posterior spinous processes into a fusion, such as claw devices or *sublaminar wires* (cables that pass under the lamina), which have always been and continue to be very risky, dangerous types of implants. But together, the techniques of lateral mass screws and cable-and-strut assembly provide a very solid and reliable method that can be used either when a fusion surgery is done for the first time or when the surgeon wants to supplement a failed anterior cervical fusion from the back of the neck rather than go into the front again.

18

Thoracic Spine Operations: Surgical Approaches to Mid-Back and Upper-Back Problems

Spinal problems affecting the thoracic region, which covers the area from the middle to upper back, are far less common than spinal problems affecting the low back or the neck. This is due, in part, to the fact that the thoracic region of the spine is fairly rigid because of the ribcage. Less movement in the spinal column means less wear and tear on the disks, ligaments, and vertebrae. Nonetheless, very significant problems can occur in the thoracic spine, such as a disk herniation or mechanical problems, including fractures that require fusion surgery.

One of the hallmarks of a thoracic disk herniation is a pinched *intercostal nerve* causing a pain that wraps around the body along the ribcage from the back to the front. Very often, the symptoms of a thoracic herniation are made worse by breathing deeply or shouting, but also by any twisting or bending movement, as with herniation in other spinal regions. In addition to nerve pinches, some kinds of trauma or differential pressure on the spine versus rib can cause pain to develop at the joint between the rib and the thoracic vertebra. A number of injuries can also cause pain at the thoracic facets, or articular joints. Whatever the problem may be, the choice of approach to thoracic spine surgery can make a tremendous difference in terms of the risk and the ease of recovery.

As can be seen below in this chapter, the factors determining the choice of approach are complex, so many surgeons who do spine work in general are hesitant to treat thoracic spinal problems. Thoracic spine patients are often seen only by subspecialists in spinal surgery who have a particular interest in, and are experienced in, thoracic spine problems; this is why many such patients must travel to a different city for their surgery. But the expanding tool kit for the thoracic region, together with all the instrumentation used in the cervical and lumbar regions, gives the specialist a full range of treatment capability for whatever type of compression, fracture, collapse, tumor, infection, or pain problem requires treatment.

Posterior, Anterior, or Lateral: Which Way?

One problem with treating herniations, tumors, and fractures in the thoracic region is that a posterior approach (from the back) is often very complicated. This is because the thoracic spinal cord carries all the neural signals for the legs, and it fills much of the space of the thoracic spinal canal. Therefore, retracting the thoracic spinal cord to access a disk or vertebral element is completely unsafe, so it is necessary instead to reach around the thoracic cord to get to any problems in the front of the thoracic spinal column.

In the neck, approaching from the front is done with very low risk and little difficulty, and is one of the very common types of cervical spine surgery. In the lumbar region, even though the anterior approach involves going through the abdomen, it is still considered a routine type of operation. In the thoracic region, however, reaching the spine from the front may mean opening the ribs, moving the heart, and passing through the area of the lungs. This makes an anterior thoracic approach more risky or difficult than an anterior lumbar approach, and far more difficult or risky than an anterior cervical approach.

Consider the problem of a significant herniated disk in the thoracic spine. Just as in the cervical spine, this herniation might pinch a nerve or nerve root, causing a radiculopathy that produces a pain wrapping around the body; or it could compress the spinal cord, causing a myelopathy that leads to leg weakness, bowel and bladder problems, or unsteadiness while walking. There is no single good answer to the question of which surgical approach to choose, because the necessary approach depends on the specific problem at hand, and several different options can be appreciated.

Thoracotomy: Opening the Chest

There are several different approaches to get to the spine in the thoracic region. The most invasive is a *thoracotomy*, which involves making a large incision between and parallel to two ribs, opening the chest wall, and either separating two ribs or sometimes removing a rib, to improve access. To avoid dealing with the heart and great vessels (aorta and vena cava), the opening is usually made from one side rather than directly from the front. Even once the chest is open, the lung is in the way, constantly moving and shifting with respiration. The anesthesiologist often has to block off the air flow to one lung to fully deflate it and immobilize it so it can be retracted out of the way.

This entry into the chest also penetrates and opens the *pleura*, or *pleural lining*, of the chest wall. Normal breathing requires the pleura to be intact, because each lung is suspended against the chest wall by negative pressure between the pleural lining of the lung and the pleural lining of the chest wall; any leak or tear may allow the lung to collapse. So once the surgical closure takes place after a thoracotomy, it is generally necessary to leave a suction tube between the pleura of the lung and the pleura of the chest wall for a day or two until all of those membranes have resolidified. Any misstep during the surgery that causes a small nick or damage to the pleural lining of the lung can lead to an air leak into the chest, which may make the recovery even more difficult and may require a more extended period with a suction chest tube.

Assuming any problems with the pleura are resolved, the mechanical force applied when opening the ribs may still lead to pain in the chest wall after the surgery. For all of these reasons, a thoracotomy should be performed only if it is the only reasonable choice. If there are no other options, bear in mind that thoracotomies are done with some frequency, and in most cases they go well and recovery is very good. However, it is better if a thoracotomy can be avoided.

Endoscopic Disk Removal: Working Through a Keyhole

One way to avoid the open-chest exposure of a thoracotomy for a thoracic discectomy is to use a video-assisted endoscopic approach. In this method, one, two, or sometimes three small incisions are made in the chest wall, and tubes are passed through each of these openings into the chest. One of the tubes is used to insert a small video camera so the surgeon can look around without actually opening the chest enough to see inside directly. A suction tool, and then some working instruments, which are long, modified surgical tools for cutting and coagulating blood vessels, drilling bone, and removing the disk, are inserted and manipulated through the other tubes (see Fig. 18.1).

One thing that is not immediately apparent when you read about an endoscopic approach is that the way the surgeon is using the tools is very different from the regular way in which a surgeon works. That is, instead of actually looking directly at what he or she is doing, the surgeon is looking at a picture on a video screen, which is essentially two-dimensional. In addition, the instruments are often very long, so that the normal feel of the tissues is lost in the extended endoscopic reach. Surgeons who do endoscopic chest operations require extensive additional training and also need to conduct a great many of these surgeries to be comfortable and skillful; for this reason, there are very few neurosurgeons or spine surgeons who perform endoscopic thoracic surgery.

The risks of an endoscopic thoracic approach are actually quite significant. It is much easier for the surgeon to make a slip or an error because of the reduced visibility and sensitivity and the use of long, awkward instruments; so, although the exposure itself is much smaller and safer, other surgical risks may be increased. The effects of these risks range from nuisance effects, such as postoperative leakage of a fatty digestive fluid called *chyle*, to major calamities, such as spinal cord injury.

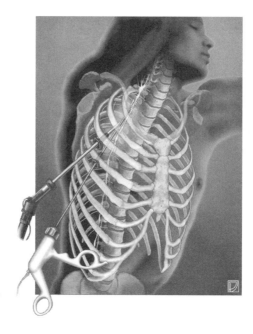

Figure 18.1 Endoscopy for access to the thoracic vertebrae. Many types of surgeries in the thoracic region of the spine can be done using endoscopic tools. This means that the instruments and a small video camera art introduced through small portals placed in the skin. The surgeon watches on a video screen while using the surgical instruments. Illustration reproduced with permission of Lippincott William and Wilkins. Reprinted from J.P. Johnson and N.P. Patel. Uniportal and biportal endoscopic thoracic sympathectomy. *Neurosurgery* 51 (5 Suppl): 79–83, November 2002.

This approach is often used to treat problems with the sympathetic nerves in the chest, in what is called a sympathectomy (lesioning or cutting of the connecting ganglion centers of the sympathetic nerves), for which the risks of endoscopy are much lower. However, if the endoscopic approach is taken for a disk removal, when heavy cutting, drilling, and biting instruments will be used near the nerves and the spinal cord, the risk goes up considerably. The open thoracotomy essentially has much lower neurologic risks than endoscopic thoracic surgery, but a more difficult recovery, and this is often the trade-off.

Transpedicular Tunneling: Sneaking Through the Back

What are the other options for thoracic disk removal? Well, one way to reach a damaged disk without going through the chest is to start at the posterior of the adjacent vertebra and to tunnel through the pedicle of the vertebra into the disk space. Using this *transpedicular* technique, the surgeon can perform a discectomy through a very small opening in the back, which often provides an attractive alternative.

Although the transpedicular approach has been known for many years, it has always posed a problem of very limited range of movement and visibility. But the advent of image-guided surgery has transformed it into a much more flexible, safe, and varied approach. Using image guidance and a computer, it is possible to track the instrument tips through the pedicle so that the surgeon can work with much greater safety and range, even without direct vision, by relying on the computer to show the placements of the instruments and the bones. The safety of an image-guided transpedicular approach is largely determined by the quality of the image-guidance system, and this is an area of active technology development.

Transaxillary and Cervical Access to the Upper Thoracic Region

Treating the upper thoracic region's first several vertebrae poses special problems. A standard thoracotomy cannot be done here in the usual way because of the position of the shoulder and the shoulder blades. Reaching this portion of the spine directly from the front is also difficult because of the great vessels (aorta and vena cava), and the top of the heart makes the surgeon's workspace very limited. If an anterior approach to the top several thoracic vertebrae is required, it may entail a very extensive operation somewhat like an open-heart surgery. The sternum is opened by a *sternotomy*, and a cardiothoracic surgeon has to move the heart and great vessels out of the way. This is certainly a very big surgery that presents many risks, so any alternative is usually preferred.

One option is a *transaxillary* approach through the underarm, a type of surgery that is very commonly used for a condition called thoracic outlet syndrome (see chapter 9). This approach allows the surgeon to come from the side of the body toward the vertebrae under direct vision, thereby avoiding the sternum, heart, and great vessels in front of the spinal column. Another alternative technique is very much like the standard anterior cervical approach described in chapter 17. If the patient's anatomy permits, simply reaching down to the top thoracic vertebrae from an anterior approach in the neck is often the simplest solution of all.

Posterolateral Maneuvers

One more option for performing a surgical decompression in the thoracic spine is to use a *posterolateral* approach, in which the surgeon starts several inches to the side of the midline in the back and follows the top of the rib around onto the targeted disk. Although this approach may entail a much more extensive incision, it does not necessarily require opening the chest or moving the ribs. As long as the problem to be treated, such as a herniated disk, is fairly posterior and accessible, the posterolateral route may provide a useful alternative to a thoracotomy, sternotomy, or transaxillary approach and to the technical challenges of endoscopy or transpedicular work.

Rescue or Removal of Thoracic Vertebrae

In the past, when a thoracic vertebra collapsed from osteoporosis, a fracture, or another injury, treatment in virtually all situations would require opening the chest. This also applied to surgery for scoliosis, or abnormal curvatures, in the thoracic spine. However, the technical problems posed by reconstructing vertebral fractures and collapses in the thoracic spine have very recently seen tremendous advances in treatment techniques that have changed this field dramatically.

Transpedicular Kyphoplasty: Minimally Invasive Repair of Collapsed Vertebrae

The first important development is the use of *transpedicular kyphoplasty* for a collapsed vertebra. A large-bore needle is passed through the pedicle into the vertebra, a small balloon is inflated to reestablish the size or shape of the collapsed vertebral body, and then a type of acrylic glue is pumped into the balloon, where it hardens and remains in place. In this way, through a small incision and the pedicle, the natural height and strength of the vertebral body can be restored without an extensive operation (see Fig. 14.9).

Thoracic Pedicle Screws: Heavy Reconstruction Outside the Chest

When kyphoplasty is not appropriate for thoracic vertebral reconstruction, such as when there is a bone fracture or an overly severe collapse, another important new development has greatly reduced the risk and extent of surgery needed to treat these instabilities: the use of thoracic *pedicle screws*.

For many years, pedicle screws were felt to be unsafe for use in the thoracic spine, because of the very small size of the pedicles and their close proximity to the very sensitive spinal cord in most of the region. Therefore, when a thoracic vertebral reconstruction was needed, a thoracotomy was often done; this, however, is a huge problem for older patients who develop spinal fractures associated with bone diseases, because a thoracotomy is fairly stressful to go through.

Thoracic pedicle screw surgery is now performed either with the assistance of an image-guidance system or by use of other recently developed approaches that allow the surgeon to move safely through the pedicle with appropriately sized screws and equipment to get a secure screw into each pedicle of interest. Then, when the deformation or abnormality in the spine is corrected, the pedicle screws can be locked together with a rod. In general, the newest screw-rod systems for this purpose have a fairly low-profile design that doesn't protrude or otherwise risk breakdown of the overlying skin (see Figs. 16.2 and 18.2).

When minimal access tubes are used to place the screws, it becomes possible to correct an extensive long deformity—such as scoliosis involving most of

Figure 18.2 Firebird scoliosis correction system from Orthofix. The advance of techniques for placing pedicle screws in thoracic vertebrae has made it possible to assemble very long constructs extending from the iliac crest and sacrum up to the high thoracic region across 17 spinal levels. After the screws and rods are in place, external wrenches and grippers are used to correct the scoliosis and then lock the correction in place. Image reproduced with permission of Orthofix.

the thoracic and lumbar vertebrae—through several small incisions. The various screws are placed, the screws are moved to ease the spine into normal alignment, and then the rods are passed under the skin to secure the screws in position. In this way, even extensive multilevel problems in the thoracic spine can be corrected without major invasive surgery. This is a very important advance for problems such as the pain from vertebral collapse or from thoracic facet or disk instability.

Vertebrectomy: Pulling It Together with Grafts, Plates, and Hooks

In the situations where a thoracic vertebral collapse is too severe to be handled with a posterior approach alone, it is still necessary to carry out a thoracotomy and often a vertebrectomy, in which the fractured vertebrae are completely removed and then replaced by a graft. In many cases, an allograft is made from a human cadaver fibula or tibia, although there are a variety of other replacement methods that use complex titanium devices or cast methylmethacrylate resins. As with low lumbar fusion, often the best outcomes of thoracic vertebrectomy can be achieved with a bone graft. A titanium plate is usually needed, however, with screws placed in the sides of the vertebrae to hold the graft in place (see Fig. 18.3).

A major area of recent innovation has been in the design of devices that can be implanted to replace vertebral bodies that must be removed. This has been very challenging in the past because a crushed vertebra from a fracture or tumor—or one that must be removed because it is destroyed by infection (osteomyelitis)—is often associated with a partial collapse of the spine. In the thoracic region, the spine tends to bend forward as a vertebra collapses. Ideally, the destroyed vertebral body can be removed and a plate or screw construct can be used to pull the spine back into a straight, full height configuration. However, this means that at the start of the operation the space left by the collapsed vertebra is relatively small, but that space gets expanded as the operation nears completion. This has made it difficult to select and trim bone grafts to replace the removed vertebral body and disks.

To solve this problem several manufacturers have developed vertebral replacement devices that can be expanded in height as the surgery progresses. The expansion can be carried out by turning a threaded device that forces the ends apart. This gradually increases the height of the spacer as the deformity is corrected by the plate or screw and rod system. As a simplification of the mechanical aspects of driving the expansion, some systems have been developed

Figure 18.3 Thoracic vertebrectomy, graft and VentroFix plate. If a fractured thoracic or high lumbar vertebra is compressing the spinal canal, the body of the vertebra can be removed in a vertebrectomy. The body is replaced by a bone graft, and the whole construct is restored to full strength with a plate and rod system. VentroFix System illustration reproduced with permission of AO Synthes.

recently that use fluid pressure to push the ends apart while maintaining a uniform gentle pressure on the end plates of the intact vertebral bodies above and below. Once the final height is reached, the device is locked at that height (see Fig. 18.4). Devices of this type can be delivered by an endoscopic approach and then expanded once eased into place.

A variety of different plate systems are used when a vertebrectomy is performed. What they all have in common is that the damaged vertebrae are fully removed, along with the disks at either end of them The graft is inserted and then screws that are passed into the sides of the vertebrae above and below the vertebrectomy secure a plate in place. The plate is equipped with a system that enables it to compress or firmly grip the graft. Usually, these kinds of assemblies

Figure 18.4 Aesculap Hydrolift vertebral body replacement. This device is typical of various kinds of replacement structures that are used when an entire thoracic or lumbar vertebral body, as well as the disk above and below it, are removed. The rough titanium surface at top and bottom can permit ingrowth of bone to help hold the device in place. After it is initially placed, a hydraulic pump system is used to gradually increase the vertical height of the device in order to fully expand the space where the damaged vertebral body had to be removed. Image reproduced with permission of Aesculap Implant Systems, LLC.

or constructs are very strong and don't require any posterior surgery. With very severe fractures, however, it is often necessary to do a posterior pedicle screw placement as well.

In the past, prior to the more common use of thoracic pedicle screws, the most common types of metal implants in the thoracic spine were hooks slipped under the lamina or around the lateral transverse processes, and these are still widely used. Although these hooks may be safer to put in place than pedicle screws in some situations, the feet of some types of hooks reach inside the spinal canal and may themselves cause problems, such as dislodging or tearing through parts of the vertebra, if a great deal of stress is placed on the instrumentation. This is why the long, hook-type implants are increasingly being replaced by stronger, short, metal constructs that involve pedicle screws and rods.

The newer techniques for thoracic spine surgery have had a tremendous impact on recovery from thoracic operations. This is because they have made it possible to greatly reduce the total amount of exposure necessary. That means smaller incisions, fewer open thoracic surgeries, and shorter surgeries.

19

Lumbar Implants and Fusion: Major Surgeries for the Low Back

The lumbar spine (or low back) is made up of the five vertebrae between the low end of the rib cage and the top of the pelvis. It is a very flexible part of the spine that carries a great deal of the body's weight. As such, mechanical problems and pains in the lumbar region can have a tremendous effect on every activity.

There are certainly many reasons that you can experience back pain, and most of them involve short-term problems such as muscle spasms, torn ligaments, or, in more serious cases, even a herniated disk. However, all of these problems are relatively easy to treat when compared with mechanical instability in the spine or with some of the irreparable failures that can occur in the ligaments and joints of the lumbar spine. When your problem is primarily low back pain that is produced by certain positions and relieved to some extent by other positions, the suspicion of mechanical back pain from lumbar vertebral instability is raised, particularly when the pain persists over an extended period of time.

The definitive test for a discogenic pain syndrome (when a disk failure is suspected to be the source of the pain) is an anesthetic discogram. This is an image-guided injection of an anesthetic into the disk to numb it. If this relieves the pain, a discogenic pain syndrome is confirmed. A similar test called a provocative discogram can alternatively be used. This involves injecting a fluid into the disk space to stretch and stress the disk, and then attempting to learn from the patient whether the pain caused by the injection of fluid is the same as the patient's usual pain. It is often difficult for patients to comment on this reliably, so the anesthetic discogram typically gives a clearer result in demonstrating that the disk itself is the source of the pain.

If an identified discogenic pain has not responded to the conservative or nonsurgical treatments described elsewhere in this book, it sometimes becomes necessary to replace the disk, most commonly by fusing it. Chapter 16 discusses the history of different fusion techniques in the lumbar spine. That history can be summarized by saying that there are many approaches and that their development has improved the practice of spinal fusion surgery to the point where it can be carried out reliably with a very low chance of failure or of making the back pain worse. Nevertheless, many of the devices that have been proposed for carrying out fusions in the lumbar spine (even the more recent ones) have their weaknesses.

Lumbar spine surgery is still an area in which different spine surgeons have different opinions, levels of training, experiences, and exposures to different methodologies. There is no definitive agreement on the absolute best methods. My own experience, however, is based not only on surgical treatment but on seeing many patients with failed surgeries and gaining impressions of the ways devices fail and the ways failure can be prevented. It is also based on the shared knowledge of several prominent spinal specialists who exchange their experiences and opinions at our specialty spine conferences. This experience has led to a series of recommendations that I make to my own patients; each recommendation can be compared with the alternatives.

Interbody Implants: Doing the Heavy Lifting

One of the important lessons from the long history of spinal fusion is that there is a tremendous benefit in actually placing some sort of implant in the disk space between two vertebral bodies if a disk is removed. Some of the earlier methods involve trying to fuse the posterior elements of the spine, leaving the anterior part floating. This often fails because of the great stress placed on whatever posterior fusion device is used. Another choice for the surgeon is to enter from the back of the spine, move the nerves aside, and insert an implant into the disk space or, alternatively, to go through the abdomen in order to place an implant into the disk space from the front.

Beating the Disadvantages of the Posterior Approach

The problem with trying to replace the disk by doing the surgery entirely from the back is that when it is necessary to move the spinal dura out of the way there is a risk of injury to the nerves or of spinal fluid leaks. Even when these two problems are prevented, the surgeon can push only a fairly small implant into the disk space from a posterior approach, and these small implants carry risks of movement, slippage, and *extrusion* (backing out) into the spinal canal near the nerves.

In addition, the disk space between low lumbar vertebrae is not flat but is more of a wedge, with the larger part of the wedge pointing forward toward the abdomen. When the implant has to come in from the back, at a small point of the wedge, it is very hard to insert something that will restore the space's normal shape; but if a flat disk implant is placed, the disk space will become flat. This can produce what is called a *flat back syndrome*: with the loss of the wedge, the whole upper body starts to tilt forward over the lumbar spine and pelvis, which can lead to chronic pain after an otherwise successful fusion surgery.

There are new methods now available that reduce the impact of these disadvantages. By shifting the approach to the spine a little farther around to the side, the surgeon can slip into the disk space by passing under the nerves. Also, wedge-shaped implants have been designed that can be rotated into position after they are slipped into the disk space.

Anterior Approaches: Exposure versus Endoscopy

Given the options, it is still the widespread practice to approach a low lumbar fusion surgery from the front, through the abdomen. With this anterior approach, the surgeon still has a number of choices in reaching the front of the vertebrae.

Very commonly, the spine surgeon works with a general surgeon or a vascular surgeon, who is responsible for opening the abdomen and providing access to the front of the spine. Between the skin of the abdomen and the spine are all the abdominal contents, and then finally the great vessels, the aorta and the vena cava, as well as their major branches, the *iliac veins* and *iliac arteries*. The surgeon who does the approach can use a *retroperitoneal* technique, which means that the abdominal contents and the sac that they are in, the *peritoneum*, are protected and moved out of the way. Or the surgeon may proceed *transabdominally*, directly through the peritoneum, and spread aside the intestinal components to create an opening to the spine. When the approach is through the peritoneum, there is a little more irritation to the intestines, which can prolong the postoperative hospital stay; however, sometimes this transabdominal approach is safer than the retroperitoneal.

Then comes the very important step of moving the aorta and vena cava out of their usual position directly in front of the lumbar spine and protecting them during the rest of the surgery. One of the serious risks of any anterior approach is an injury to either of these great vessels, which can lead to very rapid, severe, and life-threatening blood loss. For this reason, this part of the approach is usually done by an experienced vascular surgeon who is familiar with working with the spine surgeon and who should always be immediately available in the hospital, if not actually in the operating room, throughout the course of the operation. All that being said, many thousands of these surgeries are done with great safety.

Another option for the anterior approach is to use an endoscopic method, which entails making small incisions for instruments to enter into in order to illuminate the abdominal cavity and provide video-assisted guidance to carry out the operation with special tools. There are a number of good systems designed for an anterior endoscopic approach; however, even the most experienced vascular surgeons have difficulty endoscopically moving and repositioning the great vessels at the front of the spinal column, which makes this procedure relatively unsafe. Therefore, most surgeons taking the anterior approach to the lumbar spine rely on an open abdominal exposure. This often means that the abdominal incision is the most painful part of the operation to recover from, and it also means that it may be several days after surgery before the intestines are working well enough for you to eat normally. Nonetheless, when it works as intended, the open abdominal exposure results in a safe anterior approach, avoiding the risk of injury to the nerves.

Lateral Approaches—Minimizing the Impact of Getting to the Interspace

The most important change or advance in approaches to lumbar fusion surgery in the past five years has been the development of widespread use of lateral approaches. A lateral approach passes anterior to the back muscles and many of the nerves, but posterior to the actual abdominal cavity. This keeps the surgeon away from many structures in the spine (dura, spinal roots) and many structures in the abdomen (aorta, vena cava, intestines) that have been a challenge with traditional posterior or anterior approaches.

NuVasive—with its XLIF system (extreme lateral interbody fusion) and other similar systems (such as the Synthes Oracle system) involve a minimal access entry from the flank (see Fig. 19.1). The surgeon advances a tube to the lateral surface of the disk, removes the disk material and inserts an intervertebral spacer

Figure 19.1 Lateral approach for lumbar fusion implants. The patient is positioned on their side and the surgeon uses a "blunt" dissection method to pass in front of the back muscles, but behind the "peritoneal" lining of the abdominal cavity. The approach then passes through the psoas muscle and nerves to reach the side of the intervertebral disk. Image reproduced with permission of Synthes.

or graft material from the side (see Fig. 19.2). It is usually still necessary to place pedicle screws from a posterior approach but they can be placed by minimal access techniques because there is no need to open the spine from the back (see Fig. 19.3).

Although the lateral approach is attractive because is avoids well-known problems and challenges associated with posterior and anterior approaches—it is no magic cure. Although the spinal nerve roots are avoided, the surgeon must go through the psoas muscle. Here there are spinal nerves and the lumbosacral plexus (not the roots but the nerves themselves). In a posterior approach, the surgeon knows exactly where the spinal nerves roots will be, but in a lateral approach, the

Figure 19.2 Synthes Oracle lateral fusion system. A. Once the surgeon has accessed the lateral aspect of the vertebral body (Fig 19.1), the tissue dissector and collapsed retractor system are advanced into place. B. The retractor blades are opened to provide an access for placing screws and for removing the disk material. C. The access route is then used to place an intervertebral implant. D. the implant is secured in place by pedicle screws and rods placed separately from a posterior approach. Image reproduced with permission of Synthes.

Lateral view of one-level Oracle cage
and Pangea

Lateral view of one-level Oracle cage
and TSLP

AP view of one-level Oracle cage
and Pangea

AP view of one-level Oracle cage and
TSLP

Figure 19.3 Synthes Oracle lateral implant with either posterior or lateral fixation. The Oracle cage can be secured with pedicle screws—seen in lateral (A) and antero-posterior X-ray view (B). Alternatively, it can be secured with a lateral plate that is placed during the lateral access portion of the surgery (C and D). Image reproduced with permission of Synthes.

surgeon cannot predict the precise course of the nerves. They vary significantly from individual to individual in their course through the psoas muscle.

NuVasive anticipated this issue and provided an electronic nerve stimulation system to help surgeons identify nerves as the devices were advanced. This was a comprehensive new system with new types of implants, new surgical instruments and retractors, and the electronic nerve detection system. All this is combined with the advantage of quick recovery time for the patient. The new methodology was greeted with great enthusiasm and widespread acceptance among spinal surgeons, but serious problems developed causing many hospitals to halt the use of lateral approaches. The guidance was not sufficient and a dramatic increase in the incidence of nerve injuries was reported when compared with older techniques.

The reporting of complications was another shock to the system of spinal research. Initial reports showed virtually no complications and excellent outcomes, but it was later revealed that the surgeons providing data for these reports had investments in the new technology. Other reports on the same system were written using data from surgeons that had no financial conflict of interest and those reports revealed truly alarming rates of neurologic complications. The initial report from a conflicted investigator at Cedars Sinai showed a 2 percent complication rate. A later large formal report from an unconflicted group at University of Miami showed a 67 percent nerve injury complication rate—a breathtaking and unprecedented rate of neurological complication after any type of spinal surgery. Cedars Sinai then discontinued use of the product pending an investigation. Insurance companies withdrew reimbursement. Organization of a class action lawsuit was commenced. Vigorous efforts are being made by NuVasive and other manufacturers to improve the technology and training, but the damage to trust in the academic publication system has clearly been done and will be difficult to reverse.

At present, the NuVasive and similar systems have been reconfigured to reduce the risks. Some have considered using MR Neurography nerve images introduced into an image guidance system to help avoid the nerves—but nothing of this sort is in use at this time. In my nerve repair practice I continue to see new patients who developed nerve compressions and difficulty walking during lateral spine fusion approaches. In addition, the incision in the flank that is used in the approach has not been designed carefully and many patients have body wall nerves severed. This is not a problem when approaching from the back and it is not a problem with well developed abdominal approaches, but lateral fusion patients have developed troubling abdominal wall bulges that cannot be repaired when the small nerves of the body wall are cut during the course of the initial incision and approach.

Overall, lateral approaches do provide many promising advantages, but this is an area of active development at this time. Surgeons who understand the risks and know how to take steps to avoid them may be more successful in avoiding these complications. As in other areas of spine surgery, a surgeon with considerable training and experience is your best route to minimizing the risk of complications.

Bone Rings and Titanium Cages

Once the exposure is made, and the surgeon has accessed the front of the vertebral bodies in the lumbar region, the entire faulty disk is usually removed at the involved level (or levels), and an implant can be placed in the disk space. One of the key principles of placing any intervertebral implant is that the surfaces of the vertebrae have to be optimally prepared. Because the vertebral body is a kind of a box with a soft center and hard outside, the hard outside has to be preserved. If the preparation process or the actual steps of inserting the implant weaken the end plate of the vertebra, then the implant may break through the hard exterior and plunge into the soft interior, leading to a surgical failure. The surgeon scrapes any joint material and cartilage off the hard end plate of the vertebrae so that the surface is exposed and growth can take place. However, the scraping has to be done carefully so that the end plate remains thick and strong and thus capable of securely supporting the implant until fusion takes place.

There are various types of implants made from metals, carbon fiber, and other materials. However, the safest and most reliable seem to be implants made of donor, or allograft, bone. For the lumbar spine, using the patient's own bone, or an autograft, generally doesn't work because there are no available pieces of bone that are large and strong enough to be taken without causing quite a bit of trouble at the donor site. The most common type of lumbar implant is made of cadaver femur. It is a ring of bone shaped similarly to a lumbar disk. It is also wedge-shaped so that one side of the ring is taller than the other side. This assures that the normal wedge shape of the vertebral space is maintained. The ring also has roughened edges so it won't slide out of place once implanted (see Fig. 19.4).

Figure 19.4 Anterior lumbar interbody fusion. After removing most of a disk, the surgeon can spread open the collapsed disk space and then place a graft. These grafts are sliced from a femur leg bone of a cadaver donor and are machined to an optimum wedge shape. A femoral ring allograft also allows for the placement of bone fusion–promoting proteins in the central space of the ring graft. FRA System illustration reproduced with permission of AO Synthes.

The surgeon removes the faulty disk, uses a device to expand the disk space to its normal height, and then drives the bone implant into place. The center of the ring can be filled with a small amount of bone from the patient's hip or with a high-performing, synthetic bone-growth promoter such as a *demineralized bone matrix* or a *bone morphogenetic protein*. Sometimes a small retaining plate is also placed in front of the bone ring to make sure that under no circumstances will it slip forward to impact the blood vessels in front of the spine. There are also plates that can reach across the disk space on the posterior (facet) side of the space (see Fig. 19.5), adding to the rigidity.

Titanium cages have been used to replace disks, but these often overprotect the bone fusion material by preventing any compressive stress at all from reaching it (see Figs. 16.5 and 21.1). This can actually inhibit the vertebral bone from growth and fusion and may be reliable only when used along with bone morphogenetic protein. At the time of this writing, it is not clear that a titanium cage, even with morphogenetic protein, can provide a better result than a bone ring.

Artificial Disks for Natural Movement

The same approach described above can be used to implant an artificial lumbar disk. The artificial disks are designed to be held in place by the normal tension of the disk space between the vertebrae and also to permit some ingrowth of the adjacent bone into the complex material that forms the artificial disk end plate (see Fig. 21.2).

The motion of two vertebrae relative to each other is complex, and artificial disks are designed to preserve this type of movement. A problem with fusion surgery is that it always places extra stress on the vertebral levels above and below the level of the fusion, in that those levels have to work harder and move more and may experience accelerated degeneration. When an artificial disk is used instead, more normal movement is maintained, so there is not the disadvantage of accelerated degeneration in the vertebrae above and below the implant (Fig. 19.6).

Artificial disks, however, are still not appropriate in all situations. Their use is limited when the adjacent vertebral bone is not strong enough, when there is too much arthritis, or when the disk space collapse is too severe. If a back pain with movement comes mostly from the posterior elements or facet joints of the spine, using an artificial disk will not decrease movement, so the pain may persist or even be made worse. This is obviously less effective than a successful fusion surgery that is known to be able to resolve that pain. Various techniques of *arthroplasty*—treatments that relieve stress on the facets or serve to replace the facets—may be needed in conjunction with disk replacement before this

A

B

Figure 19.5 Additional fixation with anterior lumbar implants. In some cases an intervertebral implant is placed without the additional placement of pedicle screws. Another option is to use smaller devices to provide some fixation without the higher risk of pedicle screw placement. A. Techtonix tension band placed on the posterior elements of vertebrae to help hold the vertebral bodies together during the weeks in which the bone products in the intervertebral implant are achieving fusion. Image A reproduced with permission of Stryker Spine. B. When an anterior approach for placement of a interbody fusion device is done, a plate such as the Unity anterior plate from Orthofix can be attached from the same anterior access to hold the vertebral bodies in place from the front. This also helps reduce the risk that the implant will extrude ("pop out") into the abdominal cavity. Image B reproduced with permission of Orthofix.

technique can begin to replace fusion altogether. The design of some artificial disks, however, may help with facet pain as well. Some designs allow fairly free movement in various directions, while others constrain the allowed directions of movement much more.

If a back pain with movement is purely discogenic, such as pain arising from a torn annular ligament (a disk's retaining ring), then replacing the torn disk with an artificial one is an attractive option. A positive response to an anesthetic disk injection when there is no relief from a facet block suggests that an artificial disk may be the right device to use. Both the ProDisc-L from Synthes and the Charite disk from DePuy (Johnson and Johnson) have been approved

Figure 19.6 Charité artificial lumbar disc. This patient with six lumbar vertebrae has a DePuy (Johnson & Johnson) Charité disc in place at L5/L6 and at L6/S1.

by the FDA for use in single-level disorders. As with the situation for cervical disks, they have been used for multiple-level artificial disk replacement, but this is off-label use. The Medtronic "Maverick" disk is not available because of successful patent litigation by Synthes against Medtronic that has prevented the Maverick disk from being used.

The artificial disk outcome literature is another area where there are disturbing conflicts among reports from different sources. A number of prominently published reports revealed effectively no complications or failures of the lumbar artificial Charite disk, but the *Wall Street Journal* reported a number of cases of extrusion of the implant causing severe complications. It is obviously extremely unsettling if physicians and insurers are relying on the medical literature and the reporting is demonstrably false.

This has had a chilling effect on the acceptance of lumbar artificial disks because anyone can see that if a doctor tells you they are completely safe, then they are not being accurate. If you are warned of risks, did the data come from the scientific literature, from the manufacturer, or from the *Wall Street Journal?* Many insurers therefore refuse to pay for the artificial disks. Even if the literature shows they are safe, the publications are not convincing. With the elapse of time, more experience and better reporting of the complications will no doubt occur. All surgical procedures have a complication rate. The trouble comes if surgeons who are new to a technique do not realize what they must watch out for and therefore do not take necessary precautions.

More and more long term data on artificial disks is becoming available. It is already clear that they should not be used in women over 50 because the presence of osteoporosis or the development of osteoporosis is a very high risk and is expected to lead to an unacceptable high rate of artificial disk displacement. What if you are only 40 and take calcium regularly—do you expect to still have your artificial disk in 10 years? Many surgeons who support artificial disks are quick to point out how successful and important hip replacement surgery has become—but it is not yet clear that spinal disk replacement will ever be so successful. Second and third generation artificial disks are under development and this is expected to be an important area of technological advance in the future.

A completely different approach to the problem of disc replacement is the idea of inserting a soft flexible elastic implant that replaces the nucleus pulposus part of the disk but leaves the annulus ring intact. This is as opposed to the artificial disks that are fundamentally mechanical and attached to the vertebrae. There are a variety of different materials and technologies being explored for the purpose of soft disk replacement, but none of these are available for use as of 2012.

Pedicle Screws: Titanium Scaffold for Heavy Lifting

Although the anterior disk implant provides considerable immediate stability, it usually still allows enough movement in that level of the spine so that the risk of fusion failure remains a great concern. Therefore, the most successful lumbar fusion method requires that retaining screws be placed from the back of the vertebrae through the pedicles (the supports that connect the lamina to the vertebral body) as well. These screws hold that portion of the spine stiff while the implant is fusing during the several months following surgery. Of the wide variety of posterior retaining systems, pedicle screws are the most reliable.

Load Bearing and Load Sharing: When the Metal Needs to Move

There are many different types of pedicle screws, and one important distinction is between a *load-bearing* and a *load-sharing* screw. Load-sharing screws are used in a retaining system where the screws and rods together allow a small amount of movement of the affected vertebrae. This is important because bone growth occurs in response to stress, so if the retaining system is too rigid, there will not be enough pressure on the front of the bone and this will actually slow the fusion process. However, if the pedicle screws are not strong enough, particularly in a very heavy individual, the weight of the body may crush or fracture the disk implant through force from the adjacent vertebral end plates; in that situation, a load-bearing type of pedicle screw is required.

Technology is advancing steadily in the area of posterior fixation. For patients with osteoporosis whose bones may be too soft to hold a pedicle screw, Synthes has introduced a hollow screw with pores in the threaded tip of the screw (see Fig. 19.7). After the screw is placed, a bone cement can be pushed through the screw to extrude partially from the screw threads into the vertebral body to help improve fixation. However, as discussed in chapter 14, the type of glue used is critical and its distribution as it is injected has to be monitored very carefully.

Flexible and Adjustable Rods

The connection between the screws is another area of advance. Rods that can be adjusted in length as young patients grow and rods that can be reshaped either

Figure 19.7 Perforated screws (Pangea—Synthes) with bone cement injection. Many older patients have osteoporosis, which can result in relatively soft or brittle vertebral bone. This increases the risk that implanted screws could shift and loosen. This Synthes innovation allows for the injection of bone cement that passes out of the sides of the screw after injection. The result is a mass of bone cement in the vertebral body that extends into the core of the screw—this helps decrease the risk in the patient with osteoporosis. Image reproduced with permission of Synthes.

during the surgery or afterward have been developed. One of these systems involves an external magnet that essentially unlocks the rod and then relocks it a new configuration.

Yet another area of advance in the technology of rods involves flexible rods. The idea here is to provide some limitation of movement but not actual rigid fixation. It has been hoped that this will reduce the occurrence of "adjacent level disease" where the vertebral level just above a fusion undergoes more rapid deterioration because of the stiffness of the fused level below it forcing it do more work. One such flexible system is the Dynesys device from Zimmer (see Fig. 19.8). Unfortunately, this is another area of technology where there was overly rapid acceptance by spinal surgeons who understood the problem it was meant to solve. Initial reports—involving investigators with a financial stake in the product—were glowing: great success with virtually no complications. Unfortunately, later reports by surgeons without conflicts reported dramatically greater complication and failure rates. Here again, many hospital halted the use of the device and insurers refused to reimburse. With movement, the screws loosen. Loose screws promote degenerative change. Screw and bone fractures resulted. The fusion rate of the adjacent solidly fixated level decreased. The flexible rod can accelerate the very problem it is meant to correct.

What are these financial conflicts? These occur in several ways, some of them very clever and difficult for the patient to detect. They are upsetting to understand because some are clearly meant to deceive. In one approach, dozens of surgeons are asked for input when a device is under development. Then they are all treated as co-inventors entitled to patent royalties. In another scheme, dozens or hundreds of surgeons are hired as consultants to a given manufacturer or even as consultants to "distributors." A distributor is a company that has sales people that contract with the manufacturer and contract

Flexion   Neutral   Extension

Figure 19.8 Flexible links between vertebrae. At the level above a lumbar fusion, it may be helpful to reduce excess motion without fully fusing. The Dynesys system from Zimmer uses pedicle screws, but has a flexible connector instead of the usual metal rod. The result is that movement is still permitted but extra support is provided. This does place stress on the screws as movements take place, but is thought to reduce the risk of degenerative problems at such an "adjacent" level next to a fused vertebral level. Vertebral drawings from Sir Richard Owen, modified.

with the hospital. The surgeon has no financial interest in the device or the in the manufacturer, but profits by the sales of the distributor. When conflicts of interest are not declared, these kinds of commitments are difficult to follow—they are not "transparent."

Although some spine societies set rules for conflicts of interest among investigators, the usual rule is just that the surgeon disclose the conflict. The disclosure may be misleading, and the literature will probably still be read as if there was no conflict—readers assume that it is all good science if it is published. The problem here is that the executives of many of the spine societies and editors and reviewers of the journals are often financially conflicted as well. This is a huge unresolved issue in spinal surgery. There is a special society that has been set up for ethical advice wherein only surgeons with no outside financial links can join. However, a surgeon's livelihood depends on doing surgery so it is hard to see how all conflicts can really be avoided. The press and the United States Congress have been concerned with the issue. Overall, patients benefit from advances in technology. A problem with one device becomes an opportunity for technological advance for another company.

In neurosurgery, there is a process of guideline preparation in which extremely rigid rules are applied to read, review, and rank the published literature. The guideline committees—at a national and international level—decide on the quality of the literature and the evidence. New treatments are assessed as to whether there really is good reliable literature. This is the front line on a professional level—particularly because neurosurgery involves surgeons who work on brain, nerve and spine so that there is oversight from specialists who are knowledgeable about spine surgery but who may not be spine surgeons themselves. Statisticians and academics who study the medical literature for quality of research play a role at this level. However, even guideline analysis can be suppressed by conflicted senior organizational officers.

What can the patient do? This is still a troubling question. People worry that if they question their surgeon about financial conflicts their surgeon will be angry with them during surgery. Sounds like a bad idea! This is all why doctors have taken the Hippocratic Oath and this is why trust is essential. Personally, I believe that directing technological and business opportunity toward the improvement of problematic devices and methods is the answer. This does require inventors and it does require time—but that is how our societies and our medical technologies have improved over time and it is how they continue to improve.

Image-Guided Placement: Electronic, Fluoroscopic, and Human

A few years ago, the placement of pedicle screws required a very large exposure at surgery. Currently, pedicle screws are often placed through a very small incision under some sort of image guidance. The most common guidance technique is the use of X-ray fluoroscopy (see chapter 10) during surgery, but electronic, virtual image-based guidance for placement of the screws is increasingly common (see Fig. 19.9), and there are even possibilities for robotic screw placement. It is still often the case, however, that the surgeon's direct feel of the vertebral body and perceptions of the position and orientation of the vertebrae, together with fluoroscopic imaging, provide the safest and most reliable approach.

When a pedicle screw is inserted, it needs to travel through a particular, safe, posterior entry point on the vertebral body and pass through the pedicle to the front of the vertebral body. If the screw is placed a little too medially, toward the center of the spinal canal, or too low, toward the foramen (nerve canal), the edges of the screw may break through the pedicle wall and cause irritation to the passing nerves. A very gravely misplaced screw may actually injure nerves at the time of placement.

Figure 19.9 Pedicle screw placement. A computer-based image guidance system can be used to achieve accurate placement of pedicle screws (see Figs. 16.3 and 16.8). Vector Visions Spine illustration reproduced with permission of Brain LAB Inc.

A major area of advance in accuracy of spinal screw placement has come from improvements in medical imaging technology. For years, surgeons used the "C-arm" fluoroscopy system to take X-rays in the lateral or antero-posterior planes. Now many surgeons use a device called an "O-arm" from Medtronic that actually provides an image like a CT scan during the surgery (see Fig. 19.10). It

Figure 19.10 Intraoperative advanced imaging. For many years, physicians took X-rays during spine surgery to check on screw positions and vertebral alignment. Recently, these two-dimensional X-rays have been abandoned in favor of better cross sectional and three-dimensional X-ray views. A. The O-arm system (Medtronic) is an advance on the older "C-arm" (see Fig. 10.1). It uses an X-ray type tube that can make a complete circuit around the patient in order to produce a cross sectional view. Image reproduced with permission of Medtronic. B. The DViS system from Imaging-3 improves on the O-arm by completing the image more rapidly. C. The Body Tom from Neurologica is an actual portable CT-scanner. It is more bulky than the "ring X-ray" systems, but it is much faster, more precise and more capable of showing soft tissues. In CT scanning, a sharp "pencil-like" X-ray beam is used, as opposed to the standard X-ray technology in the O-arm and DViS that generate a more diffuse "wedge" of X-ray energy.

is slow and generates a great deal of radiation, but this technology will improve over time. Various smaller intraoperative CT scan rings are under development from competing companies (see Fig. 19.10).

Yet another advance in this area is advent of three dimensional X-ray technology. The C-arm and O-arm (and similar devices) place the X-ray device around the patient—which can be difficult for the surgeon to work around and can interfere with the sterile draping. However just as we can use our two separated eyes to see in three dimensions (due to parallax—the difference in position of objects when seen from two different positions), the X-ray can be taken from two different positions and then reassembled with special glasses so that the surgeon experiences a three dimensional depth perception without the CT scan. This is expected to be faster, generate less radiation, and allow the surgeon better access to the patient as the procedure goes forward with repeated imaging to guide screw placement.

Posterolateral Fusion: Hold or Pass?

In the past, the placement of pedicle screws was typically done along with what is called a *posterolateral fusion*. This is a placement of bone graft material along the bony transverse or lateral processes that protrude from the sides of the lumbar vertebrae. Posterolateral fusion provides an additional amount of stability, but it requires considerable additional exposure and mobilization of muscles.

In general, the minimally invasive insertion of pedicle screws can hold the vertebrae appropriately in position, while the large anterior disk implant can provide an adequate extent of actual fusion. The approach for placement of the screws can also take advantage of a natural plane in the tissues of the lumbar region that allows the surgeon to reach the entry point in the vertebrae without cutting or damaging any muscles. This is a tremendous improvement over the approach used a few years ago, which required extensive disconnection and disruption of lumbar muscles to place pedicle screws.

Posterior Fix-Ups on the Lamina: Treating Spondylolysis

There are less severe problems in the spine that can require some sort of fusion, including some fracturing or separation of the posterior parts of a vertebra, particularly in the condition called spondylolysis, a situation in which the lamina of the vertebra becomes separated from the superior facet and pedicle (see Fig. 8.6). Another type of problem in the posterior element arises in the various types of facet syndromes.

Repairing a Separated Lamina

To treat spondylolysis, it is often possible to reconnect the portions of the affected vertebra by roughening the separated edges and placing pedicle screws. The spinous process is then tightened toward the screws with a cable device. This can hold the structures in place sufficiently to allow them to fuse. This does not include a fusion across the disk space or across the facets. However, it is sometimes necessary to actually fuse the involved vertebrae to the adjacent vertebra below it in order to arrest the abnormal motion that can result from this problem. Recently, direct laminar screws for repair of spondylolysis have become available (see Fig. 19.11).

Options for Facet Syndromes

A common, difficult choice arises when the patient's back pain is from the facet joints themselves and all attempts to treat the facet joints fail. Although it might be tempting to simply promote fusion at the level of the joints, the fact is that the whole weight of the body is placed on the joints of the spine. Therefore, the fusion method of anterior implant and posterior pedicle screws is generally required, even if the pain is due simply to an irreparable facet joint problem.

Figure 19.11 Lumbar facet screws. When there is a limited problem with the facets or with a "spondylolysis" (separation of parts of the posterior elements of a vertebra) it may be possible to place facet screws to solve the problem with out the more extensive surgery needed to place pedicle screws and rods. This image shows the "Discovery" system from DePuy Spine Inc, Johnson & Johnson.

Another alternative is one of the various methods of facet arthroplasty. This is a late developing area of spinal surgery so that few options are widely available. One common theme has been to place pedicle screws but to connect the screws across the facet joint with a nonrigid material. This provides sufficient support to reduce some of the force borne by the facets but docs not require fusion. At present, artificial lumbar facet joints are still at the clinical trial stage in the United States.

20

Surgery to Release Nerve Entrapments in the Shoulder, Arm, Pelvis, and Leg

There is a very distinct art and science for relieving an entrapment or pinch of a nerve—a peripheral nerve—as it travels through the body after leaving the area of the spine. In the area of the spine, once we identify which spinal nerve is involved (C6 or C7, L5 or S1) there is no problem deciding where to do the surgery. From beginning to end, a spinal nerve root travels from the dura membrane to its exit from the vertebra over a course of less than an inch.

A peripheral nerve, however, can run for 30 or 40 inches—with only one small point along the nerve being the site of the pinch that is responsible for the symptoms. It's not enough to know which nerve is causing the problem, the surgeon also has to know exactly where along the nerve the problem has occurred.

A second major difference is that surgery on the neural tissues in the spine is always affected by dura membranes, spinal fluid, herniated disks, and the bone and joints of the vertebra. None of these play any role in pinched peripheral nerves. Instead, the nerve surgeon is dealing with ligaments, muscles, and fibrous canals for the most part. In addition, many problems with peripheral nerves occur simply because the nerve becomes attached to or scarred onto a neighboring structure. Scarring does take place in the spine, but it is a much more common original cause of symptoms in the nerves of the body.

Generally, a spine surgery involves drilling and cutting through bones. Nerve surgery, however, is all about soft tissues. In spine surgery, the bones can be located by X-ray and readily identified by feel. Once the correct bone area is found, the location of the neural tissue is completely predictable. In nerve surgery, the surgeon must often rely on electrical signals to locate a nerve. Instead of using an X-ray to get guidance to the nerve location, the nerve surgeon relies on the effects of a neural stimulation probe in many situations.

To release a nerve entrapment, the surgeon cuts away abnormal muscle, ligaments, or scar tissue. When lighter scarring is the issue, it is more a matter of peeling the nerve off of whatever it is adherent to. The scar tissue may be rock hard or stiff, with collagen; however, it is often "soft" scar tissue that is light and soft so that there is no actual tissue to remove. In that case the surgery is mostly a matter of peeling the nerve lose from its abnormal attachments. This type of surgery is called a *lysis* (cutting) of adhesions or it is called a *neuroplasty*, meaning that it is helping to restore or repair the nerve.

One more theme that is special to nerve surgery involves operations to move a nerve to a different location. This issue arises when a nerve follows a course that causes it to press up against a structure that can't be safely or reasonably removed. In that case, because nerves are long and have some flexibility—it may be possible to move the nerve into a new course that no longer brings it into contact with the other structure. This is called a *transposition* operation.

Carpal Tunnel Release Surgery—Open or Closed

The most common of all nerve release surgeries is a treatment for the wrist. The problem affects the median nerve as it travels from the forearm to the palm by crossing the wrist in a wide tunnel formed on three sides by the wrist bones and topped over by a roof of ligaments. In the carpal tunnel, the median nerve is also surrounded by tendons that each have their own sheaths to help them glide as they move and do their work.

The ligament that forms the roof is called the "flexor retinaculum" (or alternately the "transverse carpal ligament"). The job of this ligament is to keep the ligaments and nerve from popping up out of the carpal tunnel when the wrist is flexed. Think of the problem this way: a major flexor muscle starts on the bones of the forearm (radius and ulna) near the elbow, but it's ligament attaches to the midpoint of a finger. This allows the big powerful muscle to pull the finger, thereby generating a powerful grip, however, consider the course of a straight line that goes from the elbow to the finger. When the fingers are extended straight out, the straight line passes comfortably through the wrist. But when the fingers are flexed forward, you can see that the straight line will travel through air in a space an inch in front of the wrist. The retinaculum has the job of holding the ligaments down when the fingers are in flexion.

With all the wear and tear that occurs at the wrist, the flexor retinaculum can grow thicker and even the sheaths around the tendons can grow thicker. There is only a limited amount of space in the tunnel, so the nerve can be gradually squeezed by its thickening neighbors. It may also begin to stick or adhere to the tendons and sheaths. All of these factors, thickening of the retinaculum, swelling of tendons and their sheaths, adhesions to the various tissues—result in hand pain that affects the thumb and index and ring fingers. The pain is worsened with extension of the wrist (lifting the fingers while the front of the wrist is flat on a surface—as we do when typing on a keyboard).

Treating Carpal Tunnel Without Surgery

Treatments include wearing a splint to hold the wrist steady and unmoving and is intended to allow the swelling of tendons and ligaments to settle down, thus relieving the pressure on the median nerve. Sometimes injection of steroids into the wrist can help, but must be done with extreme care to assure against a needle actually touching or entering the median nerve and causing injury.

Open Carpal Tunnel Release

The surgical solution is among the most common of all operations—the carpal tunnel release. The basic idea is to cut through the flexor retinaculum, thus expanding the space inside the carpal tunnel and relieving pressure on the nerve (see Fig. 20.1). Fortunately, the tissues below the skin are heavy enough to keep the tendons in place even when the flexor retinaculum is cut.

It sounds simple enough, but there are two radically different ways that the surgery is done. In traditional "open" carpal tunnel surgery, the surgeon makes an incision about an inch or so in length that starts at the base of the palm and extends across the crease of the wrist to reach the end of the forearm. Then, a deeper and deeper incision is made until all the fibers of the retinaculum are cut and the median nerve and surrounding tendons come into view. At this point the surgeon can peel the nerve free of any adhesions and then close up the skin over the carpal tunnel with sutures.

Median nerve

Figure 20.1 Carpal tunnel release surgery. A carpal tunnel syndrome is caused when the transverse carpal ligament compresses the median nerve at the wrist (see Fig. 9.1). In the open surgery, the ligament is cut open to expand the space within the tunnel. Image reproduced with permission of A.D.A.M. Inc.

This surgery is very safe and reliable, but it is very important to allow time for sufficient healing of the skin and subcutaneous tissues below the skin. This usually means wrapping the hand in a big soft bandage and advising the patient not to use the hand for two to four weeks.

The biggest risk of this open surgery is an accidental injury to a small branch of the median nerve called the recurrent branch of the median nerve. This is a small branch that goes to the muscles at the base of the thumb. An injury to this branch can weaken hand movements that involve gripping with the thumb. It branches off of the median nerve in the carpal tunnel and passes through some of the tissues the surgeon has to cut through to get to carpal tunnel. Fortunately, there are a few simple measures most surgeons take that make an injury to this nerve—or to the median nerve—extremely rare. This is a simple old-fashioned surgery that works well across the vast majority of cases. Once it is well healed the problem is usually fixed permanently.

Endoscopic or Closed Release for Quick Return to Activity

The other way this surgery is done is by means of endoscopy or by related "percutaneous" techniques. The big difference for this type of surgery is that only a very small incision is made—about a quarter of an inch in most cases. This is just enough of an opening to get a specialized device into the carpal tunnel to do the job. The big advantage for the patient is no incision and an immediate return to full activity as opposed to the two to four weeks without use of the hand required by the open surgery method.

The basic idea is to get the device to puncture through into the carpal tunnel, then pass it forward inside the tunnel, along with the median nerve, and use a small blade that pops out to cut through the flexor retinaculum from inside the tunnel—so no incision is made over the carpal tunnel. It is more or less all done from inside.

There are many variations on the device used. It can be a small thin probe that works by the surgeon's sense of position and feel to get into place. There can be video and light, there can be electronic connections for nerve monitoring and stimulation as the procedure is done. In the simplest form, this is very fast—about five or ten minutes instead of the full surgery of an hour or so with general anesthesia as needed for the traditional open surgery.

So what's the downside—if any—of the closed (percutaneous) techniques? The big problem is a very significant increase in the risk of nerve injury with percutaneous/endoscopic techniques. Sometimes the problem is that sheer speed and simplicity of the percutaneous method can lead to carelessness on the part of the surgeon. Sometimes, patience and excellent care are used but the fundamentally "blind" nature of the surgery just makes it more dangerous.

Orthopedic surgeries done by endoscopy in locations in the body with large bones and tendons have a large margin of error for the surgeon. In the carpal tunnel there are very small nerves and branches from both the median and ulnar nerves that pass nearby that can have a devastating effect if injured. Very few people can easily accept losing part of the function of their fingers and hand.

What's a patient to do? Everyone is attracted to a quick easy surgery with no downtime. The important thing is to make sure the surgeon knows you are aware of the risk. Ask the surgeon what he or she does to avoid trouble with the nerves. When the endoscopic method is used by an experienced surgeon with equipment designed to minimize the risk of nerve injury, it becomes very safe so that the risk of nerve injury is just as low as with open surgery.

Cubital Tunnel Surgery—in Place or Transposed

Following right behind carpal tunnel syndrome in frequency among nerve entrapments is cubital tunnel syndrome—entrapment of the ulnar nerve at the elbow. This causes weakness in the hand as well as pain and numbness extending to the ring and pinky finger (fourth and fifth digits, in medical terms).

The problem here is that the ulnar nerve runs down the inside of the upper arm and then curves around the back of the elbow joint to get into the front of the forearm on its way out to the wrist. Because the nerve runs around the back of the elbow, there is a possibility that it will get stretched when the elbow is bent. The joint at the elbow between the ulna and the humerus bones is more or less a classical hinge joint. When the arm is extended to be flat and straight at the elbow, the distance around the back of the joint is small. When the elbow is fully flexed, the distance around the hinge joint is much longer. You can get a sense of this by first flexing or bending the elbow and then putting one finger just beyond the bump in the back of your elbow and one finger just above it. Then flex and extend your arm. The two fingers move together in extension and move apart upon flexion.

Therefore, it might seem to stand to reason that if you get pain and numbness in your hand when you flex your elbow the ulnar nerve is the problem and that the varying distance the nerve has to cover to cross the elbow is the cause. However, the actual cause of the problem may have to do with how the body normally handles the change in length of the cubital tunnel. The nerve bends and the bone more or less glides into varying positions along the nerve as the joint is flexed and extended. Consequently, the cubital tunnel syndrome may be caused by adhesions of the nerve in the cubital tunnel. When the elbow is bent, the nerve doesn't glide normally so it gets tugged at the point of adhesion in the tunnel.

These two issues—change in length of the tunnel versus decreased gliding of the nerve—lead to two very different surgery strategies. In one strategy, the objective is to loosen up the cubital tunnel so that the ulnar nerve will glide more freely. Because this leaves the nerve in its original position, it is called *in situ,* or in place, cubital tunnel surgery. The surgeon makes an incision that follows the course of the ulnar nerve as it curves around the back of the elbow, then continues down until the cubital tunnel is opened and the nerve comes into view. At this point the nerve is loosened from any attachments or adhesions, anti-scarring material may be placed, and the skin and subcutaneous tissues are then stitched closed (see Fig. 20.2A).

Ulnar Nerve Transposition to Change the Course

The other type of surgery done for cubital tunnel syndrome is called a transposition surgery. This is a more complex and ambitious operation that tries to more or less redesign the way the elbow impacts the ulnar nerve. The nerve normally travels around the back of the elbow joint, but the surgeon can move or "transpose" the nerve so it runs across the front of the elbow joint instead (see Fig. 20.2C). This reverses the functional situation from the

RIGHT ULNAR NEUROPATHY WITH SURGICAL NERVE RELEASE

Figure 20.2 Cubital tunnel surgery. The ulnar nerve can be entrapped at the elbow in the cubital tunnel as it wraps it's way around a part of one of the bones of the joint (distal humerus) called the "medial epicondyle" (see Fig. 9.4). There are two common surgical fixes. In a simple cubital tunnel release, the ligaments of the tunnel are cut open to make more space for the nerve. In some cases, a more complex surgery is done that involves moving or "transposing" the course of the nerve so that it passes in front of the medial epicondyle instead of it's natural course passing behind the medial epicondyle. Image reproduced with permission of A.D.A.M. Inc.

natural condition. Now the distance the nerve must travel is greater when the elbow is extended and less when it is flexed. One thing that can go wrong after this surgery is that now the patient has the opposite problem—the nerve is stretched and causes symptoms when the elbow is extended and gets relieved when the elbow is flexed.

To accomplish the transposition, the surgeon has to "mobilize" the nerve for several inches above and below the elbow. In addition, it is often necessary to drill away the part of the bone of the elbow joint that the nerve usually runs behind—the medial epicondyle of the humerus.

Once the transposition of the nerve is accomplished, the surgeon can just leave it running below the skin or may cover it with some of the muscle in the area. This submuscular variation on the surgery requires detaching some of the forearm muscle mass from the humerus, passing the nerve underneath, and then reattaching the muscle to the elbow so that it helps protect the nerve and hold it in place.

Releasing the Nerve Without the Move

An in situ nerve release is a small, simple operation; a transposition requires a bigger incision and changes the way the elbow works. A submuscular transposition—with or without resection of the medial epicondyle—is an even bigger operation. The more complex surgery takes longer to do, has more risks and side effects, and requires more down time after the surgery.

Choosing among the different operations—from simple to complex—is usually based on the surgeon's recommendation. However, in many cases this just reflects what the individual surgeon likes to do or was trained to do. Numerous studies have shown that the simple surgery works as well or better than the more complex surgeries.

Many specialists recommend that the simpler surgery is always the one to do as an initial surgical treatment. Transposition can always be done later if the first surgery doesn't work out. Once a transposition is done, it is very difficult to reverse if it turns out that the cure is worse than the original problem—for example, moderate pain with elbow flexion is replaced by severe pain when the elbow is extended.

Transposition as an initial surgery seems to make sense in patients whose pain comes with elbow flexion. However, an understanding that this may be due to poor nerve gliding rather than to nerve stretch shows that there is no simple way to determine that stretch is the issue.

Thoracic Outlet—First Ribs and Scalenes

Few conditions are more puzzling for patients than thoracic outlet syndrome. Here you have a problem for which 200,000 surgeries are done each year, yet many doctors say there is no such thing and no surgeries at all should be done. How can there be such a divergence of medical opinion? The answer here is partly in the mix between art and science that makes up modern medicine and partly in the conflict between the weight of tradition and the draw of advancing technology.

Everyone more or less understands that doctors are not necessarily scientists. They are knowledgeable about science, but they are also like medieval craftsmen trained as apprentices under the guidance of mentors with years of technical experience. The sum of this is that controversies in medical practice that were real and uncertain 50 years ago are often taught to doctors as controversies even though more modern research has long since resolved the controversy. The bottom line on thoracic outlet syndrome is that modern science has proven that it exists and can be treated effectively.

One other issue that affects advice on thoracic outlet syndrome is that doctors who are not familiar or are suspicious often are simply poorly trained. Doctors expect to be able to be knowledgeable about everything they encounter. When something is left out of their training, they have a tendency to believe that the condition must be unimportant rather than that their training was insufficient. In neurosurgery today, all neurosurgeons are expected to be able to diagnose and treat or diagnose and refer to a specialist when a patient has thoracic outlet syndrome. Simply sending the patient away, telling the patient they are crazy, or doing a spine surgery that is not indicated are unreasonable approaches to the problem.

Thoracic outlet syndrome involves several different types of entrapment of the brachial plexus nerves between the spine and the shoulder. The most common of these are entrapments at the level of the scalene muscles and entrapment at the first rib. This also leads to two very different surgical strategies.

Injection treatments of the scalene muscles and non-surgical treatment of nerve entrapment along the brachial plexus are increasingly successful, so surgery for this cause of shoulder, arm, and hand pain is becoming less frequent. However, if surgery is required, the advice from vascular surgeons and neurosurgeons as to how to proceed often differs considerably.

Resecting the First Rib to Free the Nerves

The surgery often recommended by vascular surgeons involves removal of all or part of the first rib. This is major invasive surgery. The patient can expect to spend time in intensive care after surgery and face major life-threatening risks during surgery. In addition, nerve injuries during first rib resection surgery is among the most common of all causes of malpractice lawsuits against vascular surgeons. The flip side of this is that some very specialized vascular surgeons are very skilled with this operation.

There are few surgeries in which the surgeon's experience has such a dramatic effect. A real specialist expert in first rib resection surgery can provide an excellent operation that relieves the pain, weakness, and numbness, that exposes you to minimal real surgical risks, and that can be accomplished with only limited time for recovery. An expert vascular surgeon with a great reputation but who only does this operation occasionally is the doctor you should try to avoid (along with any doctors with a poor surgical reputation in general, of course). Experience and excellent skill are a must for first rib surgery for thoracic outlet syndrome.

The way the surgery is done is for the surgeon to make an incision in the underarm. Then the surgeon locates and progresses along the first rib, eventually reaching up to twelve inches deep into the body working through the small incision in the underarm (axilla). Ideally, the surgeon never sees any nerves during the operation. Once the root of the rib is reached near the spine, the surgeon has to cut through the rib, disconnecting it. The scalene muscles—which attach to the first rib and between which the brachial plexus nerves pass—must be scraped off the first rib and it must be cleared of all muscle, nerve, and blood vessel contacts without injuring the lining of the lung immediately below.

Once the rib is cut in two places and freed of its contacts and attachments with all other surrounding tissues, it can be removed. The logic of this is that the brachial plexus nerves as well as the subclavian artery and vein can be pinched or squeezed between the scalene muscles that form the roof and walls and the first rib that forms the floor of the thoracic outlet area. In addition, these same structures can be entrapped between the clavicle (collar bone) and the first rib. Therefore taking out the rib opens up the space, thus freeing entrapments and compressions of the nerves and vessels.

An even more challenging variation on this operation is to carry out the surgery endoscopically from within the chest by squeezing open the space between the lung and the first rib. This is also very challenging technically, but it gives the surgeon a much better view of the location where the rib cutting is being done because the video camera can be passed deep inside the body to locations where there is no viable line of sight.

The main reason that first rib surgery seems to fail about 50 percent of the time when nerve symptoms predominate is that there are often adhesions or scarring that is entrapping the nerves. In these situations, removing the first rib may have no beneficial effect. The surgery can go very well, but no improvement results.

Complications of first rib surgery include damage to nerves and blood vessels, increased pain after surgery, and a punctured lung. When a punctured lung occurs, air can leak out of the lung into the space around the lung. This is a bit puzzling for the patient to sort out, but an air leak from the lung can be a serious emergency if it is not recognized in time. The leaking air can fill up the space around the lung and around the major veins, squeezing everything dangerously. This condition is called a pneumothorax. It is treated by placing a suction tube inside the chest near the lung so that leaking air can be suctioned out while the lung heals.

Less Invasive Surgery by Removing the Scalene

The alternate approach to thoracic outlet surgery has far lower risks but is generally offered only by a small number of specially trained neurosurgeons (and a few vascular surgeon or plastic surgeons with a special interest in this). This is usually a scalene resection surgery and is far more similar to the other types of nerve release surgery than to the drama and risks of a first rib operation.

In a supraclavicular scalene surgery, the surgeon approaches the anterior scalene muscle from an incision at the base of the neck, above the collar bone. In some cases, a very simple operation is done. The anterior scalene muscle is identified, separated from surrounding tissues, and cut. This has the effect of removing or expanding one wall of the thoracic outlet area. Problems with this simple operation are often due to the issue of scar tissue entrapping the nerves. Simply cutting the anterior scalene muscle may not fully relieve the nerve compression. The surgery is quick and simple with minimal risk and quick recovery, but may not be sufficient. The overall success with simple anterior scalene cutting is not much better than with first rib surgery although the major risks are much lower and the recovery is much easier.

Most effective is the newer procedure involving resection of the anterior scalene muscle and nerve releases (neuroplasty) for the involved nerves. This can also be done with a more cosmetic minimal access approach—an important issue for most patients with the incision in the visible low neck.

The anterior scalene resection usually needs to involve complete removal of about two centimeters of the length of the muscle so that the body does not regrow a short stiff muscle reconnection across the resection site. This addresses a problem in the past that has caused recurrence of symptoms. At the time of surgery, the surgeon cuts through the anterior scalene muscle and the two ends retract widely, giving the appearance of a good decompression. However, over the following weeks, the two cut ends will tend to heal by reconnecting. The reconstituted muscle is often shorter and stiffer than the original muscle and this leads the patient to experience initial improvement, followed by recurrence and worsening.

The most significant risks in the anterior scalene resection include nerve and blood vessel injuries. On the front surface of the anterior scalene, the surgeon must find, avoid, and protect the phrenic nerve. This nerves operates the diaphragm and so plays an important role in breathing. Injury to the phrenic nerve on one side usually is just barely noticeable. This is because we breath by using all of our intercostal muscles between the ribs as well as the diaphragm. Even the scalene muscles can help by pulling the first rib up toward the neck.

An injury to both the right and left phrenic nerves is very noticeable and gives the patient an anxiety-provoking sense of being unable to get a deep breath. For this reason, right and left surgeries should not generally be done on the same day for a given patient unless excellent phrenic nerve function on the side operated on first can be definitively verified before proceeding to do surgery on the other side.

Once the anterior scalene is resected, the major brachial plexus elements at this location—the upper, middle, and lower trunks—must each be identified and fully released from any fibrous bands or tight muscle components. These are large nerves in the surgeon's direct view so injury is relatively unlikely.

During most nerve surgeries of this type, a dozen or more monitoring electrodes are placed around the arm and shoulder. This allows the surgeon to use an electronic probe to check hidden nerves. The probe will trigger the nerve and the monitoring EMG electrode will immediately show the response. In this fashion, the surgeon can locate nerves while they are still hidden from sight. This is most important for some of the smaller nerves such as the *long thoracic nerve* or *dorsal scapular nerve* that pass through the middle scalene muscle on their way to feed the muscles of the scapula and low neck.

A neuroplasty surgery can also be done through the underarm (axilla). This is different from the *transaxillary first rib resection* since the objective of the axillary neuroplasty is to immediately identify the nerves of the brachial plexus and free them from their entrapments that may occur between the collarbone and the axilla.

This can also include treatment of the *axillary nerve* that operates the deltoids. This nerve emerges from the posterior cord of the brachial plexus where it separates from the radial nerve (innervation of triceps and wrist/finger extensors). It then travel through the *quadrangular space* between four crossing muscles near the shoulder blade. Because most of the nerves of the brachial plexus are long and large, the axillary nerve stands out because it is small, short, and fixated by its passage through the quadrangular space. When it is irritated or compressed, the result is difficulty raising the arm. This is also a cause of shoulder pain that can be very confusing. Orthopedic surgeons treat various shoulder problems such as rotator cuff tears and impingement syndromes with a variety of open surgeries and endoscopies. One reason all of these may fail is that the actual problem is an axillary nerve entrapment.

Piriformis Surgery—Tendon, Muscle, and Nerve

Among the most common reasons for failure of a lumbar spine surgery is the situation where the lumbar spine was not the site that should have been operated on. The most important reason that this can take place is that the radiating leg pain of sciatica is due to a direct compression of the sciatic nerve by the piriformis muscle as opposed to a cause in the spine. The piriformis muscle and the sciatic nerve exit the sciatic notch of the pelvis together and the nerve can be compressed and irritated by the chronic muscle spasm that can affect the piriformis muscle (see Fig. 20.3).

Since everyone has back pain every now and then and because everyone has a few abnormalities that will show up on a lumbar MRI, it is very important not to jump to the conclusion that a given case of sciatica is caused by a spinal problem. This point is still true even if there is some back pain and even if there are some abnormalities in the lumbar spine.

It is even more likely that the piriformis muscle is the cause of the sciatica if there is no back pain and if the lumbar MRI is either normal or if doesn't show any abnormalities that could reasonably be expected to affect the L5 or S1 spinal

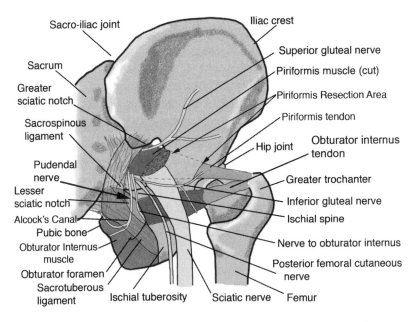

Figure 20.3 Piriformis release surgery. Several of the nerves that pass through the sciatic notch can become entrapped by the piriformis muscle when it becomes subject to chronic unresolvable spasm (see Fig. 9.8). This problem is corrected by cutting the piriformis muscle. A section of the muscle is removed so that the two cut ends will be widely separated leaving a large open space for the nerves. In some entrapments of the pudendal nerve or obturator internus nerve, the surgeon also cuts out a portion of the sacro-tuberous ligament and in some cases cuts the sacro-spinous ligament as well. Drawing by Aaron Filler.

nerves. When there is also soreness in the mid-buttock and aggravation by sitting, the piriformis syndrome moves to the top of the list as the possible cause of the problem.

Piriformis Treatment by Stretching and Injection: Is There a Role for Botox?

If the piriformis syndrome is later proven by imaging such as MR neurography and by image guided injection of the piriformis muscle, then treatment options directed at the piriformis muscle need to be pursued. Injections of the piriformis muscle can be carried out accurately by MRI guidance or with less accuracy with ultrasound, X-ray, or electronic (EMG—electromyography) guidance.

When a piriformis syndrome is suspected, the most common method of resolving it is the use of a program of piriformis muscle stretches. Fortunately, this is one painful nerve condition that can often be relieved by stretches and physical therapy. However, when this approach fails to relieve the syndrome, then injections to relax the piriformis muscle with anesthetics may break the cycle of muscle spasm that causes the nerve pain.

Another injection option is *Botox (botulinum toxin type A)*. Botox is a purified component of the highly toxic material that causes botulism; it comes from the bacteria *Clostridium botulinum*. Botox, which is made from a part of the natural toxin, is used in millions of cosmetic procedures. For these, it is injected into facial muscles to relax them for months and thereby smooth out facial wrinkles. It is also used to treat various types of disorders that involve muscle spasm—some in the eyes, some in the neck, and also for the treatment of piriformis syndrome.

The toxin works by attacking, blocking, and then leading to the destruction of the receptor proteins on the surface of muscle cells that are the connection point between nerve and muscle. With these receptors damaged or destroyed, the nerve can't cause the muscle to contract and a paralysis results. In the doses used medically, the paralysis is usually very local—just near the site of injection, it is partial, and it is temporary—lasting a few months. Ultimately, the body regrows new receptors on the muscles, the nerves find them, and the system starts working again. In some situations, the Botox treatment can just be repeated. In other situations, the muscle spasm may resolve so that additional injections aren't needed.

Although sometimes it seems as though just about everyone is having botox injections, it also seems that there are numerous reports of complications. What's the truth here? Both facts are true. Botox can cause allergic reactions, it can cause excess weakness, it can even cause pain much worse than the problem it was meant to treat. This is a particular problem for botox injections in the piriformis muscle because the muscle is large, much larger than facial muscles.

Overall there is about a 5 percent risk of some sort of complication. In addition, even in patients with proven piriformis muscle spasm as a cause of their pain problems, only about one-third of patients get a very significant positive result.

How does it all add up? First, botox probably should only be used if there has already been a successful injection treatment with anesthetic only. In that situation, before any exposure to the risks of botox, it is already proven that the patient does have a piriformis syndrome and that the sciatic nerve symptoms can be relieved by relaxing the muscle with anesthetic. Second, since some patients get permanent relief with one or two anesthetic injections, it would also be clear the anesthetic alone was insufficient. As in other areas of medicine, the risks make more sense when it is already proven that botox has a reasonable expectation of providing a significant benefit. If you have already had botox injections for cosmetic or other reasons and they have all gone well, there is usually very little risk with a botox piriformis injection.

Old and New for Piriformis Surgery Methods

For patients who don't get better with stretching and exercises, and who only get short-term relief with injections, piriformis surgery can be the correct choice. There are a variety of other surgical choices, however, that the patient may have to sort through.

Piriformis surgery is done in four very different ways that vary greatly in risk and success rate. There are two older traditional surgeries that each have bad reputations and two newer methods that have better success and outcomes.

The traditional orthopedic surgery for piriformis syndrome is a very simple procedure that is based on the way that a hip replacement surgery is done. At the beginning of a hip replacement surgery, the orthopedic surgeon has to detach the tendon of the piriformis muscle from its attachment point on the greater trochanter of the femur. It therefore seems obvious to the orthopedic hip surgeon that if a patient has a problem with the piriformis muscle, it is only necessary to do the first steps of a hip replacement—make an incision on the side of the hip and cut the tendon—and then that's the end of the operation and the surgeon closes the skin.

This makes the whole issue seem very trivial from the surgeon's point of view. The problem with this surgery is that most of the time, the problem is more complicated than simply relieving tension on the piriformis muscle. First, there are variations from person to person; for example, in as many as 20 percent of individuals, part of the sciatic nerve passes through the piriformis muscle rather than passing near it. If this condition is not detected before surgery (it is usually easily diagnosed in an MR neurography scan), the tendon release becomes very dangerous. Once the tendon is cut, the muscle starts to retract into the pelvis and this will tend to pull the segment of nerve along with it. The result can be a severe weakness or paralysis of the leg. Because the surgeon only has a view of the tendon attachment, he or she has no idea whether the tendon release will be safe. This high rate of a major complications leads most orthopedic surgeons to want to avoid doing this surgery. It also results in a very large and unsightly incision on the lateral thigh and can cause disruption of some of the muscles that pass over the hip joint. In general the recovery is good, but only about 50 percent of piriformis patients will be improved.

The second traditional type of piriformis surgery is usually offered by neurosurgeons. It gives the surgeon a very good view of the sciatic nerve and the numerous other nerves near the sciatic notch, but the operation very often results in a permanent difficulty with walking and running that may be worse than the original problem. This surgery involves a large incision—about eight or ten inches in length—that cuts through all of the gluteal muscles—the gluteus maximus and gluteus medius and the gluteus minimus. Once the opening is made, the surgeon has an excellent view of all the critical structures and can do detailed electronic testing of nerve function—even making direct measurement of the speed of nerve conduction from point to point in the field in order to detect and verify areas of nerve malfunction. The piriformis muscle can be completely and safely resected, even when it has the split muscle/split nerve configuration. The problem is that once all the gluteal muscles are cut through, they often don't heal properly. Too many small nerves within the gluteal muscles get cut by the opening and the internal muscle scarring from the repair also interferes with function. Recovery from the surgery itself is often long in time (many weeks or months) with ongoing problems with walking and running.

Third, the newest option is endoscopic piriformis surgery. In this method, the surgeon can't do any electrodiagnostic testing, but the view of the sciatic nerve is good and the opening incision is small. It also is not very effective for dealing with nerve adhesions or if additional nerve elements—such as the nerve to the obturator internus—need to be released by neuroplasty. This type of surgery is relatively new, and it still poses a high risk of multiple nerve injuries. Many of these injuries have occurred in the very first patients to have the procedure. With time, endoscopic piriformis surgery can be expected to improve in safety and quality. As with all endoscopic techniques, there is a very high skill level and a great deal of experience required. Nonetheless, endosopic methods have worked for the wrist but have generally been failures near other types of nerves elsewhere in the body, so the future of this procedure is not assured.

Neurosurgeons generally will not use endoscopes because any bleeding that occurs during a surgery can obstruct the view of small delicate nerves. In the abdomen, the space is inflated with air and there is an excellent video view of the gall bladder or appendix during endoscopy. Any blood drips away to the bottom of the abdomen and doesn't interfere with the view. In endoscopy of a joint, the orthopedist can flush constantly with irrigation fluid to wash away blood and keep the view clear. In the area of the sciatic notch, however, bleeding can completely block the view of the endoscope, while suction, irrigation, and imprecise cautery can't be used safely without an unacceptable risk of nerve injury.

The fourth type of piriformis surgery is being offered increasingly by neurosurgeons and some specialized plastic surgeons and offers the best balance of methodology overall. This is a minimal access transgluteal open surgery. The incision is small—about an inch and a half—(which is similar to the opening used for endoscopes), so recovery can be rapid. Instead of cutting the gluteal muscles, the surgeon gently spreads them to pass in a special retractor system that maintains an excellent direct view of the nerves and muscle. The surgeon has direct access so most electrodiagnostic methods can be used to aid in nerve identification and nerve protection during surgery. Because of the direct access, all of the advanced neurosurgical methods of brain surgery can be brought to bear on this complex area of nerve surgery. There is good scientific reporting of the outcomes, and this type of surgery has success rates of 85 percent or better and much lower risk of major nerve injury (less than one in a thousand) than the tendon-cutting or endoscopic methods. Recovery from this kind of surgery is just a few days, without any known loss of full activity in walking, running, or athletics.

Pudendal Nerve Entrapment—Ligament and Canal, Muscle and Nerve

One of the last frontiers in surgical treatment for nerve pain problems is in regard to disorders of the *pudendal nerve* that cause pain, numbness, and functional problems in the *perineum*—between the legs—and involve rectal, genital, and urinary area neurologic symptoms. Urologists, gynecologists, and gastrointestinal specialists have been slow to get involved in nerve surgery, while neurosurgeons (and orthopedists) have generally stayed away, considering this to be out of their usual area of work and training.

Nonetheless, and despite the emotional and psychological overlay that can go with genital and rectal pains, pudendal nerve entrapments are still nerve entrapments. Most of the pudendal nerve surgical issues are very similar to those that apply in other areas of neurosurgical treatment of nerve disorders.

The pudendal nerve travels a complex course and is subject to nerve entrapment in four distinct areas. Each requires a different type of surgery or at least a different focus. Using just one type of surgery on one part of the nerve only works if the patient happens to have the one type of entrapment that relates to that approach. For this reason, a physician evaluating or treating patients for pudendal entrapments must be capable of correctly diagnosing which part of the nerve is involved and doing the necessary steps to achieve an release of the entrapment (see Figs. 9.8 and 20.3).

Pudendal Transposition at the Sacro-spinous Ligament

The most commonly done procedure offered by urologists is an approach from the low posterior pelvis just off the midline. The surgery is intended to cut through one or two of the major supporting ligaments of the pelvis—the *sacro-tuberous ligament* and/or the *sacro-spinous ligament*. The sacro-tuberous ligament runs from the sacrum to the ischial tuberosity (sit bone), while the sacro-spinous ligament runs from the sacrum to the ischial spine. The basis of these surgeries is in the fact that the pudendal nerve emerges from the pelvis through the greater sciatic notch (along with the sciatic nerve and piriformis muscle) and then does a U-turn. It loops across the ischial spine (or, if medially placed in a given person, across the sacro-spinous ligament) and then heads back into the pelvis through the lesser sciatic notch. The idea of cutting the sacro-spinous ligament derives from the fact that in some patients, the nerve is pulled into contact with the ischial spine or the sacro-spinous ligament as it does it's U-turn. The nerve can be transposed and released but cutting through the sacro-spinous ligament so that it can avoid doing the U-turn. The pudendal nerve is put into a new course that never exits the greater sciatic notch and therefore doesn't need to reenter the lesser sciatic notch.

The sacro-tuberous ligament covers over both the pudendal nerve and the sacro-spinous ligament when viewed or approached from the back of the pelvis. It has to be cut to expose and get access to the sacro-spinous ligament when this approach is used. One of the big risks of this surgery arises because in some patients, the pudendal nerve is actually adherent to (attached along) the deep surface of the sacro-tuberous ligament. In that situation, the urologist can sever or injure the pudendal nerve during the approach. Other problems with this operation result from the fact that even if transposed, the pudendal nerve may be impinged by structures just deep to the sacro-spinous ligament or it may become encased in scar tissue that forms as the ligaments try to regenerate.

The most common reason for failure of this surgery, however, is simply that this type of entrapment seems to be responsible for pudendal nerve entrapment in only about 10 percent of cases or fewer. The surgery offers no help at all if the entrapment is at another point along the nerve and can actually make some of the other types of entrapment worse. However, for those patients who have the entrapment at the sacro-spinous ligament, this surgery can be very effective.

One other problem that can arise from ligament-cutting surgery for pudendal entrapment is destabilization of the pelvis. The sacro-spinous ligament and the sacro-tuberous ligament play major roles in resisting rotation of the sacrum relative to the pelvis at the sacro-iliac joints. Particularly when surgery is done on both sides, the loss of stability can limit athletic activity and can affect walking. For this reason, some surgeons now offer repairs of the sacro-tuberous or sacro-spinous ligaments for those patients in whom instability develops. The repair typically involves a tendon graft sutured in place over the released/transposed nerve.

Alcock's Canal Surgery

Another older type of surgery offered for pudendal entrapments is directed at the *Alcock's Canal* portion of the nerve along the inside surface of the *obturator internus muscle*. For this operation, the surgeon makes an incision just off midline between the legs and extending up onto the buttocks. This provides a good safe access for the surgeon, but this will only be an effective treatment if an entrapment of the nerve in the Alcock's Canal is the sole and definitive cause. There is no access to any other part of the nerve, so the surgeon must be quite certain in advance that this is the correct cause.

Transgluteal Approach for Piriformis-Pudendal and Obturator Internus Syndromes

The most recent addition to the methodology of pudendal surgery is a transgluteal approach through the upper buttock that gives the surgeon access for treatment of any one of the four major pudendal nerve entrapment areas during a single surgery. In this approach, a small incision is made in the mid-buttock (about an inch and a half in length) and the surgeon gently spreads a path through the gluteal muscles so that a special retractor can be inserted. The retractor can then be swung into various positions to provide access to each of the four major areas of potential entrapment. This allows for the surgeon to do the single type of release required, but it also allows for direct intraoperative inspection of each of the four potential entrapment areas.

First, the surgeon can carry our a piriformis muscle resection, with a focus on the deep, upper portions of the piriformis muscle that can entrap the S2 and S3 spinal nerves that form the pudendal nerve. The surgeon can also release any entrapment affecting the pudendal nerve as it exits the greater sciatic notch along with the piriformis muscle.

Second, this approach also provides access to the "U-turn" area of the pudendal nerve at the ischial spine and sacro-spinous ligament. Unlike the traditional urological surgery for this area, the transgluteal approach gives the surgeon a view from the side—effectively on the deep side of the sacro-tuberous ligament. This means that the sacro-tuberous ligament does not have to be cut to get to the ischial spine. If the surgeon finds that the pudendal nerve is resting against the sacro-spinous ligament under tension, the sacro-spinous ligament can be notched to make more space—with full safe access to protect the pudendal nerve—or it can be cut if necessary. If the pudendal nerve is adherent to the undersurface of the sacro-tuberous ligament, the nerve can be released by a neuroplasty procedure.

Third, the nerve to the obturator internus is also accessed just below the greater sciatic notch. This proves to be the key to the surgery in more than half of patients with pudendal nerve symptoms. Often there is no actual entrapment of the pudendal nerve itself. Instead, the obturator internus muscle is in spasm and this is causing the pudendal irritation. By releasing an entrapment of the nerve to the obturator internus, the obturator internus spasm can be relieved and the pudendal symptoms resolved.

Fourthly, the surgeon working from the transgluteal access can open up and release any adhesions affecting the pudendal nerve that occur at the opening or entry of the lesser sciatic notch. The pudendal nerve can then be followed and released along its course on the medial surface of the obturator internus muscle—which includes the portion in the Alcock's Canal.

The main advantages of the newer transgluteal surgery is that it allows the surgeon access to a variety of different pudendal entrapment or irritation locations, uses a very small incision, and can be uses to treat adjacent problems—such as piriformis muscle spasm or obturator internus spasm—that can be the actual cause of the pudendal symptoms. By leaving the sacro-tuberous ligament intact, it reduces the risk of instability of the pelvis, even if the sacro-spinous ligament needs to be cut. The newer surgery employs detailed electronic monitoring of all the nerves in the area and so it greatly adds to the safety of the surgery. Because of the smaller incision and non-destructive passage through the gluteal muscles, the recovery is fast and post-operative pain is minimal.

Peroneal Nerve Entrapment Surgery

The peroneal nerve at the knee can be entrapped above the level of knee as it runs along the inner surface of the biceps-femoris muscle, or it can be entrapped as it wraps around the head of the fibula in the lower leg (see Fig. 9.7). A surgical incision along the course of the peroneal nerve can give the surgeon access to both of these areas.

A special situation arises when a major injury to the knee has caused the peroneal nerve entrapment. In these injuries, the fibular head can be fractured off along with the attachment of the biceps tendon. An orthopedic surgeon can repair the attachment of the biceps tendon by re-attaching the fibular head to the fibula. In some cases the fibular head is intact, but the biceps tendon attachment is torn off of the fibular head. The tendon is re-attached by placing anchor screws in the fibular head and then using the screws to attach thick sutures that are sewed into the tendon. This allows the surgeon to pull the tendons back onto the fibular head.

In either of these repairs, the patient often starts with an injury to the peroneal nerve suffered at the time of the initial trauma. However, after the repair surgery, the body generates a very significant amount of fibrous tissue as part of the healing process. Unhelpfully, the peroneal nerve nearby can be caught up in the healing scar. The result is that the biceps tendon heals, but the peroneal nerve function deteriorates further. This can lead to a weakness of elevating the foot—a "foot drop."

To avoid the peroneal entrapment caused by healing—a nerve surgeon sometimes helps with the orthopedic procedure. The peroneal nerve is first released from the injured tissue, the orthopedic repair is completed, and then anti-scarring materials are placed around the nerve. A second surgery to release the nerve later is sometimes needed if the healing is too energetic and overcomes the anti-scarring barrier. By doing a nerve release along with a repair, the foot weakness can usually be corrected completely.

This type of injury at the knee is often a sports injury from soccer, football, or skiing. A similar type of injury and healing problem can occur at the ischial tuberosity where the hamstring tendon can be torn. When it heals or is repaired the sciatic nerve can become entrapped. A nerve release of the sciatic nerve at the time of the hamstring/ischial tuberosity repair can avoid progressive problems with the sciatic nerve. Injuries of this type can happen to athletes such as runners and jumpers. This is also something that happens to horseback riders who are thrown from the horse and land on the ground in a sitting position.

Nerve Decompression for Diabetic Neuropathy

One controversial new area of nerve surgery is to help relieve nerve pain that is due to *diabetic neuropathy*. In diabetic neuropathy, a problem develops with the internal chemistry of the nerve. Normally, the nerve efficiently carries nutrients and proteins up and down its internal length. In diabetic neuropathy, this and other nerve functions don't work normally. The patient begins to develop pain and numbness—particularly at the end of the longest nerves—such as the sciatic nerve components that travel all the way to the foot. There is still no good medical treatment for this if it develops.

Some specialists have reported that by decompressing the space around the smaller nerves in the lower leg, the symptoms of diabetic neuropathy can be decreased. The surgery itself is very simple. Incisions are made along the lower the leg to pry open and enlarge the natural spaces along the length of the nerves. This is still an area under active evaluation. However, the first formal studies to look at outcomes from this do seem to confirm that some patients are helped by the release surgery.

21

Genes, Designer Proteins, and Biomaterials: The Role of Biotechnology in Spine and Nerve Surgery

It is hard for the mind to fathom the notion that even after the arrival of the twenty-first century, spine surgeons still rely on hammers, chisels, power drills, and saws to repair and reassemble the spine. It certainly may not stay that way forever, since a host of changes are already starting to arrive. The next 20 to 30 years will almost certainly see the near complete replacement of the hammer and chisel by genes and "designer proteins" that help the spine to repair itself.

In many ways the breadth of new technology and the rate of change of its application are extraordinary in spinal surgery. The complex interplay of advancing neuroscience, materials design, mechanical engineering, and advanced biological modifiers makes this a surgical field with incredible dynamism.

Biomaterials and Synthetics for Bone Growth

One of the first tests of the biotechnology and biomaterials approach to repair the spine is to understand how growth takes place in the spine and to look for ways to replace the hip bone graft. Bone grafts are unattractive for a couple of reasons, although in current spinal surgery they continue to play a significant role.

Induction and Conduction: Graft Versus Growth

Traditionally, different types of bone grafts have been considered from the point of view of their structural usefulness and their tendency to fuse successfully. A more modern approach also distinguishes among materials by the way they affect bone growth. A material is *osteoconductive* if it just provides a framework into which bone-producing cells can grow. An *osteoinductive* material actually acts to cause bone to grow. *Osteogenesis* itself is accomplished only by the actual *osteoblastic* cells of the patient that help form the definitive bone.

An autograft—bone taken from the patient's own body—has the significant disadvantage of requiring additional surgery at the site where the graft is taken from, often causing as much pain and disability as was relieved in the original location of surgery. But autografts offer all three necessary properties for bone repair: they are osteoconductive (providing a framework), osteoinductive (containing hormones that can promote the growth of bone), and osteogenic (containing the cells that produce the bone in its final form).

The alternative to an autograft has been an allograft, taking the bone from a deceased donor. However, this has its disadvantages because it is still not possible to eliminate completely the risk of transmission of a wide variety of potential diseases, from HIV to hepatitis to West Nile virus. Risks are low but nonetheless have to be considered. Further, an allograft is only osteoconductive because all of its living growth promoters have been carefully and completely removed as part of the sterilization process.

In fact, an allograft is not even fully effective in a conductive role because it now lacks many of the structural proteins that provide a scaffold for new bone to grow on. When an allograft is used, it is therefore helpful to improve its osteo-conductive properties and also provide it with some osteoinductive capabilities.

Further, if it is possible to use some other method to hold the vertebrae in position structurally, it may be possible to substitute designed or synthetic materials for the allograft. This is particularly true if the synthetic material can improve on the osteoconductive properties of fully prepared allograft.

Demineralized Bone Matrix: Less Autograft Needed

One of the successful new biomaterials used to induce or promote surrounding bone into activating new bone growth is *demineralized bone matrix* (DBM). Essentially, if you melt away all the calcium in a bone, there is still an elastic, rubbery, protein core left. By synthesizing these core proteins and placing them in the space where bone growth is desired, the body will naturally react and send its own bone-forming cells, or osteoblasts, to crawl along the DBM that is implanted. These cells will then go about their job of pulling calcium out of the blood and depositing it to form new bone. In fact, when optimally prepared, DBMs have proven to be very effective, even when compared with autografts, for rapid and successful bone growth at sites of fusion surgery. However, in general, DBM is limited to an osteoconductive role.

Calcium, Coral, and Plaster of Paris

The calcium in bone provides two functions. First, it is available to provide the hardness that will resist compression, and second, it provides a matrix in which cells can lay down the proteins required for growth to take place. There are other biological materials, including coral and some other purely synthetic calcium-based materials, that can be used in place of human bone. Calcium sulfate can be mixed up in such a way that it can be poured into a space and turned into a hard, white, calcium material, essentially, plaster of Paris. Unfortunately, like plaster of Paris, this kind of material can shatter when compression is applied.

Textured Titanium Implants

Other important advances in purely synthetic material to replace bone include the development of textured titanium surfaces. Such materials provide some of the structural support and also help to promote a strong interaction between synthetic and natural material. Instead of the surface of the metal implant being smooth, it actually has a surface that, when seen under the microscope, is rough and complex. The advantage here is that natural bone growth will essentially grow into the titanium, providing a bonding between bone and metal (see Figs. 21.1 and 21.2).

Elasticity in New Bones or Disks: Carbon Fiber, Polymers, and Hydrating Gels

One of the problems with any metal implant, and certainly also with plaster of Paris, is that it has a different elastic behavior, or modulus of elasticity,

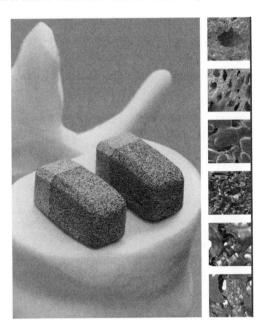

Figure 21.1 Titanium PlivioPore intervertebral implants. Various types of porous titanium can be formed for use in vertebral implants. The pores allow bone to grow into the interior of the implant to fuse through them. The metal resists the kinds of collapses and biological reaction that can occur with bone implants and some plastics. It can also simulate the "modulus of elasticity" of bone because the porous cast allows for some slight deformation. Image reproduced with permission of Synthes.

Figure 21.2 Textured titanium and polymers. A variety of new types of disk replacement technologies are being developed. A. Cast poly-lactic acid (PLA) implant will dissolve away as bone grow into the fusion site. Illustration reproduced with permission of the *Journal of Neurosurgery*. Reprinted from D.W. Cahill, G.H. Martin Jr., M.V. Hajjar, W. Sonstein, L.B. Graham. and R.W. Engelman. Suitability of bioresorbable cages for anterior cervical fusion. *Journal of Neurosurgery* 98 (2 Suppl):195–201. March 2003. B. Dr. Charles Ray of Raymedica has introduced a prosthetic disk nucleus. (PDN) which restores the natural elasticity of the nucleus pulposus but keeps the ligaments intact and preserves normal motion. Illustration reproduced with permission of the *Journal of Neurosurgery*. Reprinted from H.J. Wilke, S. Kavanagh, S. Neller, C. Haid, and Claes L.E. Effect of a prosthetic disc nucleus on the mobility and disk height of the L4-5 intervertebral disk postnucleotomy. *Journal of Neurosurgery* 95 (2 Suppl): 208–14, October 2001. A variety of titanium and plastic artificial disk replacement devices have also been developed, including C: Medtronic Maverick (Illustration reproduced with permission of Medtronic. Inc.), D: Spine Solutions ProDisc, and E: Link SB Charité Artificial Disk. Illustrations D and E reproduced with permission of *Journal of Neurosurgery*. Reprinted from V. Traynelis, Spinal arthroplasty. *Neurosurgical Focus* 13 (2):A10, 2002.

than the natural tissue or bone. Therefore, when you put one of these hard stiff materials up against bone, the result of wear and tear may be to grind away at the bone. So materials that mimic bone's natural elasticity or bendability, as well as its hardness or resistance to compression, are very attractive.

Another important issue in calcium-based implants is absorbability. Some calcium materials such as tricalcium phosphate will be more rapidly absorbed by the body, while other forms more similar to bone such as hydroxyapetite are absorbed only on a much more gradual basis and may actually slow the formation of definitive living bone.

One area of material design that holds some promise is carbon-fiber technology, which provides for very light, strong materials that are used on some types of advanced airplanes. Any carbon-fiber implant also has the advantage of being transparent on X-rays, so that the natural process of new bone growing through the implant can be more readily observed on an X-ray or CT scan without the implant itself getting in the way of the imaging. These materials also can be fabricated to have an elasticity similar to that of bone (see Fig. 16.7).

Unfortunately, because carbon-fiber materials are not as strong as titanium, the implants have to be more bulky in order to carry the weight and do the job, and this cuts down on the surface available for bone growth. In the future, advanced carbon-fiber material design may make these implants more usable on a widespread basis.

There are other polymer materials that are similar in strength to bone and that do not entail the introduction of nonbiologic materials such as pure carbon and epoxy. Two examples that are already in increasingly widespread use are PEEK (polyethyletherketone), which is relatively nonabsorbable, and *PLDLA (poly LDL lactide)*, which is absorbable. These materials are chemically similar to what has been used in surgery for years as suture material.

A completely different type of design solution has to do with replacing the center of a degenerated spinal disk. The natural material in the center of a disk is an elastic gel, the nucleus pulposus. In some instances, this material hardens, dries, fractures, and bulges, leading to a condition that may mandate removing the natural nucleus and replacing it with an artificial one. One form of artificial disk nucleus is essentially a bag filled with material that will hydrate when exposed to the body's water. This bag is slipped into the annulus through a small opening. Once inside, it takes in water, expands, and develops an elastic behavior that restores normal function to the disk. The trick here is to build an elastic, deformable material that will last over the years and will spread so that it evenly distributes pressure on the end plates of the vertebrae above and below.

By segmenting the hydrogel material into a series of adherent flat sheets, the hydrogel can be engineered so that most of its expansion and elastic resistance to compression will be directed upward and downward to the vertebral end plates that it sits between rather than bulging outward to deform the annulus. Various hydrogel-based disk replacements are starting clinical trials at this time, but none of these are FDA approved for use.

Proteins and Genes for Bone Growth

Ratcheting up the level of technology beyond materials design, we enter into the realm of genes and gene therapy and their potential for causing bones and disks to repair themselves. The types of signaling proteins that will cause bone to grow have been known to science for decades; however, finding just the right way of delivering, applying, and using these signals has been a huge challenge, and such an approach has only very recently been bringing success in the actual treatment of patients.

Bone Morphogenetic Protein

The most important type of new proteins developed to promote bone growth are the *bone morphogenetic proteins* (BMPs). BMPs are manufactured to simulate natural proteins that occur in human bone and now can be produced purely synthetically in the laboratory (see Fig. 21.3).

In 1965, orthopedic surgeon Marshall Urist discovered these proteins and appreciated early on that they could be used to promote bone fusion in surgery. Not until the advent of genetic engineering, however, was it possible to produce large enough quantities of BMP with sufficient purity.

Now FDA-approved for some spinal uses, BMPs can be placed at the site of intended fusion to make the surrounding bone cells begin to grow and produce additional, new bone. Among two of the biggest problems with this are

Figure 21.3 Proteins and bone fusion. (1) OP-1 protein is implanted at the site of fusion embedded in a collagen carrier. (2) OP-1 attracts stem cells from the bloodstream to prepare for bone growth. (3) The OP-1 protein provides instructions to the stem cells to commence work in forming new bone. (4) The activated cells release other bone growth-promoting signal proteins. (5) Osteoblasts and osteoclast cells mature and begin the work of depositing calcium to generate strength. (6) The bone remodels its own shape to optimize its ability to meet mechanical stress. OP-1 illustration provided by Stryker Biotech (note—OP1 is no longer a Stryker product).

the following: (1) the BMPs act only for a short time before they wash away, and it may take weeks or months for the full amount of bone growth to take place; (2) if a very large amount of BMP is used and great care is taken to assure that it doesn't wash away, the opposite problem may occur, which is that too much bone growth occurs and the new bone formation actually causes new nerve compression as a complication.

One other theoretical problem is the concern that a biologic growth promoter will actually induce cancerous growths. After nearly 40 years of research on BMPs this possibility has been fairly well laid to rest. Yet another concern relates to the inflammation that can be caused by any foreign protein if the body attacks it, and, similarly, there is the possibility of allergic reaction to a material partially encapsulated in your bones. In general, however, the body's natural processes will digest away any BMP applied within a few weeks.

A variety of complex methods are under development for providing a continuous but controllable supply of BMP over the extended period required for a solid fusion. Some approaches involve very advanced methods from the field of nanotechnology in which tiny devices slowly release the BMP. A different approach involves encapsulated, genetically engineered living cells capable of remaining alive for months and producing a steady supply of the protein to the site. Once bone fusion is adequate, however, these cells have to be removed or somehow "switched off."

The first FDA-approved commercial BMP product (InFuse—Medtronic) uses a much simpler "medium tech" solution. The BMP (recombinant human BMP-2) is soaked into a collagen sponge material. The thin sponges are placed at the sites where fusion is needed. The BMP leaches slowly out of the sponge over weeks. The sponges also help assure that the BMP stays mostly near the intended site of action before they themselves are digested away by the body.

There is a similar protein from Stryker called OP-1 (rhBMP-7) that is made in a putty form. It is FDA approved on a more limited basis called a "humanitarian device exemption" or HDE approval. This means that the evidence provided by Stryker to the FDA was not completely convincing as to safety and efficacy but that they did show that it was helpful in some patients who have many factors that increase their risk of failed fusion.

The approval problem had to do with the design of the research study conducted by Stryker, and there have been continuing disputes between Stryker and the FDA over OP-1 that have resulted in criminal charges against the former president of Stryker (asserting that Stryker hid information about the amount of OP-1 being used and in the way the Stryker sales force marketed the product). The criminal indictment was dropped in September 2011 in exchange for a $1.3 million penalty paid to the government for reporting and marketing errors on

Stryker's part. These events demonstrate the heightened concern of federal regulators regarding spinal surgery devices. The relatively small fine (considering that Stryker has annual business volume of nearly $7 billion) does suggest that this case did not prove to be an overly serious violation.

Gene Therapy: Vectors to Put the Proteins in Their Place

Yet another high-tech approach to providing BMP on an extended basis draws on the realm of gene therapy. In this approach, it is possible to design a modified virus that can go into the cells in or near the graft and cause them to begin producing extra amounts of BMP. Unfortunately, however, we don't have an easy way to turn the genes off after they have been put in place by the virus; moreover, this approach involves being exposed to an engineered virus for the purpose of promoting a fusion, which doesn't seem likely to be attractive to patients anytime in the near future.

Genes can also be delivered by *synthetic vectors* (see Fig. 2.1), which are temporary carriers that don't pose any risk of spreading or causing infection, and there is active work into the development of these as well. When a gene is put into production in the cytoplasm (general interior) of a cell by a synthetic vector instead of being placed in the nucleus by a virus, it will be digested within a few weeks. Synthetic vectors are a developing field (and also an area in which I have been granted patents and have done research and development work).

Osteogenic Proteins for Disk Regeneration

Aside from the bone morphogenetic protein, another group of proteins, called osteogenic proteins, is showing great promise for actually helping the disk regrow and repair itself. These proteins are being investigated, both because they show promise in helping the annulus grow back into a nice, strong ring, and because they also can help the disk itself regenerate so that its normal height is restored and it becomes more resistant to bulging or other breakdowns.

One area of advance in this field concerns molecules that can amplify or increase the concentration of useful proteins and factors at a fusion site. A clever molecule has been designed that is first used in its expanded form to allow the attachment or adherence of large numbers of fusion-promoting molecules. The carrier is then shrunk so that it packs a large number of active agents into a physically smaller space. This allows for very high-concentration delivery and slowed diffusion or migration away from the site where fusion promotion is needed.

From Hammer and Wrench to Reconstructing DNA

Yet another type of advanced technology for disk repair is the use of *stem cells* to regrow disks; and, in fact, the natural cells of the nucleus pulposus are unusual cells that have a wide variety of potential for growth with other tissues. One way of getting the disk to regenerate itself may be to harvest some of the nucleus pulposus cells. Some cells could be saved for other purposes, but a portion of these cells could be treated with gene therapy to cause them to regrow or help form a new disk. Just as with the bone morphogenetic proteins, however, the risk is that there will be too much growth (in this case cartilage formation rather than bone formation), which could cause significant problems in the spine and nerve tissue as well. Stem cells are also being investigated as a way to promote the growth of bone in fusions.

So at one extreme we have a hammer and chisel to create and place a bone graft, and at the other extreme is putting together synthetic virus replacements and high-tech designer proteins in the Petri dish of the future to carry out bone and disk replacement.

Electronic Fusion Stimulators and Robotics

A very different approach to encourage bone cells to form naturally is to use electromagnetic fields, which seem to affect the way that cells grow and move without relying on designer proteins or genes. Electronic stimulators are in use now and involve either placement of a stimulator within the body at the time of surgery (small wires are placed right along the area where the bones are to grow, leading out to a battery that's implanted below the skin) or, in a somewhat less dramatic approach, placement of an electrical field generator outside the body, which is used to direct and encourage bone to grow. This technology is advancing more slowly, and it is not clear whether it can be improved on in the future, but it certainly is another promising area whereby the body is redirected to repair itself rather than relying on the mechanical approaches that predominate current treatments.

Finally, a very futuristic approach to correcting and rebuilding mechanical problems to the spine involves active robotic-type devices that can control and adjust the way that vertebrae move relative to each other by monitoring movement and applying appropriate counterforces and corrective forces. This is a level of technology that goes well beyond the material, engineering, and robotic science of today, but it remains an open frontier for the design of new ways of repairing and avoiding further breakdown in the spine.

22

Risks, Outcomes, and Choices

Aside from finding out exactly what is wrong, what needs to be done, and how the work should be carried out, you face an array of choices and risks, as the potential patient, that can significantly affect what results you can expect from your treatment. Choices can be daunting or overwhelming to some; however, many people find that making informed choices provides a sense of empowerment. You can't know the future, but you can take some responsibility for choosing the path you will take.

Risks and Complications of Surgery

Throughout this book, I have discussed, where relevant, the various possible dangers that accompany some of the therapies and surgeries for spinal problems. The purpose of this section is to review many of the types of risks that can be faced in the course of any surgery, spine operations in particular, and even in nonsurgical treatments for spine problems. In the end, it is impossible for such a review to be totally comprehensive because a wide variety of individual risks reflect the given patient's medical history, the particular requirements of a patient's treatment, and the way in which a particular practitioner or surgeon goes about the treatment.

Nonetheless, there is also an extensive set of common concerns that the prospective spine patient may benefit from understanding. This discussion is intended to be helpful, therefore, in the mutual obligation of the patient and the physician to explore and understand the risks of spine treatment. First, it is important to understand that there are always risks, and that these can be cataloged and listed in a standardized fashion. Second, there are measures that can be taken to reduce these risks, and if any complications do develop, there are steps to be taken to minimize their impact and to achieve the patient's best possible recovery. And third, it has to be made absolutely clear that simply knowing about a risk does not make the risk go away.

Occasionally, a patient becomes obsessed by a particular risk and possibly won't even proceed to treatment when that risk exists. For this reason, I very often encourage my patients to consider the choices that they make when they travel in an automobile. As everyone knows, we can be killed, paralyzed, or injured in our cars at any time doing just about anything. Any of these things can happen in an instant for no reason that we have any control over, and yet we choose to drive in our cars and accept the known risks because we see the benefits of driving. It may be that our choice is entirely rational, that we know the risk percentages and compare them with the benefits; or it may be a kind of psychological sleight-of-hand whereby we hear the risks, decide to accept them, and tuck them away so that they don't come into our consciousness.

The existence of surgical risk is rarely a good reason not to proceed. There are situations, however, in which the surgeon may inform a patient that the risks are so high that the patient should not proceed, placing the decision in the patient's hands. Sometimes this advice is given with great concern. Sometimes the patient may not accept it and seeks another opinion. Sometimes even high risks in surgery or other treatments are taken because of the consequences of not choosing any treatment at all.

Overall, complications and other possible negative outcomes can be divided into generalized risks, which anyone faces when having a surgery, and specialized risks, which pertain to the particular type of operation being carried out. In addition to the important issue of understanding the risks, there is the closely parallel issue of understanding the possible positive outcomes, that is, how to predict the benefit of treatment. Because decisions will be made by balancing potential benefit against risk, this chapter also includes a discussion of how benefits are assessed.

Blood Loss During Surgery

Among the concerns of any surgeon planning an operation are problems, such as bleeding, that commonly occur as a normal part of surgery. If bleeding risks are anticipated in advance, they are easily managed. When there is an expectation of ongoing bleeding, advance stockpiling of the patient's own blood (autologous units) or the use of a special suction device can avoid the need to use donated blood. When the elements of a particular surgery pose a risk of injury to a major blood vessel, the ready availability of vascular surgery specialists in the hospital reduces the risk of any serious blood loss. Injuries of a major blood vessel occur at an extremely low rate and should not be considered as a reason not to proceed with surgery.

Routine Blood Loss

Bleeding always takes place during cutting of tissue, drilling and scraping of bone, and removal of disks. A wide range of techniques is used, so the same operation in the hands of two different surgeons may involve virtually no blood loss or may involve extensive blood loss. As a general rule, the size of the incision and exposure have some relationship to the amount of blood loss, but other details of the particular surgery also affect it considerably.

There are a number of surgical situations in which bleeding starts and the length of time before it can be halted affects the amount of blood that is lost. Sometimes, for instance, it is necessary to open or tear blood vessels that are against the surface of a very sensitive neural tissue, and it is not possible to stop the bleeding until the neural tissue is protected first. A similar situation exists in the preparation of bone for fusion: the surgeon has to remove some of the bone's protective surface to promote new growth, but the bone then begins to bleed, and the normal methods to stop bone bleeding also tend to inhibit fusion.

Transfusion: Details about Replacement

Steps such as preparing for *transfusion* (the intravenous administration of blood) can be taken ahead of time to minimize the risk to the patient when significant blood loss is expected. In general, if the need for blood transfusion is anticipated, the surgeon will recommend an autologous blood donation, in which you donate blood ahead of time for use in your own surgery. Your blood is obviously the safest to use, because blood that is donated by another individual would have to be tested and matched to yours.

When there is insufficient time before a surgery to donate your own blood, when there are health reasons why it can't be done, or when the surgeon encounters unanticipated bleeding, transfusion can be carried out with blood donated by someone else that has been carefully cross-matched to your own blood. Matching involves not just blood type but also many finer factors and markers in the blood that determine its compatibility. Although donated blood is tested, there is always a small risk of disease transmission due to the limitations of blood-testing methods. The only down side of donating your own blood is that you need significant advance warning, because you can donate only a limited amount of blood at a time, and your body must rebuild its own supplies and strength after your blood is removed.

Cell Savers: Rescue, Reuse, Recycle

Surgeons rely on suction tubes to draw blood away from their area of work and to maintain a clear view by preventing blood from filling the operating field.

This is obviously essential because there are many structures that have to be seen clearly in detail throughout the operation. In most cases, the blood that goes up the suction tube amounts to disposable waste, and as long as this is a small quantity, that is probably safest and best. But for surgeries in which a large amount of blood loss is anticipated, it is possible to manage the blood loss with a device called a cell saver that works to clean and transfuse the blood as it is lost.

A cell-saver machine collects the blood from the suction tube into a medium that prevents clotting and includes various filters to cleanse the blood cells of any contaminants. After the cells are washed, they are prepared for transfusion back into the patient. In general, these machines are effective only when a significant amount of blood is lost, enough to necessitate a transfusion, and the method is most appropriate when that blood loss is expected to be steady and extended. For spine surgeries, a cell saver is most often needed in a lumbar fusion surgery or in a multiple-level laminectomy.

Major Hemorrhage: Being Prepared

One other small step the surgeon can take to minimize your risk in the case of unexpected blood loss is to assure that your autologous units or some fully cross-matched units are actually in the operating room during your surgery. This step guarantees that they exist, that they can be located, and that they can be put to use promptly if needed.

Similar concerns affect the choice of location for your surgery. In the past, virtually all spine surgeries were carried out in a hospital. Currently, discectomies are often done in outpatient surgicenters. In some locations, even fusion surgeries are done in this way. The patient should understand that the choice of a surgicenter over a hospital does entail some risk for more extensive operations.

Preventing and Treating Infection

Another area of common surgical risk is infection. This risk cannot be completely eliminated because there is always some bacteria somewhere in the environment, and they cannot all be eradicated. Fortunately, the body has excellent natural defenses against most bacteria, and in addition, the vast majority of surgeries carried out in the United States begin with intravenous antibiotics given on a preventive, or prophylactic, basis at the start of surgery. The antibiotic is usually in the bloodstream by the time the initial incision is made.

There is some risk of allergy to antibiotics, but the administration of general anesthetic provides a great range of possibilities for treating any possible allergy. This is because virtually all of the life-threatening consequences of a severe allergic reaction can be easily and immediately treated by the anesthesiologist using the life support equipment already in place in your body for the general anesthesia. Certainly, if the allergy is known in advance, then an appropriate alternative antibiotic will be selected.

The most common types of infection after surgery are very superficial, that is, at the level of the skin closure. Superficial infections involve some redness and perhaps some drainage of white or yellow fluid, called pus. Any redness developing in the area of the wound over the two to three days after surgery is usually easily treated with an oral antibiotic and is not a cause for great concern. Deep infection, happily, is quite rare but is a risk that cannot be reduced to zero. As long as there is adequate awareness and attention to the potential for deep infection after surgery, the commencement of strong antibiotics at the first sign of trouble can usually halt it quite easily.

Urinary Tract Infection

If a surgery takes longer than one to two hours, it is typical for a urinary drainage catheter or "Foley" to be placed in the patient so the bladder does not become overly full. Although the catheter is usually placed with sterile techniques, its presence can allow the introduction of infection. This risk cannot be eliminated completely, so a postoperative *urinary tract infection* is fairly routine. Therefore, if itching and burning with urination develops after surgery and testing of the urine confirms a urinary tract infection, this should be treated with antibiotics.

Pneumonia: Challenges to the Lungs

Another type of postoperative infection problem is a *pneumonia*, or lung infection, which can develop when the reexpansion of the lungs after surgery isn't complete. During general anesthesia and machine-assisted ventilation, portions of the lungs can slightly or partially collapse, a process called *atelectasis*. Normally, the lungs reexpand rapidly after surgery. However, when an area of the lung does not fully expand, the normal flow of air and fluid in and out of the lung segment is decreased, and naturally occurring bacteria can cause a local infection in that section of the lung. Most pneumonias are identified by chest X-rays and are also easily treated with antibiotics.

Use of an *incentive spirometer* after surgery is a routine way of reducing the risk of pneumonia. This is usually a small plastic device with a suction mouthpiece and a little plastic ball or other marker inside. After surgery the patient is told to suck on the tube repeatedly to try to get the ball to go higher and higher in the plastic chamber. In this way, the patient works to reexpand the lungs.

Bone Infection: A Difficult Task for Treatment

Occasionally, an infection after surgery extends down deep into the core of the surgical site, which can pose a number of more serious risks. If an infection gets into the disk space after a disk surgery or even after a discography injection, for instance, it can be extremely painful and can be destructive to the vertebral bodies above and below the disk. An infection that enters the bone is termed an *osteomyelitis*. Infections of the disk space (called *discitis*), which has relatively little blood supply, and infections of the bone are often very difficult to treat and may require weeks or even months of intravenous antibiotic therapy.

For these reasons, all deep areas involved in the operation are washed out with antibiotic irrigation just before wound closure is started at the end of the surgery. Careful attention needs to be paid if new pain develops during the days after surgery, particularly when there is fever or any abnormalities are seen in specialized blood tests that can detect infection. If a deep infection does occur, a new operation may be urgently necessary to clean the infected area and wash out any accumulating products of the infection.

The pus that is formed in a deep infection that does not drain out to the skin may become an ominous problem when it is sealed deep near the spine. This is because infected tissue and its products can press directly on the dura (membranes surrounding the spinal cord) or nerves, causing weakness, numbness, and other neurological injury. This rare but quite serious complication is called an *epidural abscess*. A similar type of infection after an opening of the dura can spread between the dura and the innermost lining of spinal membranes, the arachnoid. An infection in this space is called a *subdural empyema* and can produce the weakness and numbness without producing as much pain as an epidural abscess. Both of these complications are extremely rare occurrences.

Spinal Fluid: Can You Get Meningitis?

Occasionally, an infection actually enters into the spinal fluid space, which is classified as a *meningitis*. The word "meningitis" carries great concern because some of the contagious types of meningitis are very severe. A meningitis from surgery, however, is usually very different in that it tends to be very easily treatable and is certainly not contagious to anyone else. The risk of a meningitis is very small unless the dura is actually opened. This limits the problem in part to those unusual surgeries done inside the dural membranes (see chapter 15), but it also remains an issue when there is an inadvertent tear in the dura during a routine surgery, particularly if there is a spinal fluid leak that reaches through wound closure in the skin.

Drainage of crystal clear fluid from a spine surgery closure site therefore always warrants immediate attention by the surgeon, particularly if there is a fever as well. One additional sign that a meningitis is developing is a stiff neck that starts a few days after a lumbar spine surgery. For obvious reasons, a stiff neck after a cervical spine surgery is not a reason to consider meningitis.

Implants: Bacteria Hiding in Plastic and Metal

Another important postoperative infection issue arises from the spinal implants themselves, because any implanted material that is foreign to the body can provide a refuge for bacteria. You have to consider that from a bacteria's point of view, blood is a noxious, dangerous substance full of antibacterial poisons and shark-like white blood cells eager to swallow and digest any foreign organism. But anywhere in the body that doesn't have an active blood supply would be a great place to live and grow, and implants can fit the bill perfectly.

An otherwise effective antibiotic treatment may leave a small amount of surviving bacteria clinging to the implant. Then when the antibiotics are stopped, the infection will recur. In general, there is no need to remove metal implants after an infection, but it may be necessary to remove plastic or latex implants and some types of donor bone implants in order to fully halt the infection. These are additional reasons, when any implant is placed, that all precautions are taken against infection, antibiotics are given before and immediately after the surgery, and irrigations with antibiotic solutions are used during the operation to try to reduce the risk.

Anesthesia: Medical Care During Surgery

Simply receiving anesthesia exposes a patient to certain unavoidable risks, some of them merely annoying, and others potentially life-threatening. The various types of anesthesia include *local anesthesia*, which numbs a designated area of the body; *intravenous sedation*, in which a medication is given that makes the patient drowsy or sleepy; and full-scale *general anesthesia* in which the patient is entirely unconscious and relies on the anesthesiologist for breathing.

Intubation: Injury to the Mouth and Throat

The vast majority of spinal surgeries are carried out using general anesthesia. While under general anesthesia, the patient is dependent on a breathing tube that is attached to a *ventilator* machine. The difficulty of inserting the breathing tube correctly at the beginning of surgery presents some risks of injury to the teeth, throat, and tongue. Although these injuries certainly can occur, they are extremely rare and are more often nuisances than serious, long-term problems. For some shorter surgeries, use of a *laryngeal mask* instead of a traditional *endotracheal tube* (the tube that connects the ventilator to your lungs by passing down your trachea) can allow the anesthesiologist to do the job well without risk of vocal cord irritation or injury. For voice professionals such as singers, teachers, and trial attorneys, this may be an important consideration, since the development of hoarseness after surgery may have a particularly significant impact.

When a patient is having surgery for spinal cord compression in the neck, the traditional method of placing a breathing tube may be unsafe: The anesthesiologist administers a medication that effectively relaxes or turns off all the muscles in the body and then extends the patient's head and neck backward to get a clear view down the throat. When there is spinal cord compression, however, this maneuver itself can cause compression of the spinal cord. In this situation, the anesthesiologist may choose to use a fiber optic endoscope for the intubation and may even do the procedure with the patient partially awake. An anesthetic spray prepares the way in the throat, and the flexible endoscope is threaded down into the airway and into the trachea. The anesthesiologists can see video from the tip of the endoscope and can use control wires to bend the tip around corners. Once the endoscope is in position, the endotracheal breathing tube is slipped down over it and into place without having to extend the patient's neck.

Positioning: Padding for Pressure

Because the surgical patient will be lying in a single position without any movement for a number of hours, careful attention has to be paid to properly situating the patient during the course of the operation. Most hospitals have an elaborate positioning routine involving particular types of padding, which are placed over all of the patient's affected pressure points to protect against nerve compression, development of sores on the skin, and any traction or pressure on other sensitive structures. This is particularly important in longer surgeries such as spinal fusions.

Blood Clots: Maintaining the Flow

One of the great risks with surgery is the formation of blood clots in the calves. A blood clot of this type, called a *deep venous thrombosis*, can break loose and float up into the lungs, which can be life threatening. Measures taken to reduce the risk of blood clots generally include having the patient wear support stockings, which help to prevent blood from pooling in the veins of the legs, or air-compression stockings, which continuously squeeze the legs while the patient is motionless under anesthesia. Such stockings may also be used during the postoperative period while the patient remains in bed and is moving very little. In addition, after surgery it may be helpful to use medications that thin the blood, such as heparin, or even a non-steroidal anti-inflammatory medication such as Toradol.

If a blood clot starts to develop in the calf, the patient most commonly notices a new pain in the back of the calf muscles. A venous thrombosis can be detected by an ultrasound imaging test, and if it is found, medical treatment may be needed to prevent the growth of the clot, reduce the risk of its spread to the lungs, and speed its natural breakdown.

Cardiovascular Risks: Keeping an Eye on the Heart

Prior to surgery, virtually all patients are seen by an internist, who reviews their general medical history. Any heart or lung problems are addressed, tests are performed, and assurances are made so that anesthesia can be administered without posing excessive risks. During the course of anesthesia, careful attention is paid to the patient's blood pressure to ensure that it doesn't fall too low as the body is relaxed; an overly low blood pressure places risks on the neural tissue that is being operated on during the surgery. Fortunately, the modern operating room has a wide array of elaborate monitoring equipment that greatly reduces many of the cardiovascular risks of surgery, although these risks cannot be completely reduced to zero.

Postsurgical Pain: Making It Through the Day After

Any surgery will result in some pain afterward. In general, depending on the extent of the operation, the amount of pain that the patient will experience can be reduced by careful attention to details during the surgery; however, for larger surgeries, it is often quite difficult to eliminate significant postoperative pain completely.

Temporary Tissue Pain

Doctors will commonly inject a local anesthetic around the area of surgery so that the immediate pain after an operation can be greatly reduced. Other special measures, such as placing an epidural catheter (a tube that leads from an external medicine administration port through the skin and into the spinal canal) to maintain general pain reduction during the days after a spine surgery, may also be helpful in difficult situations. For the most part, however, it is possible to use routine postoperative pain medications.

Narcotic medications are often administered through a *patient-controlled analgesia* (PCA) device. The patient pushes a button on the PCA device to administer multiple, small doses of narcotic medication through an intravenous line. This device reduces the risk that too much narcotic will cause an increasingly drowsy patient not to breathe adequately, because if the patient becomes drowsy, he or she stops pushing the button; thus, only a sufficiently aware patient can self-administer medication. Of course, one problem with this strategy is that when you go to sleep at night, you may awaken with no pain medication at all in your system and be in quite a bit of pain. To prevent this, PCA machines often have a setting to provide a continuous, low-level, background dose during the night.

As soon as possible after surgery, the patient is switched from intravenous to oral pain medication and is then usually ready to go home. When surgery is done in an outpatient setting, injections of local anesthetic, long-acting anesthetics, and strong anti-inflammatory medications play a very important role in assuring that the patient is comfortable enough to go home without having difficult postoperative pain problems.

Increased Pain from Unintended Results

Surgery is not necessarily a perfect technical enterprise, and there is a matter of art in surgery just as there are variations from patient to patient and a matter of unpredictability in the individual aspects of the human body. It can even happen that the pain for which an operation is undertaken will actually worsen after surgery. This is clearly an unintended result but may occur if the diagnosis was wrong, procedures were not carried out completely as intended, or an accidental injury to a nerve, bone, or joint took place during the operation.

When an increase in pain or the development of a new pain after surgery cannot be explained by routine aspects of the surgical approach, it is very important for the surgeon to carefully consider the symptoms, investigate the possible causes, and take measures to alleviate it. In most cases, increased pain after surgery or development of a new, persistent pain that does not resolve along with the normal pain from the incision or operation site should lead to additional tests. Many postoperative pain problems can be corrected, even if an additional surgery is required to do so.

Among the biggest risks to preventing the correction of inadvertent problems is the expectation of perfection on the part of both the surgeon and the patient. Everyone involved should strive for and desire a perfect result, but both parties also need to be prepared to undertake the hard work of correcting a problem if one occurs so that the best ultimate outcome can occur for the patient. Dealing with complications and unintended results has to be a matter of trust between the patient and the surgeon, because if that trust breaks down, everybody suffers. When any kind of mistake is made, the surgeon has to be willing to communicate the details to the patient and to be aggressive about identifying the problem. This is because the purpose here is to minimize the patient's harm or suffering. The patient, in turn, has to cooperate with the doctor in identifying and treating the problem to minimize any additional risk. If the development of postoperative problems after an unobserved or unanticipated event leads to defensive behavior, failure to carry out tests, and disputes, these get in the way of solutions. It is often the case that months of litigation with no ultimate settlement leave the patient in pain and the surgeon in frustration, when cooperative attention to the problem at the start could have resolved it in short order.

Special Risks for Neural Tissue

Because spine surgery involves work on hard, bony tissue immediately adjacent to soft, sensitive neural tissue, there is certainly plenty of opportunity for injury, damage, or irritation of nerves to take place. Other chapters in this book discuss nerve injury in terms of its assessment and recovery.

Nerve Injury or Compression

The simple surgical facts of moving nerves aside and scraping, cutting, or drilling bones immediately adjacent to them places the nerves at risk. Risky situations include not only the directly observed contacts between bone and nerves but also relatively unobserved contacts. A surgeon correcting the misalignment of two vertebral bones, for instance, needs to anticipate the effect of that correction on any nerves near those vertebrae. The surgeon's experience and skill, of course, is generally directed toward minimizing or reducing such risks as much as possible.

In the course of surgery, vertebrae may be repositioned in ways that don't actually injure nerves but do place pressure on them. This can often be corrected at the time, but if it is not discovered until after surgery, additional nerve decompression can be required. Pressure on a nerve may cause pain, numbness, or weakness but does not necessarily mean a permanent injury, only the need to further decompress the nerve. Nerve compression can also recur after removal of herniated disks if a new herniation occurs; again, a repeat surgery has to be considered as a possible treatment for the problem.

Spinal Cord Injury or Compression

The spinal cord is relatively intolerant to compression or injury and may not recover if significant injury occurs. Aside from other nerve compression or injury, spinal cord injury is the most-feared complication of spine surgery. Fortunately, it is extraordinarily rare, probably occurring in less than one in 100,000 spine surgeries on the whole. Although cord injury is of concern, it is far less of a risk to the patient than, for example, the risk of death from a motor vehicle accident. Most of the impact of this risk is on the design of surgery, and it is not necessarily a significant consideration for a patient who is considering whether or not to undergo a spine surgery.

Surgical situations in which the spinal cord could be injured are rare. These may include unexpected mechanical failures or other catastrophic and unusual events, and do not represent a risk of routine operations. There is virtually no risk of spinal cord injury in a lumbar spine surgery because the cord does not extend to where most lumbar spine problems happen, below the level of the L1 vertebra. In a cervical or thoracic spine surgery, however, there is a significant risk of pressure or injury to the cord, so all operative techniques are carefully designed to eliminate or reduce that risk.

Special Risks for Bones and Joints

As the nature of problems in the vertebral column often involves the overgrowth of bone and similar obstructions, spine surgery is generally designed to remove parts of bones and joints that are pinching spinal nerves. The downside of this is that removing these elements may lead to decreased spine stability and function.

Instability: Weakening the Joints

In general, decreased stability causes a risk of spinal pain, and in the most severe situations, instability may actually pose some risk to the neural tissue. Spine surgeries are designed to minimize resulting instability, and postoperative X-rays are taken to investigate any new pains that might suggest it or simply to make sure that there is no reason for concern. If there is an occurrence of instability after surgery, it may often require an additional surgery, progressing from the original and smaller decompressive surgery into a second, more extensive fusion operation.

Failed Fusion: When Bones Don't Join

One of the most common risks of fusion surgery is that the fusion fails to become complete. When two bones are in abnormal contact with each other but are not fused solid, they can form a kind of false joint. The technical term for this is a pseudoarthrosis, which is often quite painful. To correct a failed fusion or a pseudoarthrosis, a new surgery may often be needed to remove any fibrous surfaces that may have developed and prevented further fusion. New fixation devices may need to be implanted to hold the bones in place, or a different bone surface may need to be approached. For instance, a posterior cervical fusion may be carried out to treat an anterior surgery that failed to fuse.

Fracture: Excess Stress

Sometimes the reduction or removal of bone to achieve decompression of nerves weakens the bone to a point that, rather than the spine becoming unstable at a joint, the bone's structural elements fracture. This kind of problem also may require subsequent treatment with fusion surgery, as well as careful attention to any risks posed by the lack of stability. Typically, a postoperative spine fracture is heralded by a new onset of pain with movement after the surgery and should be adequately identified during routine X-ray evaluations, including flexion and extension or movement X-rays.

Special Risks with Implants

Any foreign material placed into the body can carry with it a special set of risks that require attention prior to, during, and following surgery. Some of the risks with spinal implants have to do with the type of material and the body's response to it, as well as the way in which the material responds to treatments that work properly for natural tissue but may not be as effective for an implant.

Allergy and Inflammation

A primary issue in the design of any medical implant is to be sure that the material is well tolerated by the body. The design is often based on identifying materials that do not stimulate allergy; however, an allergic response to an implant may still occur in individuals who are more sensitive to unusual materials than others. Sometimes this risk can be anticipated in an individual who has many allergies to environmental stimuli, and a test can be carried out on the patient's skin prior to surgery to ensure that the intended implant material does not cause an allergic response. This is particularly important with any protein material, such as BMP, that tends to be more *allergenic* (producing of allergic response) than other types of material. In addition, patients who have metal allergies may not be able to tolerate the placement of metal implants for stabilization.

Inflammation, however, may be a normal part of the body's response to resorbable materials, which are often used in spine surgery. These materials include everything from sutures to antiscarring materials to implants that are intended to dissolve over time. The natural process of dissolving these resorbable materials may involve inflammation.

Rejection: The Body May Not Accept Foreign Material

When any material is implanted in the body, whether it is a synthetic, an allograft from a cadaver, or a transplant from a living donor, *rejection* may take place. Rejection is a vigorous attack on the foreign material by the body's immune system, which leads to inflammation, pain, and displacement of the implant. If rejection of an implant is observed, attempts can be made to suppress the response, but this situation often requires removal and replacement of the implant with something else.

Dislodgment: Getting the Mechanics Right

When large titanium implants are used in the spine, an important concern is that the implants may shift to an undesired location if the fusion fails. In the case of a titanium interbody cage placed for an anterior lumbar fusion, failure of the fusion could result in the cage's migration, either into the path of a nerve root or into the abdomen. This kind of *dislodgment* is rare, but any graft in the lumbar or cervical regions of the spine has the potential to move. The plates and screws used in both neck and low back fusions will generally stay securely in place while the bone is supposed to be solidifying. If the fusion fails, however, the hundreds or thousands of repetitive motions per day of the bone against the metal may loosen the screws and plates and begin to shift or move them.

Essentially, most of the implants that are used to support spinal fusion are intended to withstand about four to six months of movement against them; by that point, the bone should be fused or another operation should be planned to address the failed fusion. If movement continues after that date, the stress and metal fatigue will progress, and the material may fracture. Instrumentation is usually placed in such a way that it does not pose any risk even if it fractures, but dislodgment is certainly an issue to be monitored when there is a fusion failure.

Mechanical Failure

Spine implants that stay in place should be able to carry the loads that they were intended to, aside from the situation of failed fusion. But metal, although it seems to be very hard and strong, will actually fragment and break when subjected to repeated movement stress. Even with a properly progressing fusion, some implants may eventually prove inadequate to the stresses applied and may be subject to failure or fracture or, being harder than their surroundings, may lead to fracture of the bone around them. This risk of mechanical failure may lead to the need to replace a device or redo an operation. It is also one reason, in many cases, that a cadaver bone implant is preferred to titanium, because the cadaver bone will be transformed by new bone cells and will have hardness and elasticity similar to normal bone tissue.

Successful Outcomes

As discussed at the beginning of the chapter, in order to assess a risk, you have to know what the benefits are, which means being able to understand accurately the expected, good outcomes. It proves to be very challenging, however, to find out just how well people do after they've had spine surgeries.

Certainly, to start with, all the different types of people and types of spine surgeries must be separated in order to compare apples to apples, but when that is done, it is often surprising to see how little is known about outcomes. For technical reasons, it can be difficult to measure outcomes in the first place, and surgeons have also been slow to go about obtaining this information. Many insurance companies are now very concerned with finding outcome data so that they can determine whether there are procedures that are ineffective that they should not be paying for.

Double-Blind Randomized Trials

An important issue in collecting outcome data is the question of who assesses the outcome and whether there will there be any bias inherent in that assessment. For instance, a common problem is that a surgeon who reports the results of surgeries may tend to overestimate the success of his or her own work. To prevent this bias, outcomes are often assessed by an independent third party by using standardized testing questions or measurements. Ultimately, it is best if the person who is collecting outcome information doesn't even know exactly what treatment was administered to the patients.

A methodology that is used in assessing some types of treatment, such as new medicines, is called a *double-blind randomized trial*. If it is not yet known whether a new medication for a particular condition actually works, it seems reasonable to take 20 people with a particular condition and assign them at random to receive either pill A, which is the medication, or pill B, which is essentially a sugar pill, or a placebo. The individual patients don't know whether or not they have received the medication, and the doctors administering the treatment and performing the assessments don't know either (which is why it is called "double- blind"), thus eliminating reporting bias from all participants. In this unbiased fashion, we can find out how the patients do and then find out later what they were given. Then it can be determined whether the condition of those people taking the new medication was improved more than the condition of the people taking the placebo. The result of a double-blind randomized trial is very reliable.

This kind of high-quality test, however, usually cannot be applied to assess the success of surgical treatments. If there are twenty patients with a certain condition, and ten of them receive a designated surgery, what about the ten who are not going to have the real operation? In a sham or placebo surgery, a patient would be opened up in the operating room for a few hours and then closed up, with nothing actually done to the spine. It could be considered unethical, however, to conduct a placebo surgery for the purposes of a double-blind trial, because even though there may be uncertainty about the value of the particular surgery, there is no uncertainty about the fact that any kind of surgery exposes the patient to risks. The patient would certainly need to be fully informed, and certainly very few people would agree to participate in a study if they knew there was a chance of receiving this sort of nontreatment. For these and other reasons, surgical outcome studies generally can't rely on this scientific method of assessing and validating their results.

This approach can be used, however, for comparing two competing surgical treatments for the same condition. But if they are significantly different treatments, such as open surgery versus percutaneous, or through the skin, surgery, then the patient will easily know which treatment he or she has had, and this certainly would be apparent to the surgeon doing the treatment as well, therefore, the study will not be truly blinded.

Prospective Cooperative Studies and Cohort Studies

A typical kind of surgical outcome study involves the comparison of various treatments in an agreed format but without the "blinding" used for medicine studies. One type of study in this category is a *prospective cooperative study*, which means that a plan is made beforehand and then patients with a particular condition are enrolled and treated in the study with their informed consent. It generally involves patients from many different hospitals and institutions in order to have large patient numbers and to capture the effect of variation in technique between different doctors. The patients are, for example, given medication, or treated with surgery, or assigned a waiting period before treatment. After the study is carried out, a comparison can be made between the groups of patients to evaluate the relative outcomes of different treatments.

A *cohort study* involves a large number of patients at multiple locations and institutions who may not have exactly the same disorder or exactly the same surgery. This was the sort of study used to evaluate pedicle screws. In essence, it asked about overall outcomes in patients having various types of lumbar fusion surgery for various reasons, but distinguished those who received pedicle screws from those who did not. Although there were many factors in all the different surgeries and all the different outcomes, it was very clear that the typical condition of fusion patients receiving the screws was much better than those who did not receive them. This showed that the "hypothesis" that pedicle screws hurt spine patients could not be true.

Retrospective Reviews

Another common way of assessing outcomes, which is considered to be of lower quality, is a *retrospective review*. This means that a surgeon or another researcher looks back at the results reported for patients who underwent treatment in the past. For instance, a surgeon performs 100 lumbar microdiscectomies, reviews his results, and then writes that 80 percent of those 100 patients said that they had a really excellent outcome, 5 to 10 percent said that they were no better after the surgery, and 5 percent said that they were worse. The problem with a retrospective study is that there is extensive room for bias to enter into an after-the-fact selection of which patients to include in the analysis; also, because the study is not planned in advance, collection of the actual outcome results may be of poor quality.

Surgical Series

Often, a single surgeon will carry out a procedure on a series of individual patients and then report the results that he or she has achieved with that procedure over time. Even though there may have been a prospective intention of reporting what would be done, the fact that there is only a single participant reduces the quality of the study if formal measures are not taken to assure that the outcomes are carefully reported. Single surgeon series may be appropriate and unavoidable when new procedures are first developed, and they play an important role in identifying new treatments that deserve to be subject to more formal and extensive analysis. In general, the quality of a surgical series can be greatly increased if standardized questionnaires are used before and after the surgery to allow the patients to report their own progress with regard to subjective issues, such as pain and function, along with the collection of any available objective outcome measurements.

Surgeons' Impressions

Much of the informal kind of outcome information that is given to patients comes from individual surgeons who provide a kind of generalized personal impression of how their patients have done. Essentially, you ask your doctor, "How have your patients done with your surgeries?" and the surgeon says, "They have done very well." This is the most common way that outcomes are reported to patients and risk decisions are made. This is true in part because, unfortunately, there really are not any adequate, solid outcome data for the vast majority of spine surgery procedures.

In evaluating a potential surgery and requesting direction toward any available outcome data, you need to consider the fact that the published data may show you only that specialists at some advanced medical center have achieved a certain outcome. What you also need to know is whether this is a procedure that your own surgeon has carried out frequently; whether your surgeon has become expert at it and is using the latest techniques; and whether your hospital is supplied with the best support and monitoring methods. All of these factors can affect whether the reported outcome in another setting reflects your own surgeon's results.

Perhaps the best situation is when your surgeon has collected high-quality outcome data on the procedure that you may undergo. Then, if your condition is sufficiently identical to most of the other patients in the study, you can get some kind of statistical prediction of the likelihood that your surgery will have a certain outcome. Short of this, in real life, you can come away only with a kind of a thumb nail impression of what you should expect.

This brings us back to the analogy of the risks of a motor vehicle accident and the benefits of being able to drive. The benefit assumes that no accident will happen, and the risks are something that you therefore accept. We understand overall what a surgery is intended to reasonably do and what it accomplishes for some patients. The statistics on your precise likelihood of success and the precise likelihood of particular complication ultimately can't make the decision for you. That decision is made on an emotional basis, with as much objective input as possible. On this basis, it is considered that you are able to give truly informed consent. This simply means that you know why a procedure is being undertaken, what you might be able to get from it, and that there are risks. Beyond that, the interaction of detailed outcome reporting and risk assessment can make only subtle impressions in your decision-making process.

Choosing a Surgeon

You can find a specialist spine surgeon near you by using any one of several Web sites, such as www.spineuniverse.com, www.neurosurgery.org, or www.spine. org. Finding a surgeon on one of these Web sites may confirm their credentials and location, but you should rely on advice from your doctor about which spine surgeon is most suited for your particular problem. A very experienced senior surgeon in your area may be practicing with the same techniques he or she learned 20 years ago but will bring great insight and technical finesse to bear on your problem. A newly trained surgeon can probably be counted on to know all the latest methodology, but won't have as much experience with any surprises or unexpected challenges that might occur during surgery. That is relative, of course—ten years of training doing hundreds of surgeries per year is plenty of time for a surgeon to see and learn most of what there is to know.

Often the choice of a surgeon has a great deal to do with his or her personality or style. Strong testimonials or referrals from previous patients you may know can also be important. In most cases, your own doctor will have sent a variety of patients to a variety of surgeons over several years and will have a useful perspective. Spine surgeons who work in multi-surgeon groups with internal educational conferences can also be a good bet because they are constantly exposed to the opinions, techniques, and findings of other surgeons.

Board Certification

Many guidebooks give advice on how to choose a surgeon and suggest standard questions. Is the doctor board-certified in the specialty? This is a reasonable question and can be asked of the staff prior to making your appointment. Board certification means that your doctor has completed all of the required training and tests for his or her specialty. For a neurosurgeon, this means six to eight years of formal training in a formally accredited US neurosurgery training program. After training, once the neurosurgeon has passed an elaborate written examination, he or she becomes "board eligible" and is allowed start a neurosurgical practice to care for patients without further supervision. After two years of practice, senior neurosurgeons from the American Board of Neurological Surgery (ABNS) do an extensive review of every surgery performed by the surgeon in his or her first two years of practice and request detailed information on any complications or failures experienced by the surgeon's patients. Additional board-eligible years may be required.

Once a satisfactory two-year record is complete, the surgeon goes through an even more intensive oral examination in which various members of the ABNS question the surgeon to test his or her skill in making a diagnosis, in choosing the best approach for surgery, and in handling any surprises that may emerge suddenly during an operation. Passage of the examination makes the surgeon board-certified for a period of ten years after which a new examination is required to assure that surgeon is keeping abreast of the latest developments.

Are there surgeons in practice who are not board-eligible or board-certified? Yes, there are. This is because most states don't formally require any training beyond the most basic one-year hospital internship. It is up to a hospital to decide whether to give "privileges" to a given surgeon based on its review of the surgeon's training. If a hospital has many choices it will demand the highest level of training. If a hospital has been unable to attract any surgeon in a specialty of interest, it may lower its requirements. There is only minimal regulation of these choices.

Fellowship Training for Neurosurgeons and Orthopedic Surgeons

The full training for a spinal neurosurgeon is the longest training for virtually any work on this planet: up to fourteen years after college. The four years of medical school are followed by up to eight years of training to be a neurosurgeon; then, although any neurosurgeon can do brain surgery, it takes an additional year or two of advanced fellowship training to learn to handle all of the most advanced new equipment for spine surgery.

Spine surgery is offered by most neurosurgeons, but fellowship training in spinal neurosurgery may mean that a particular surgeon is able to handle any of the most difficult and complex problems. Often the most senior and experienced spinal neurosurgeons do not have fellowship training because it was not widely available for neurosurgeons in training until the early 1990s.

One measure of the quality of many types of medical Fellowships is whether or not the training program was approved by the ACGME—American College of Graduate Medical Education. For orthopedic surgeons, they may have gone through an ACGME accredited Fellowship. Neurosurgeons who have done a neurosurgical spine fellowship will have at least equivalent levels of training, but the field of neurosurgery has not endorsed the existence of ACGME accredited spine fellowships, so a neurosurgical spine specialist—although Fellowship trained—will not have an ACGME credential for this.

Orthopedic spine surgeons almost always have spine fellowship training. This is because routine orthopedic surgical training doesn't include very much exposure to spinal surgery; most orthopedic surgeons do not do spine surgery. In general, orthopedic spine surgeons have specialized in lumbar surgery for disk problems and for patients needing fusions. However, the more experienced orthopedic spine surgeons offer a full range of standard and complex surgical treatments for the neck and low back.

Surgical Experience

Next you may want to ask your surgeon about experience with the particular type of operation that has been recommended to you. Some operations involve new technology, and no surgeon has done very many. Others are "old" operations that every neurosurgeon or fellowship-trained orthopedic spine surgeon has already done a hundred times during training. There are some operations, such as endoscopic thoracic spine surgery, that require a very high level of specialized skills, so very few surgeons will offer to do these procedures. When your surgeon recommends a new type of implant or new type of operation, it is fair to ask why the surgeon has made that recommendation. It is also useful to ask which fraction of all the surgeon's operations are the type that has been suggested to you.

When to Get a Second Opinion

No doubt you've chosen your surgeon because every bit of information you can find suggests that he or she is the best expert available. In some cases, the choice may be determined by your health insurance plan, but you should expect that your plan has chosen to work with a capable expert. At some point, trust becomes essential. You have to believe that the advice you're getting from your doctor is good and correct.

There are situations, however, when you need to seek an opinion from a second specialist. Often enough, this second opinion is required by your health plan. Sometimes you may pursue the second opinion on your own because of some nagging uncertainty you have about what has been recommended. Sometimes it's just a matter of your difficulty in accepting what has been advised-you're worried about the thought of having surgery, but the doctor says there is no other choice.

It certainly is reassuring if the second doctor tells you that he agrees completely with the recommended plan and that your doctor is excellent. However, what if the second doctor disagrees? If it's a second opinion required by your insurance plan, you may be forced to accept the less expensive alternative, for example, "Your back hurts—learn to live with it." The fact is that if you see three different doctors, you may get three different opinions. For this reason, you have to put just as much thought into choosing your second opinion doctors as into your choice of your original surgeon.

You might think that if there is a difference of opinion that the various doctors could have a discussion and work out the best recommendation, but unfortunately, doctors who disagree don't usually like to discuss the disagreement with each other. Each may feel that his or her opinion is based on years of experience and the other doctor is wrong. What do you do in this situation? It is a good rule of thumb that that when there is a disagreement, you probably have a choice. In the end you may just have to go with the doctor you like best or the one you feel has the best credentials.

Trust and Confidence

While all of these questions are helpful, your choice has to be based ultimately on trust in your surgeon. You should develop a sense that your surgeon knows you, understands what your problem is, and is truly concerned with helping you get your problem repaired. Once you've achieved that level of trust that you have a caring physician who is knowledgeable and capable, you can relax and accept the choices recommended by that doctor without taking on every detail of the operation yourself. In the end, no matter how much you read or study about the surgery, you can't really begin to gain a full enough understanding to be confident in all your choices. This is why belief and trust in your surgeon is the best way to achieve peace of mind as you approach the day of surgery.

23

Recovery After Surgery

There is a tendency to think about recovery after surgery as a kind of global event where something happens to you and then time passes, and then you are over it and return to your usual activities. To an important extent, this is true. However, it may be helpful to understand the different components of recovery, because any one of these components may go faster or slower than the others and may affect the overall recovery time.

Time for the Surgical Wound to Heal

Everything about the recovery first assumes that the surgery went well and that no further surgery is required. Additional surgery can be warranted after a disk surgery when a new piece of disk herniates, X-rays taken after placement of instrumentation reveal a problem with the instrumentation that wasn't recognized during surgery, or there are complications such as substantial bleeding after surgery, wound infections, or spinal fluid leaks. So when none of these problems happen and the essential purpose of the operation was accomplished, the recovery has a lot to do with what the surgeon had to do to get to the location for the actual surgery and what had to be done to close up and get back out.

Fascial Strength

For surgeries on the back of the neck, the upper back, or the low back and in a number of other locations in the body, some of the greatest mechanical stresses go to a key fascial layer. This will generally be a dense, heavy layer of ligaments and muscle, which usually comes together at the midline and may even attach to the tips of the spinous processes of the vertebrae. The surgeon typically has to go through the fascia to get to the area of the problem on the spine, the disks, or the nerves, and on the way out the fascia has to be closed.

Closing, for the most part, still relies on sewing with thread. There are a variety of types of suture threads that are used. Most commonly, these are absorbable sutures, which are braided material that gradually dissolves over weeks and months. Sutures are intended to maintain their full strength for at least two weeks, and then to deteriorate over the subsequent six to eight weeks, so that there is no material remaining. This is meant to give the body's fascia time to start to reform itself, so that as the sutures are dissolved away, the fascia regains its natural strength.

Muscle Spasm

There are some ways in which this process can go badly. First, if vigorous stress is applied to the fascia before it is fully healed, the sutures may tear and a gap may form between the edges that may interfere with natural healing. If the fascia doesn't heal in its proper position with full strength, it tends to lead to muscle spasm. The reasons muscles go into spasm is that they are accustomed to pulling on fixed structures in proper locations. When the muscle encounters an abnormal amount of movement or an abnormal position or interaction, essentially the muscle becomes confused at a neuromechanical level, and this leads to spasm or abnormal activity as the muscle struggles to reach its normal position of length and tension.

Occasionally, it is necessary to repair fascia; however, most spine surgeons take great care to put a significant number of very heavy stitches into the fascia to make sure that it is solid and has sufficient strength to resist mechanical forces until healing is complete. This is really one of the main reasons why heavy lifting and strenuous activity are often discouraged after a back surgery. The muscles themselves, in addition to the fascia, often are attached to areas of bone on the vertebrae to which the surgeon must have access. When the surgeon closes, these muscles are laid back down onto the bone and then must rebuild their attachment. Muscle spasm, once again, is a common problem as these attachments reconnect.

Skin Strength and Cosmetic Issues

Just like the fascia, the skin itself is a critical focus of the closure. Here, however, there are two competing concerns. The first is to provide a strong, resilient closure, usually with an absorbable suture, so that the patient is not left with bumps under the skin from permanent sutures. In contrast, it is also often important to try to achieve the best cosmetic effect. However, the lumbar spine area is not the most cosmetically prominent area of the body, so it is often the case that a surgeon concerned with major spinal repair does not attend to the cosmetics of a low-back incision. This is more acceptable than it would be for an incision on the neck or face, but it is something to consider beforehand: whether you want the surgeon to take extra time for the cosmetic closure, or whether you would rather have your surgery over as quickly as possible to get safely out of the operating room, which is an important concern as well.

The wound closure will look best if the skin edges are carefully aligned so that they are at exactly the correct place when the closure takes place, rather than having one edge shifted relative to the other. When the edges are shifted, the appearance of the closure deteriorates somewhat, and you may get little bulges or "dog ears" at each end of the incision. Besides the alignment, the thick, leathery part of the skin needs to be closed with a strong, light suture, so it doesn't spread, and then the surface cutaneous layer needs to be closed neatly as well.

There are three major types of superficial skin closures. Through-and-through suture closures, often made with a nylon, nonabsorbable type stitch, give a very tight, waterproof seal usually with relatively little skin reaction, but may leave scars from the little punctures from the sutures. These punctures remain in the skin as long as the suture is in, so the skin does not really truly seal and must be kept dry for more than a week. Even after the sutures are removed, an additional day or two is required to allow the skin to heal. Staples are an alternative to through-and-through suture closures with thread. These are very rapid for the surgeon to place, but similarly involve skin punctures and may leave "railroad track" marks along the edges of the wound.

Next there are subcuticular closures, where the superficial skin sutures are threaded below the skin surface, so that there are very few or no punctures through the skin (see Fig. 13.1). This can be done either with a nonabsorbable nylon-type suture, which has very low reactivity but still needs to be removed after five days to two weeks, or with an absorbable suture, which stays below the skin and then dissolves away without the need for removal. The benefit of the absorbable subcuticular stitch is that the skin closes rapidly, and within a few days it is safe to get the wound wet.

Finally, the most superficial layer may be closed with Dermabond, which is a super-glue sealant that forms an instant seal so that the wound never needs to be protected from getting wet. When the super-glue sealant is used, there is actually no need for a dressing at all. The super-glue tends to crack and peel, so it may not last for more than a few days, but by that time, the superficial skin layer usually has grown across and formed its own natural seal.

Scarring and Drainage

As the surgical wound matures, there may be tension on its edges. If that is the case, and if the wound edges spread apart at all, new tissue will need to grow in to fill the space that's opening up. This will usually be an abnormally red-appearing skin, which will leave a more noticeable scar. That's why close apposition (edge-to-edge alignment) of the wound is important. In fact, this is why wounds are often pulled extra tight so that they bulge upward a small amount—even if there is a little bit of give in the tissue, the superficial edge remains closely in line to avoid formation of that thin line of abnormal-appearing scar tissue.

In many cases in a spinal surgery, the surgeon may feel that the edges of the bone and muscle within the wound are not completely, safely dried, that is, that there is still a small amount of oozing or bleeding that may be occurring. This is not necessarily a problem if it is dealt with appropriately, but it can become a problem if there is excessive bleeding and the blood begins to form a deep clot that presses on the nerves. For this reason, it's often a surgeon's choice to leave in place a drain, which is a small tube that punctures through the skin into the inside of the wound, so that as any fluids accumulate, they pass out through the drain into a sterile, sealed suction container. When a drain is placed, it may be left in for as long as one to two days, at which time any abnormal oozing or bleeding should stop. If oozing continues past this time, further surgery may be required. A drain cannot be used if there has been a spinal fluid leak during the surgery, because it will only cause the spinal fluid leak to worsen.

Once the drains are out and the skin is sealed over, as the weeks pass after the surgery the wound still may have a raised appearance and will look best only once it is flattened. It's helpful to apply a silicone patch, which can be purchased in most drugstores, over the wound, which essentially helps to remind the skin to flatten to achieve the best cosmetic result. Ideally, if the initial incision is made in a skin-line, is perfectly aligned, and has subcuticular closure and good alignment, the final scar from the incision should be difficult to see.

Time for the Bones to Fuse

A whole separate consideration comes into play when your surgery includes some sort of fusion that requires regrowth of bone, because this process is slower and also depends on which bones are involved. A lumbar spine fusion may take anywhere from three months to two years to achieve full strength, whereas a bone fusion in the neck may fuse solid within four to eight weeks. What has to happen for a bone fusion to take place is that the live, natural bone in the remaining vertebra has to grow into the bone graft, whether it's bone from the person's own hip, a synthetic bone-like material, or donor bone from a cadaver. The natural process involves bone-dissolving cells called *osteoclasts* that cause graft bone to melt away. This is followed by the work of *osteoblast* and *osteocyte* cells that form and support bone that move into the area cleared by the osteoclasts. X-rays taken will begin to show blurring of the initial sharp margin between graft and vertebra until the edge between them begins to disappear.

External Support and Internal Fixation

During the early stages of fusion, if there is considerable movement between the natural vertebra and the graft, scar tissue may form between them that can permanently prevent fusion. Therefore, it is important for the graft and the vertebra to be held in contact with relatively little movement until the contact becomes "sticky" in a sense and begins to seal out any intervening tissues.

The two options for keeping the contact points stiff are either an external brace or internal fixation with screws in place. Internal fixation with screws is very helpful, because it gives a solid lock right at the site where it's needed and is usually much more effective than the brace. In fact, internal fixation is usually so effective that, at least in the neck, bracing is not needed, although many surgeons still recommend a brace as an additional measure, in case of a fall or a car accident during the recovery period.

Because of internal fixation with screws and plates, the vertebral column where the graft has been done may give the feeling of being very solid and rigid right from the start. However, this can go too far, in that if it is too rigid, there may be so little stress conducted to the bone that it grows more slowly, actually delaying the fusion. This is why, particularly when titanium cage implants are used, the fusion process may be extremely slow and take as long as two years.

When Can You Drive After a Spine Surgery?

Before you begin to drive after surgery, you of course want to be over the general stiffness and soreness, which usually takes one to two weeks. But you do not want to be in a driving situation where you need to turn your head but you don't, because of postsurgical stiffness. Similarly, you don't want to disrupt the healing process by making sudden turns with your neck or back. That's why, for cervical spine surgery, there usually is a recommendation of waiting six to eight weeks before driving, although with solid internal fixation a surgeon may allow a patient to resume more activities earlier. For lumbar fusions, often the wait for resuming driving or other physically intensive activities is as long as three to six months. Surgeons do vary considerably in their recommendations on this point, and there is no fixed and agreed standard.

Time for Strength to Return

External bracing, in particular, has the effect of reducing movement and may lead to weakness of the muscles. So once the fusion has taken place or the crux of recovery is under way, the muscles may be slightly atrophied, and it becomes important to gradually increase activity to build the muscles back up to their normal strength. Then, once the skin closure, the fascial closure, and the bone fusion are solid, you can begin to increase activity, such as a full range of normal work and possibly even physical therapy, although the latter is often delayed until healing is well advanced. Physical therapy can help maintain motion while healing is taking place, but active strengthening has to be undertaken with caution when it may run counter to the needs of growth and repair of the fascia, the skin, and the bones.

When Healing Doesn't Progress: Time for a Reevaluation

It is important for patients to understand that whether it takes four days or four months, there should be a steady improvement in the symptoms or problem for which the surgery was originally performed. If there is no improvement or even a worsening of symptoms, it is reasonable for the surgeon to begin to investigate the cause of the delay. There may be another round of imaging or injections. This sort of evaluation is routine because it is well known that in 2 to 4 percent of patients, disks reherniate, fusions don't solidify, or other unanticipated problems arise. This is obviously frustrating and disheartening when it occurs. For this reason, it is important to accept this possibility in advance of the original surgery. It doesn't necessarily mean that anything was done incorrectly or was missed at the time of your surgery.

The small percentage of cases in which further treatment is required simply reflects variations in the human body, conditions of recovery, and a variety of subtle aspects of diagnosis and surgical treatment. Although this is frustrating, it is important to remain focused on the ultimate objective of correcting the spinal problem. Most of the causes for failure to heal or improve can be successfully and definitively treated. If there is a reherniation of disk material, the additional material is removed, and it is highly unlikely to occur a second time. If the fusion fails, the surgeon will need to supplement or restart the fusion process, possibly with an additional surgery.

Return to Normal Activity

The objective of most spinal surgeries is to return you to your normal level of activity. A professional football player who has a solid successful fusion may actually return to playing football. The simple fact of having spine surgery does not mean that your active days are over.

There are certainly many cases in which the spine surgery is not fully successful in this way. This may mean, for instance, that the surgery relieved 80 percent of the symptoms, but some pain still remains that stops you when you try to reach full activity. Also, when a fusion surgery is carried out, there are a certain number of patients who will have only very slow progress toward a complete fusion or in whom the fusion will actually fail and require further surgery.

However, those situations aside, most spinal surgeries are designed to preserve or restore the strength and functional capability of the spine. There are many different spine surgeries and many different individual situations, so there is no single time line that applies to all spine surgery patients. This is an area where postoperative evaluation by your own doctor is critical. Physicians vary on their expectations and time scales for recovery as well.

At the minimum, some patients can return to work a few days after a cervical fusion surgery or microdiscectomy with no need for any special physical therapy. This is really the goal for all spinal surgeries. However, as a general rule, many spine surgeons advise their patients to expect to take off work for two to four weeks and to take things easy during that time. Aside from lumbar fusions, most surgeries result in significant recovery of full tissue strength within six to eight weeks in a normal, healthy individual. Age is also a factor in this. Patients in their teens and twenties heal and recover strength much faster than most patients in their seventies and eighties.

Once your physician feels you are ready to resume work, either on a limited or full-fledged basis, you still have to remain vigilant. When a particular movement or stress seems to cause excessive pain, then that is a good reason to ease off and progress more slowly for a while. Eventually, though, you may feel that your spine is really up to strength. You gradually add on stresses and it does well. What remains is the process of recovering your full preinjury or presurgery strength. The issue of strength is mostly about rebuilding your muscles, although many people experience a generalized fatigue after surgery as the body devotes its excess energy to tissue healing.

This last phase of recovery may be entirely under your own direction or it may involve physical therapy. In general, physical therapy for postoperative spinal patients is postponed until recovery is well under way, and it is definitely not needed for all patients.

Physical therapy is most helpful when you need instruction and guidance on restoring lost range of movement or in designing a safe but intensive program of rebuilding your capabilities. A typical physical therapy program may include up to three visits per week with a therapist and may continue as long as three months. A program like this is very time consuming and should not be undertaken without thought for how it will affect your daily life. This is an area where various physicians have strong opinions, and it is wise to discuss this with your surgeon in advance of the surgery.

Overall, the final stages of healing of the body's tissues actually requires that you resume full activity. Bones grow to meet mechanical stresses. Similar principles affect muscles and ligaments. In the end, your body should take over the work of healing completely. The surgeon has stepped in to make sure the body can heal itself and that the best conditions for healing are in place.

The surgery is similar to the jump through hyperspace in a science-fiction movie. Before the surgery, the body is struggling to heal against mounting failures, and the situation is going from bad to worse with no end in sight. The surgery stops the deterioration and sets the body back on course to heal on its own. Once the surgery recovery is over, the body picks up again with normal healing—under much improved conditions. The surgery has altered the conditions. You've traveled through a strange and previously unimagined world of carbon fiber and titanium, genetically engineered proteins and computers with flashing LEDs guiding drills through your body, all monitored by people doing something that is apparently so complicated and fraught with risk that it requires up to fourteen years of training after college just to be considered fresh-faced beginners. All this has taken place, and now, we all hope, you have been rapidly but gently set down on the other side, returned to your normal reality where healing relies on walking, eating well, and getting your rest.

This is a view you can take as you consider the whole process of surgery. The surgery is a precise, corrective step applied by a doctor who understands the problem in full detail. The objective is to achieve a remarkable and lasting recovery that your body cannot achieve on its own. A full understanding of this partnership should lead to a successful outcome.

24

Health Insurance and the Cost of Surgery

Planning for a necessary surgery is most commonly determined by the medical need, the certainty of the diagnosis, and the risks and benefits of the surgery. However, financial considerations may play an important role in a number of aspects that affect the timing of the procedure, the choice of physicians to perform it, and even precisely what type of procedure is done.

For the most part, the American health care system is designed in such a way to minimize, or at least to create the appearance of minimizing, the impact of health care finance on the selection and provision of care. However, because of the very large cost of some of these procedures, this impact certainly becomes a consideration. Understanding the ways that the costs are generated, how they are controlled, and how your insurance covers different parts of them is complex. This chapter is intended to provide some of the vocabulary and lay out some of the groundwork to help you to be an informed consumer and to understand the financial options that are available.

How Much Does an Operation Cost?

Determining the cost of an operation in advance can be difficult. It is helpful, at least, to understand the various components that contribute to the cost so that you can understand where there are some choices that you may be able to make and why there may be some uncertainty.

CPT and ICD-9: Outlining It All in Codes

One of the aspects of surgical pricing and billing that may seem very confusing and mysterious is the use of codes for all aspects of the process. The codes are used because many of the people involved in billing and finance have relatively little specific medical knowledge. Coding is a way of creating a bridge between the medical people who understand the specifics of care and the financial people who understand the financial side. In the United States, this process is carried out to an extreme degree, so that virtually every aspect of care is converted into numerical codes, which then allow the financial people to determine how the different types of procedures are billed.

The two biggest classes of codes in current use are the *CPT* and the *ICD-9* (International Classification of Disease, Ninth Revision, Clinical Modification), although there are a few others. (The ICD-9 is being replaced by ICD-10 codes in 2012.) The CPT (current procedural terminology), provides a numerical code for virtually every type of operation or intervention, such as an injection, an MRI scan, or even a doctor visit. The CPT codes are very specific, and there may be as many as fifteen individual codes to describe different parts of a single operation.

However, medical practice is constantly changing whereas code updates are infrequent. Because of this, you may have a procedure for which there is no exact CPT code. In this case, the surgeon is supposed to choose a similar code that comes close to what was done. The insurance company may prefer a different code and the bill may go back and forth while the surgeon and insurer reach agreement on which is the most appropriate code.

For a doctor's visit, numerous codes may be used to determine the length of the visit, the detail of the exam, and the number of possible diagnoses that the doctor had to consider. In a sense, the designers of these codes tried to determine how much thought went into decision making about diagnosis and treatment during your office visit. Widespread adoption of the Electronic Medical Record (EMR) system makes automated coding very common as well.

The ICD-9 codes are numerical descriptions of the different types of diagnoses and medical problems from which patients can suffer. These also are fairly detailed, and although the ICD-9 is the ninth version of the ICD codes, this system was never originally designed for the detailed billing use that it now serves. Because of this, the ICD-9 codes are often general and vague and do not necessarily pertain specifically to an individual patient's condition. Similarly, numerous different ICD-9 codes can be used interchangeably, as they all may apply to a given condition.

Administrators in health care finance use the ICD-9 codes to determine whether a particular CPT code is justified. If a patient has a diagnosis denoted by a particular ICD-9 number, a computer can tell whether it is OK to approve them to have certain CPT code-numbered procedures performed on them. If the ICD-9 doesn't match up with the proposed CPT, the insurance company computer will deny approval of your procedure. In theory, a mismatch only prompts the administrators to turn to their medical directors in an attempt to analyze the problem. However, you may just see a denial while the insurance company waits for an appeal.

Using a computer is a simple way to make sure that the right things are being done for a given diagnosis. This also causes problems, however, if your diagnosis doesn't happen to be correctly described by the ICD-9 codes or if the procedure that you need is a little different from what's commonly described in the routine CPT codes. Another huge flaw in the system is that most doctors know relatively little about these codes and rely on office staff to read what they write and come up with the codes. If a wrong code is entered, an insurance rejection will result.

Other important acronyms are the *RBRVS* (resource-based relative value scale) and *RVUs* (relative value units). This is an attempt by the US government's Healthcare Finance Administration, the American Medical Association, and various other professional societies to determine the amount of "medical energy" it would take to carry out any given CPT code. This is supposed to reflect the amount of training for the doctor, the amount of time it takes to do a procedure, the risk the doctor faces, the risk the patient faces, the amount of thinking involved, and the complexity of the procedure. All of these factors are meant to be incorporated in this numerical value scale, and then the numbers are used by Medicare and the Healthcare Finance Administration to predict how much should be paid for each type of CPT code. Although these codes don't tell you the absolute cost, they do show how at least one organized group of collaborating doctors at a high level assesses the relative value of different CPT codes.

In general, Medicare expects to get about a 75 percent discount off the doctor's usual and customary charge, so if a particular CPT code has payment by Medicare of about $800, their expectation is that the physician will be charging four times that amount, or about $3200. If the doctor then says, "Well, since Medicare will pay only $800, I will just charge $800," Medicare will turn around and say, "Well, if you are charging $800, we still want our 75 percent discount, so we will now only pay you $200." Therefore, a kind of a cost structure is laid out by the RVU system and by the amounts that Medicare pays. The amounts that Medicare pays also vary from city to city because they try to account for different costs of living, rents, salaries, and real estate values, so the given RVU price for a certain CPT can't predict the Medicare allowable payment without knowing the complex additional formula.

These RVUs and RBRVS scores turn up in most payments from insurers even when they have no involvement with Medicare. This is because an insurer may convince a physician to join its contracted PPO (preferred provider organization) by offering to pay the doctor, for instance, 1.5 times Medicare, five times RBRVS, or some similar formula. An HMO, for instance, may try to get participating physicians to accept just 60 percent of the Medicare rate. This allows an entire complex fee schedule agreement to be encapsulated in a single number that shows the multiple compared with what Medicare would pay in that locale.

It is also the case that a given CPT code may have different values and different charges depending on whether it is used on its own or whether, for instance, a particular surgical step is part of a larger, more complex surgery. The concept is essentially that the doctor did all the evaluations and brought the patient to the hospital, did the preoperative work and the opening, and there is a certain amount that will be paid for doing a laminectomy, a certain amount for a foraminotomy, and a certain amount for a discectomy. However, the payment that Medicare gives for that procedure reflects the entire process of the preoperative visit, the hospital stay, exposure, closure, the posthospital care, and the postoperative visit, so when additional CPT codes are used during that procedure, Medicare may only pay 50 percent or 25 percent of its usual payment for the additional codes and give its full payment in the first, main, or largest code.

Surgeons' Fees

One of the major components for the cost of your hospital stay is certainly the surgeon's fee. For a routine, small-scale spine operation with a two-day hospital stay, the surgeon's fee may come to only about 10 percent of your total bill. This is because surgeons' fees for simple spine operations will run anywhere from $2000 to $8000, but a hospital may charge as much as $35,000 to $100,000 a day for admission. If the surgery is done in an outpatient surgicenter, the price may be $10,000 to $15,000, even for a fairly brief procedure.

Surgeons' fees have developed over time and reflect what is called a "usual and customary charge;" only no one really knows exactly what a usual and customary charge should be. The best guide is to look at the Medicare payment for a given procedure and multiply it by four, which brings you into the ballpark; however, doctors are not supposed to discuss their fees and charges with each other because this would be a form of collusion or price fixing. Although this does give you a ballpark figure, you may find that a surgeon who is the world's leading specialist in a particular type of procedure charges higher than the predicted amount for this particular procedure and much lower for an operation for which he or she has no special experience.

There are other unusual variations that affect surgeons' fees, such as their participation in different hospital groups. It is not uncommon for a university to offer leading, world-famous specialists to insurance companies at relatively low fees in order to compete with another university in town. This sort of good deal also can arise when a particular organization has both a hospital and employed surgeons feeding income into it. It may be in the interest of the organization to reduce its surgeons' fees to attract patients, but then make up their income with higher hospital charges. This works because the hospital charge is a larger part of their income than the surgeons' fees. As discussed next, however, the surgeon's fee may have very little resemblance to what you or anyone actually has to pay for the operation.

Other Physicians

In the course of a surgery and hospitalization, there may be a number of other consultants and participants who also generate charges. Almost invariably, there will be an internist or some other physician who does a preoperative examination. This is an important step in bringing together your general medical information and assuring that there are no surprises. Surgeons specialize in their own areas, and although they are, of course, medical doctors, they may rely on internists, cardiologists, or other specialists to carry out a complete preoperative evaluation.

Also, quite important in the procedure will almost certainly be an anesthesiologist, whose fees will be generated in the course of administering anesthesia. The anesthesiologist usually does not do the preoperative evaluation but expects to verify that it all has been done in good order in advance of the surgery. In addition, there may be fees from radiologists because X-rays may be taken during the operation and/or scans may need to be reviewed.

Subsequent to the surgery, a pain specialist may be consulted who generates fees in several visits; the internist or neurologist who evaluated the patient prior to admission may visit the patient in the hospital for follow-up visits, and this may generate additional charges; and if any complications arise such as concern about the cardiac situation, the pulmonary situation, or infections, there may be cardiologists, pulmonologists, and infectious disease specialists, in addition to physical medicine and physiatry specialists who will plan physical therapy. All of these specialists may generate separate bills or, in some situations, may have their services offered as a package by the hospital.

Hospital and Surgicenter Facility Charges

As noted earlier, the facility fee (hospital or surgicenter) usually generates the largest portion of the expense of surgery. Also, hospital charges for regular admission may be anywhere from $25,000 to $35,000—or even $100,000 per day at hospitals such as Cedars Sinai. Surgicenter outpatient fees are in the range of anywhere from $5000 to $15,000 for a procedure. These fees will often include not only the hospital bed but also the length of time in the operating room and all equipment and supplies used during the procedure. The hospital is trying to cover its cost for its physical plant and for payment of the salary of the nurses and for the various other hospital-employed professionals involved in the course of the procedure.

Your insurance coverage for your physician may be quite different from your insurance coverage for your hospital. Sometimes, as with a large university group, it is very difficult to separate the surgical and the facility or hospital fees. In other situations, such as when a private practice surgeon is used, the fees of the hospital and the surgeon are completely independent, as they are quite separate entities from a financial or business point of view.

Equipment for Recovery

After surgery, equipment such as braces or other special therapy machines may be required. These usually entail relatively modest costs, but certainly should be considered as well. It is the practice of some doctors to employ a wide variety of special postoperative equipment, including electrical stimulators, cold packs, and refrigerated units. Some of these can be very elaborate and potentially expensive, and there is tremendous variation in medical coverage for these kinds of devices. It is probably best to make direct inquiries with your own insurance company to learn in advance what sort of postoperative recovery aids are covered under your policy.

Postsurgical Therapy

Following surgery, there may be courses of physical therapy as well, which will generate additional expenses. Beyond physical therapy, some surgeries may require additional treatments to complete or achieve their final expected effect, and this is something else that should be factored in. Usually, these are relatively small charges compared with the cost of the operation itself, but if they are not covered by your insurance plan, they may become an important consideration.

Who Pays for What Parts?

Now, aside from having awareness of all the different charges and how they are assembled, there is tremendous variation in what part will be paid by an insurance company and what part will be paid by the individual. This is determined by the nature of the health plan, and given a particular type of health plan, there are various complex terms that can determine how much payment is available for a given treatment.

HMO, PPO, Indemnity, POS, and Medicare/CMS/HCFA

The various types of medical payers fall into an alphabet soup of different categories that are organized in different ways to achieve different effects, controlling costs by either limiting or expanding the array of choices available to a patient. One of the best known is the *HMO*, or health maintenance organization. The idea of an HMO is that instead of allowing patients to make medical purchases and then seek reimbursement, one can effectively have the insurance company directly agree to purchase the services in bulk for its members. Because of the resulting purchasing power, the HMO is able to buy hospital days and surgical procedures at a kind of a bulk-rate discount. The surgeons and the hospitals agree to discount their rates in order to guarantee a flow of patients.

Why would the flow be guaranteed? Well, essentially, a private practitioner with no contracts has to compete against all other doctors for patients, and for the most part patients will choose a doctor based on reputation if costs are the same. However, if a physician chooses to do a large volume at a low price, it may actually be difficult to attract patients: If you were choosing and you had infinite resources, would you choose the doctor who prefers to treat a small number of patients per day, spend a thorough amount of time with them, but has the highest fees, or would you always look for the doctor who is the cheapest in town and does the most operations per day? You have to ask yourself that question because the low-cost, high-volume doctor is exactly what the HMO is looking for.

In some cases, very good doctors are included in HMO plans. This happens when a physician is associated with a hospital or group of doctors that make that choice collectively. It also happens because some doctors choose to accept a limited number of HMO patients. Further, HMOs have to compete for new members, and price is not the only issue—they need to make a credible case that they offer quality care. Because of these considerations, an HMO may work for you but requires particular care in choice of your doctor if any choices are allowed in your plan.

The upside of the HMO is that everything in the preceding part of this chapter about fees for hospital care, doctors, other doctors, consultants, and equipment is essentially wrapped up in a way that eliminates any financial worry for the patient—that is, if the procedure is approved and meets the guidelines of the HMO. Health maintenance is also called managed care because HMOs may choose to review carefully what is being done. If the HMO decides that a procedure is not warranted, you may not be allowed to proceed with it unless you pay the bill personally in full. But as long as the procedures are approved by the HMO and the individual uses the doctors and facilities that participate in the plan, the costs are usually extremely low. Instead of facing expenses of hundreds or thousands of dollars, the cost to the patient may be $10 or $20. Why should they even bother with the $10 fee? Well, the idea is that many people will refrain from frivolously using a service that costs them even $10, which they would go ahead and use if it were completely free.

One of the reasons people have tended to shy away from HMOs is the feeling that the subscriber doesn't have any choice about who will be his or her doctor. When the doctor arrives, the patient pretty much has to take whoever it is, without much say in the matter. This is sometimes an uncomfortable situation. It is always the suspicion that because it is the cheapest care it may not be the best, even though there may be very excellent doctors provided by an HMO through complex contract mechanisms. There is also the worry that the HMO won't approve the procedure based on financial imperatives rather than based on purely medical ones.

Another common type of payer plan is a PPO, or preferred provider organization. In this case, the physicians and hospitals that participate have again agreed to a fee discount, but usually not as sharp as the discounts for an HMO. Here, the patient often has a wider choice of doctors, and there may be a far greater variety of good-quality physicians and facilities that participate because a less severe discount is demanded of them. People choose PPO plans because of the greater choice, and, therefore, it is in the interest of the PPO plan directors to have as many good doctors as they can in order to be attractive to people who are looking for choice.

One of the older or more traditional types of payment plans is called an *indemnity plan*, which really just means that you go out and see your doctor, he decides what treatments you need, and he submits the bill to your insurance company. There is no review; there may not be special contracts with different providers and prearranged discounts. Indemnity plans usually require the patient to pay a larger proportion, often as much as 40 percent of the total charges, which can be quite an extensive amount of money, although as seen later in this chapter, limits are placed to protect the patient financially even in an indemnity plan.

Another type of health care is POS, or point of service. Here, a patient has a choice of going with an assigned HMO provider, selecting a PPO physician, or choosing to proceed on an indemnity basis, depending on the specific medical problem being treated. The idea is that for the majority of routine problems, such as a urinary tract infection, a simple arm or leg fracture, or even an appendicitis, there are a wide variety of physicians who can readily and easily take care of the problem. In these situations patients are often less concerned about exactly which specialist does the procedure and are usually happy to use an HMO doctor. If, on the other hand, there is a more unusual problem, such as a difficult spine problem that doctors seem puzzled about, the patient may choose to go on a PPO basis to a recognized specialist; if it is a very puzzling problem where even the specialists seem to disagree, the patient may want to be able to go to an out-of-town, recognized leader in the field outside the arranged plan but still to have some significant coverage. A POS plan allows the patient to make that choice on an event-by-event basis.

Medicare is available in the United States to individuals over 65 and to others with some varying amounts of disability. It is supervised by the US Center for

Medicare Services (CMS, formerly called the Healthcare Finance Administration, or HCFA). Physicians may or may not participate as providers in Medicare, although the vast majority of physicians do participate. Medicare sets allowable fees based on the RVU structure described earlier in this chapter and is very aggressive in assuring that physicians may not pursue collecting any funds above and beyond what Medicare feels is allowable. Typically, Medicare pays about 80 percent of charges and leaves about 20 percent to be met by the patient. Medicare also has not, in the past, offered any significant coverage for prescription medications.

In some cases, your physician may advise you to undertake a procedure for which Medicare offers no payment at all. If you are appropriately notified of this fact in advance (under advance beneficiary notification) and you choose to proceed, you may face a bill for which you alone are responsible, despite your Medicare coverage.

Medicare may be supplemented by various types of secondary insurance. However, there is one key aspect of this to keep in mind—a Medicare secondary will usually help with the patient portion of the bill only if Medicare itself receives a bill and pays its part. If Medicare recognizes the provider and recognizes the procedure but has a payment rate at or near "zero" this would seem to require the physician to work for free. In that situation a secondary may be very helpful in persuading the provider to offer the service.

However, a different scenario comes into play when a physician is opted out of Medicare. In this situation, Medicare cannot be billed by the physician at all and therefore, paradoxically—your secondary will not pay either.

Uncontracted Providers

For very high-quality subspecialty care, particularly in the area of surgery, some patients may encounter uncontracted providers. These are doctors who do accept insurance payments but do not have any discount contract with any of the insurance companies. Usually, physicians will act as uncontracted providers only if their services are in such demand that they have no motivation to provide discounts to bring in more patients.

The main impact of the lack of a contract is that even after the insurance has paid some portion of what it considers to be the allowable charge, the patient portion may be large. For example, two physicians in town offer a procedure for which they post a charge of $1000. One of them is contracted and the other is not. The contracted provider has agreed to do this service for patients with a particular health plan for just $500. This plan pays 90 percent and the patient pays 10 percent; therefore, the insurance will pay $450 and the patient will pay $50. For the practitioner with no contract, the insurance will still pay just $450, but the patient will face the unnegotiated patient portion of $550. The uncontracted physician may not expect to collect the entire $550. He may negotiate with the patient and accept $100 or $200. The patient may choose to pay the $200 instead of paying just the $50 in order to have access to the more expensive doctor with the better reputation.

Doctors who are uncontracted may also negotiate with the insurance company on a case-by-case basis. If the doctor feels that the $450 paid by the insurance company is not adequate, and no other doctor offers that procedure, the insurance company may negotiate with the doctor for a one-time case rate and may pay $700. So the uncontracted arrangement introduces uncertainty, but it allows subspecialists with advanced special training and skills to charge a higher rate than those providing routine, standard services.

The Insurance Payment Process

Once a surgical procedure is completed, the surgeon dictates a report. The billing process usually involves matching the ICD-9 code that describes the diagnosis and all the CPT codes that are employed in the procedure with the information in the operative report or hospital report. The reports document or support the claim that each of these billed procedures was carried out. All of the professional fees are collected on a standardized form, usually called an HCFA 1500, and the facility charges are collected on a UB92 form, and these are sent to the insurance provider. In some cases, the patient receives the bill initially, but it is common practice to bill the insurance company first.

If the information in the claim matches completely, insurance companies will usually generate a response, called an *explanation of benefits (EOB)*, within 45 to 60 days. The initial response may be to point out that there is one digit wrong in the birthdate and that therefore the claim will not be paid and must be resubmitted. Then, another 60 cycle may occur before an actual initial payment comes out. The insurer may pay only a fraction of what was expected without any clear explanation. The doctor will then do an appeal and point out that under insurance law and preauthorization, a certain payment was expected under the contract. Finally, after an elapse of six or seven months, the final payment to the doctor or hospital may be received from the insurance company. Only at this point will the doctor know what the patient portion truly is and be able to turn to the patient and bill the patient portion or negotiate what the patient portion will ultimately be, whether it can be paid all at once or in a payment plan, or whether there will be no fee at all.

For most medical practices, the patient and not the insurance company is ultimately financially responsible for paying the bills. Sometimes a physician's office that is frustrated by nonpayment or long delayed payment by the insurance company will begin aggressively billing the patient. This is done in the expectation that the patient will then complain to the insurance company about its poor response to the initial bill. The patient is paying a premium to the insurer and is the actual customer.

In general, for Medicare and for many of the insurance plans, doctors are expected to collect some sort of patient portion of the payment. The position of Medicare is that if a doctor does not collect the 20 percent from the patient, then the doctor is engaging in Medicare fraud. Accepting insurance only as payment in full may be considered as a criminal offense by the physician.

This may seem strange to the patient, but the thinking from the point of view of Medicare is that the patient portions are included to provide a relative disincentive to patients to consume care that they may not completely need. If the doctor routinely waives the patient portion, Medicare may suspect that the doctor is encouraging patients to consume what becomes, to the patient, free care that they would not otherwise normally consume. This is why it is viewed as fraud. Because a doctor may essentially face criminal prosecution, fines, exclusion from Medicare participation, and even jail time for voiding the patient charge, many doctors are understandably hesitant to do this.

Ideally, though, a clean or complete charge is generated electronically by the doctor's office, the insurer responds within ten to fifteen days, paying the expected amount, the bill is received by the patient, and, with a simple discussion, the patient negotiates a reasonable payment and the procedure cost is dealt with. The hospital charges must be arranged in parallel with these.

Covered Charges and Allowable Charges

For any given procedure described by a CPT code, you can rapidly verify that the procedure is usually covered by your insurance. One set of exceptions to this concerns the wide variety of procedures that do not have formal codes, either because they are new or because the codes are not sufficiently specific. For these, the insurance company will need specific evidence of what a particular procedure was and why it was done to support the payment. Another category of treatments excluded by many insurance companies is for cosmetic surgery as opposed to surgery that is considered medically necessary because of a medical problem. And finally, there are procedures that the insurer may consider experimental or novel, terms for which there is no specific definition, and it is very often a matter for dispute when anything other than the most routine procedures are carried out.

For every charge posted or applied by any doctor for any CPT code, the insurance company will determine an *allowable charge*. This essentially is what they will allow after their discount, so if they insist on a 60 percent discount or 75 percent discount, their allowable charge will be 25 percent of the physician's usual charge. The insurance company may also assign a fixed price that they consider to be a usual charge from their own point of view, whether or not the doctors in the community agree with the insurer on what that amount should be. Then they determine what percentage of the allowable charge they will pay, for instance, 80 percent; under contract, the patient must pay only the remaining 20 percent of the allowable. The doctor is not able to go to the patient or the insurance company for any amount beyond the allowable charge. If the doctor is not contracted, then the allowable charge may still determine how much the insurance company will pay, but this scenario won't be helpful for limiting the patient expense.

What Is the Patient Portion?

As described previously in this chapter, it is difficult to predict the patient payment portion for surgery, and in advance of a surgery it is almost impossible. This may lead to uncertainty when you are in a plan other than a contracted HMO or PPO plan. It is usually possible to have a general agreement with the physician or hospital or to negotiate an advance cash or credit card payment to limit the patient portion prior to the surgery. Nonetheless, it is very common for patients to simply wait until their full insurance amount is paid and then to carry out negotiations after the fact.

Deductibles and Out-of-Pocket Maximums

A number of other factors may affect how much the patient actually pays, even in the PPO or indemnity setting, including the existence of deductibles and out-of- pocket maximums.

A deductible means that even though the doctor is charging $1000 and the insurance company usually allows $500 and would usually pay $450, if there is a $500 deductible on your policy, the insurance company may pay nothing and the full $500 falls on the patient. The deductibles are usually on an annual basis, so that once the deductible is paid, then the full insurance coverage is triggered for any subsequent claims that year. This is why patients who have had a surgery and possibly need an additional one will often try to get the second one done before the end of the year, when a new deductible will apply.

The exact meaning of an insurance policy's out-of-pocket maximum may vary considerably and usually applies to the total amount of the 10 or 20 percent portion of the allowable that the patient pays. If these portions accumulate past a certain amount, there is usually a maximum, whether it is $5000 per year or $2000 per year, depending on the plan, and beyond that the insurance company will pay 100 percent of allowable charges. This does not mean that they will limit charges that go beyond what is allowable or covered.

When Is a Procedure Experimental?

Often one of the greatest areas of dispute is over whether a procedure is experimental and, if it is, whether or not insurance should pay. This is often a very emotional issue for patients with cancer who are considering new types of chemotherapy that may not be fully proven but which have evidence supporting their success. In these situations, the patient may feel that being denied the payment will make something unreachable in terms of expense and turn the situation into a death sentence. This is an extreme situation, but it characterizes the nature of the problem. Similarly, there may be a diagnostic procedure that is new and that the insurance considers experimental.

There is no specific standard to define what is experimental and what is not, so that even if a procedure has been available for eight or ten years and there are 20 to 30 publications concerning its usage, including formal outcome studies, an insurance company may still try to claim that it is experimental in hopes of avoiding payment. This is often a subject for disputes and for appeals when payment is denied. Often, a letter of medical necessity from the physician that explains the procedure is sufficient to demonstrate to a medical director why a new procedure is being carried out.

It is important for patients to keep in mind that some insurance companies will deny anything that can be denied in the hope that patients will simply not appeal. But when an appeal is carried out, there may be a considerable rate of success. There are other issues that an insurance company may see as a liability to be avoided that they will be intransigent about. Although it is difficult to predict the outcome, very often it is worth the trouble of an appeal when any sort of payment is denied.

President Obama's Health Care Reform

At the time of writing of this second edition, it is not at all clear how much of the Obama legislation will eventually come into effect. Among the most important provisions is one that is intended to prevent insurers from looking at preexisting conditions in deciding on what expenses to pay and who to cover. Other effects include allowing young people up to age 26 to remain on their parents' health insurance, and improving the completeness of coverage for medication expenses.

There are plans to try to review inefficient and expensive types of care—and spine fusion surgery is high on the target list for review. However, very little of this type of reform will take place until the larger outlines of the plan are settled.

In the area of preventive care, the Health Care Reform has mandated that there should not be deductibles and patient portions for preventive care. In treatment and routine visits, the idea has been that a patient portion is necessary in order to discourage patients from consuming unnecessary resources. In prevention, however, it seems to make sense to drop this discouragement.

This scenario reminds me of a type of problem that plagued the UK National Health Service when I first worked in the United Kingdome before the Thatcher reforms in the 1990s. A patient would have to pay about 80 pence ($1.20) for a bottle of Tylenol (paracetomol in the United Kingdome). However, if it was prescribed by a physician, it was free. A patient with a headache could call out an ambulance to their home (free) and be taken to their General Practitioner's (GP) office for an urgent visit (free) so that they could obtain a prescription to make the Tylenol free. Cost to the patient—zero. Cost to the system to save the patient from having to pay 80 pence for the Tylenol—about $2500. Free care like this can obviously bankrupt the health care system. If unchecked, it can help bankrupt the whole country, as the Euro crisis that developed in 2011 revealed starkly.

The GP was allotted a budget based on how many patients from the local district were assigned to his or her care, and the GP would have to pay for the visit and ambulance (and the medication) out of that budget. If the GP ran out of money, his or her office would close for the rest of the year until the next year's budget came out. How did Margaret Thatcher fix this particular problem? She made it possible for a GP to "strike off" (discontinue service) for patients who seemed to be excessively expensive to take care of. This created new problems because some physicians struck off many patients, thus leaving them with a great deal of funds to work with but relatively little work to do. And so on as it went.

The United Kingdom has gone through a long process of discovering problems and developing fixes for its health care system over more than 63 years (since its founding in 1948). Overall the UK system is relatively efficient and effective—although it is supplemented by a widely used private system. Most UK citizens take great pride in "The Service" as they call it and consider it to be the best in the world. The main take-away point regarding US health care reform is that there will be good and bad, mistakes and breakthroughs—possibly over the next 100 years as we all work together to hit the right balance.

Epilogue: Knowledge and Resilience

Experiencing a spinal problem that might require surgery and grappling with the information contained in a book such as this are processes that teach us about our own beliefs about our bodies and our health. The questions that arise are major ones. Why does the body break down? Is it better to promote the body's natural healing capabilities or to replace them with titanium and plastic and get on with life? Is there a reason that certain joints and body elements tend to fail while others work perfectly for eight or more decades? To whom do we talk about these design flaws? Can anything be done to remedy them or at least to head off the impact of the impending consequences? Are spine problems injuries or are they signs of routine wear and tear? At least you don't really have to ask "Why me?" because spinal problems affect virtually everyone.

Problems with the spine are unsettling because the spine is near the core of our active selves. We naturally expect our bodies to act effortlessly to accomplish our intentions for physical action, but a problem with the spine can be a disheartening disruption. Because of the centrality of the spine, it is more distressing when it begins to fail than, for instance, when there is a problem in the hand or foot. It is harder for the mind to isolate a problem in the spine as a small mechanical problem to fix rather than as a challenge to continuing your life as you know it.

What do we expect in seeking surgery to repair the spine? Does it call to mind Bob Dylan singing "Forever Young" as you struggle to hold off the accumulated wear and tear of life? Perhaps instead it's Smashing Pumpkins singing "Today," just a matter of an injury suffered in a moment of excess—you want to get fixed up and back to full speed without a worry for tomorrow. A successful spine surgery can have that effect of turning back the clock and reanimating a person who seems to be losing the spring and confidence of youth or of repairing the bruised wings from an injury to launch someone back into flight.

As I have tried to make clear, there are no guarantees of success when a spinal surgery is in prospect. However, with the wide array of technological advances now in use, there is a very great likelihood of success and cure. Further, the improvements and capabilities that are promising to arrive over the next decade will bring more and more of spinal breakdowns into the realm of the routine repair.

Overall, you should approach the treatment of your problem with confidence. I strongly recommend that you identify a doctor you can believe in and then use that belief to help you through the choices and concerns. If you can do these things, then you're well on your way to enjoying the benefits and opportunities of a swift and sure success.

» Glossary «

ablation: The use of heat to lesion or destroy some tissue.

absorbable suture: Suture material that can be placed below the skin that the body will absorb by itself over time.

acupressure: The use of focused pressure points to relieve pain and tension in the body.

acupuncture: The placement of needles in locations over the body's surface to manipulate the body's pain system.

adductors: Group of muscles in the medial thigh innervated by the obturator nerve that pull the leg inwards.

adhesion: A location where two anatomical structures that normally glide past each other are instead fixated to each other.

Alcock's Canal: A region on the inner surface of the obturator internus muscle where the pudendal nerve passes through fibrous tissue on the muscle surface.

allergic: A reaction by the body to foreign material, that may cause various levels of body abnormality.

allograft: A graft material such as bone taken from another individual in the same species.

allowable charge: The amount of money an insurance company prefers to pay its contracted providers for a given procedure.

analgesic: A medication that relieves pain without producing numbness.

anaphylactic: Severe allergic reaction, that may be life threatening.

anatomical variants: Differences in anatomical structure that occur among individuals.

anesthetic discogram: An injection intended to temporarily block the pain, originating from the annulus of a disc.

anesthetic: 1. General: Medication that tends to produce deep, painless sleep. 2. Local: Medication that reduces sensation as well as pain.

aneurysm: An enlargement in a blood vessel, that may expand and rupture.

angiogram: A type of radiologic study for viewing blood vessels, that can include either an injection of intravenous contrast or that may be conducted with out an injection by MRI scanning based on the physical properties of blood flow (MR Angiogram).

anisotropic diffusion: The tendency of water molecules to preferentially diffuse more rapidly along the length of nerve and muscle cells relative to the rate of diffusion from side to side in these cells. This forms the basis for the ability of diffusion tensor MRI to visualize the internal structure of neural and muscle tissue.

ankylosing spondylitis: An auto-immune condition, that can lead to progressive natural fusions of the vertebral bodies and forward angulation of the neck.

anneal: To fuse together, typically applied to a heat-based process; in the spine, attempts to repair the annular ligament.

annular tear: A disruption or tear in the annular ring or the annulus fibrosis around the disc space.

annulus fibrosis: A complex ring of dense fibers that surrounds the nucleus pulposus of a spinal disc.

anterior scalene muscle: A muscle running from the lateral processes of the cervical vertebrae to the first rib, that may be injured in a whiplash syndrome and that can compress the nerves of the arm in the brachial plexus.

anterior: Toward the front of the body.

antibodies: Natural molecules developed by the body that can recognize and adhere to various target proteins (antigens) and then direct the blood cells to attack and destroy the target.

anti-convulsants: Medications to prevent seizures.

anti-emetics: Medications to prevent nausea or vomiting.

anti-inflammatory: Medication to reduce inflammation or irritation in a tissue.

anti-scarring agents: Medications or implants intended to prevent undesired adhesions and formation of fibrous tissue or scar—also "adhesiolytic."

aorta: The largest arterial blood vessel in the body, beginning in the heart and then descending into the low lumbar area.

AP or anterior-posterior X-ray: An X-ray in which the beam is sent from the front of the body to the back, that produces an image as if the body is viewed from the front.

aquatherapy: Physical therapy or exercise therapy carried out in a pool of water.

arachnoid: Thin membrane inside the spinal dura but outside the spinal fluid as well as small amounts of fibrous tissue within the spinal fluid space.

arbitration agreement: Agreement between a patient and a physician to settle disputes by arbitration rather than standard litigation.

Arnold-Chiari malformations: Congenital abnormalities at the base of the skull and the posterior parts of the brain, that come in type 1, type 2 and type 3; with type 1 being mild, causing headache; type 2 causing significant abnormalities; and type 3 being in many cases, fatal near the time of birth.

arthritis: Inflammation affecting the joints.

arthropathy: Any degenerative abnormality affecting the joints.

arthroplasty: Replacement of a joint by an artificial material.

articular processes: A part of the vertebra, that extends from the lamina and supports a surface of a facet joint.

ASIS: anterior superior iliac spine—A bony prominence on the front of the iliac crest of the pelvic bone.

assignment of benefits: An agreement by a patient to allow any insurance payments for medical care to be paid directly to the doctor rather than to the patient.

atelectasis: Collapse of portions of the lung, that can take place during routine anesthesia.

autograft: A grafted tissue taken from one place in the body to be used for a surgical purpose elsewhere in the same person.

autoimmune: An error of the antibody immunity system that leads the body to mistakenly attack its own normal cells and proteins

autologous: Blood transfusion using the patient's own blood.

autonomic nervous systems: A set of nerves in the body that control sweating, skin temperature and functions in the gastrointestinal system.

AxialLIF: A spinal fusion procedure in which a large screw is passed up from beneath the coccyx to fixate the center of the first sacral vertebral body (S1) to the center of the lowest lumber vertebral body (usually L5).

axilla: The underarm.

axis vertebra: The C2 vertebra.

axonal transport: A natural process whereby chemicals and proteins are moved along the length of a nerve.

axons: Elongated portion of a nerve cell that projects from the cell body out toward to the endpoint such as on muscle.

basal ganglia: A portion of the brain that is involved in controlling smooth movement.

biceps brachii: A muscle in the upper arm that pulls the radius toward the humerus and shoulder resulting in flexion at the elbow. It is innervated by the musculocutaneous nerve with predominantly C6 components.

biceps-femoris: A two part muscle in the hamstring group in which the long head originates from the ischial tuberosity at the base of the pelvis and is innervated by a branch of the tibial portion of the sciatic nerve and the short head originates from the femur and is innervated by the peroneal portion of the sciatic nerve. Both insert on the fibula and act together to flex the knee.

biofeedback: A system that allows an individual patient to see visual or auditory signals that reflect their own level of physiologic or brain activity.

BMP, Bone morphogenetic protein: A natural or synthetic protein that acts to promote the grown of bone.

bone graft: A piece of bone placed at a site where bone fusion is intended to grow.

bone spurs or osteophytes: Abnormal extensions of the normal contour of a bone or vertebrae, associated with degenerative change.

bone spurs: General term for osteophytes which are abnormal bone overgrowths that can put pressure on neural tissue.

Botox: Trade name for preparations of botulinum toxin—a protein from the bacteria *Clostridium botulinum* which can cause sickness if ingested, but which is used medically to selectively paralyze selected muscles.

bovine: A product deriving from cattle.

brachial plexus: A group of nerves between the cervical spine and the shoulder, that carries the connections that operate the arms and hands.

bradykinins: Chemicals released by the body at the site of injury.

bursitis: An irritation or inflammation of a fluid filled pouch adjacent to a joint or bony prominence. The bursa of the greater trochanter of the femur or the bursa of the ischial tuberosity are sometimes affected.

C-arm: A type of X-ray machine that has a transmitting X-ray source and a receiving fluorescent screen and electronics joined together by a C-shaped arm. The system captures continuous motion and is used for guidance by surgeons placing screws in bone.

cage, fusion: A hollow titanium cylinder or box, that holds two vertebrae in place and carries bone graft material in its interior.

calcaneum: Latin name for the heel bone.

cancellous bone: The loose, open, lattice of bony material within the center of many bones.

carbon fiber: Material used in aeronautics and increasingly in medicine, that provides a rigid, lightweight structure.

carotid artery: One of the main arteries running up the neck and into the face and brain.

carpal tunnel syndrome: A compression at the wrist, that causes a pinch of the median nerve affecting the thumb, 2nd and 3rd fingers of the hand.

carpal tunnel: A structure within the wrist that carries the tendons and the nerves into the hand from the forearm.

cartilage: Soft connective tissue that often occurs in joints and in areas of the face.

CAT scanning: X-ray based system for producing cross-sectional images for medical examination.

catheter: A tube used for delivery of fluids or withdrawing fluids.

caudal epidural: An injection into the epidural space placed through the sacrum.

caudal: Toward the lower end of the body.

causalgia: A nerve-based pain associated with nerve or bodily injury.

cautery: The process of using targeted heat or chemicals to stop bleeding during surgery.

cell saver: A machine that aspirates blood lost during surgery and cleans it for re-transfusion back into the patient's body.

central canal: A structure in the center of the spinal cord that conducts cerebro-spinal fluid.

central nervous system: The brain and spinal cord.

central pain: Pain that is based primarily in abnormal function within the spinal cord or brain.

cerebellar tonsils: The lowest end of the brain that may, in some conditions, extend through the level of the foramen magnum.

cerebellum: A posterior and low portion of the brain involved in the smooth coordination of movement.

cerebral cortex: The upper, superior covering over the brain involved in higher level integration and thought.

cerebral palsy: An associated condition with birth in which abnormal levels of spasticity prevent normal limb movement.

cerebrospinal fluid: A clear fluid that bathes the brain and spinal cord.

cervical plate: A device used to secure and hold cervical vertebrae in place during the time that they are fusing after a surgery.

cervical spine: The vertebrae in the neck.

cervical: Associated with the neck.

chelator: A chemical that removes metal ions from solution.

chest tube: A catheter tube placed through the chest wall to help re-inflate a collapsed lung.

chiropractic: A process of manipulation of the vertebrae and spine to achieve relief of pain or muscle spasm.

chronic pain: A symptom that last continuously over weeks and months as opposed to an acute symptom of recent onset or short duration.

chyle: A fluid produced in the digestive tract that carries nutrients from digestion up the thoracic duct and into the neck, where it flows into the venous system.

claudication, neurogenic: A progressive pain and weakness of the legs that occurs as the person walks, but which is relieved by a short rest. It is caused by narrowing or stenosis of the spinal canal.

claudication, vasogenic: A progressive pain and weakness of the legs that occurs as the person walks, but which is relieved by a short rest. It is caused by narrowing or stenosis of the arteries to the leg.

clavicle: The collarbone that extends from the top of the sternum in the mid chest to form a joint with the acromion portion of the shoulder blade (scapula).

clotting factors: Chemicals in the blood that allow the blood to form clots and halt bleeding.

coblation: A heat-based process for evaporating disc material.

coccyx: The lowest portion of the spine.

cohort study: A research evaluation of a clinical technique, that follows a large number of patients with similar conditions to assess the affect of different treatments.

colitis: An inflammatory disorder of the bowels that often has an autoimmune component.

collagen: A protein that provides fibrous strength in the body. It is prominent in ligaments and tendons but also plays an important role in bone.

collarbone: The clavicle bone (see above).

Complex Regional Pain Syndrome (also:Reflex Sympathetic Dystrophy): Type of pain that does not respond to the usual medications and that involves the autonomic nervous system.

complications of surgery: Adverse events arising during or immediately following a surgical operation that are directly caused by the steps of the operation.

compression stockings: Stockings worn to prevent the pooling of blood in the veins and to reduce the risk of deep vein clots (thrombosis) in the legs.

concordant: The experience of pain during a disc injection procedure, implying that the pain is similar to the pain the patient usually experiences from their condition.

consent form: Statement of understanding by the patient of the nature of a medical intervention giving the permission for the treating physician to proceed.

contrast agent: An injected material that helps distinguish the appearance of two or more tissues during radiological imaging tests.

cortical bone: The hard outer aspect of bone.

cortical responses: Electrical activity on the surface of the brain (cerebral cortex) detected by an evoked potential monitoring system.

costovertebral: The area of the thoracic spine where the rib meets the vertebra.

Cox II inhibitors: Nonsteroidal anti-inflammatory medications that are less irritating to the stomach than the routine non-steroidal anti-inflammatory medications.

CPT: Current procedural terminology. A code system for providing a numerical description of the various components of medical care.

cranial: Toward the head or associated with the skull.

cranium: The skull.

crosslinked: The joining together of proteins or of mechanical surgical implants in a way that increases the structural strength.

cryotherapy: The use of cold to accomplish medical treatments. Freezing a small sensory nerve may be an effective means to treat pain in some situations.

cubital tunnel: An area in the distal humerus (upper arm bone) through which the ulnar nerve passes as it crosses the elbow. In general, the area of the "funny bone."

cyst: An abnormal enclosed fluid space within the body.

decompression: Operation to relieve pressure on a structure

deep venous thrombosis or DVT: A blood clot within a vein.

deep: Further away from the skin.

deformity: Abnormal shape or structure of a region of anatomy.

degeneration: Loss of functional or structural integrity of an anatomical structure associated with aging or continuous use.

deltoid: A muscle in the shoulder that elevates (abducts) the humerus relative to the shoulder girdle. It is innervated by the axillary nerve and originates from the clavicle and scapula.

demineralized bone matrix: A supplement to bone fusion made up of the fibrous proteins of bone.

demyelination: The loss of the normal lining of an axon so that conduction of nerve signals is greatly slowed or blocked.

dens: The portion of the C2 vertebra pointing upward.

dermatome: An area of the skin innervated by a single spinal nerve root.

DEXA scan: Dual energy X-ray absorptiometry used to assess bone density to diagnose osteoporosis.

diagnosis: The identification of a medical condition that explains a patient's symptoms and predicts the necessary treatment.

diagnostic imaging: The use of medical imaging to achieve a diagnosis.

diaphragm: A major respiratory muscle that separates the chest space from the abdomen. It is innervated by the phrenic nerve which travels down from the neck crossing the surface of the anterior scalene muscle.

diffusion tensor imaging (DTI): An advanced type of MRI scanning that collects and displays information about the internal architecture of brain and nerves. This also includes related techniques of HARDI (High Angular Resolution Diffusion Imaging) and Q-Ball techniques under the broader category of Diffusion Anisotropy Imaging.

disc bulge: An abnormal expansion on the margin of a disc, typically still well contained by the annulus.

disc herniation: The escape of a portion of the nucleus pulposus through or partly through the annulus fibrosis.

discectomy: Removal of all or part of a spinal disc.

discitis: Infection within a disc space.

discogenic pain: A pain syndrome deriving from an abnormal spinal disc.

discogram: An injection used to evaluate the health of a spinal intervertebral disc, particularly to identify annular tears.

distracting stimulus: A sensory stimulation applied in order to distract the patient typically from pain carried by the same nerve.

dorsal root ganglia: A collection of neurons associated with the processing of sensory information. Found within the sensory portion of the spinal nerve, just as the nerve exits the spinal foramina.

dorsal: Toward the back.

double-blind randomized trial: A type of medical research study in which neither the patient nor the physician knows whether a treatment or a placebo has been given. Considered to help avoid bias in the evaluation of results of an experiment.

dura: A hard, leathery membrane that surrounds the brain and the spinal cord.

dysphagia: Difficulty swallowing.

electrodiagnostic monitoring: The use of real time evoked potentials and electromyography during surgery to guide the operation and detect nerve reactions arising while the surgeon is operating. Often uses sterile monitoring electrodes and sterile stimulator contacted directly to nerves to test them.

electrodiagnostic tests: Electromyography, evoked potentials, and nerve conduction velocity testing, that can be used to evaluate the health and function of nerves or the muscles innervated by them.

electromyography: Monitoring the electrical function of muscles using needles placed into the muscle or monitoring electrodes on the skin surface.

electroneural interface: A system for detecting nerve signals to drive a robotic system. Used in new generation advanced computer based robotic limb replacements developed since 2010.

electroneural interfaces: Advanced microchips designed to have direct contact with nerves.

eloquent: Complex neurological function.

embolization: Passage of a solid material through the blood stream that may result in blockage of some blood vessels.

EMG: Electromyography.

endorphins: Natural morphine-like substances within the bloodstream.

endoscopes: Tubes used by surgeons to obtain a view within the body without making a large incision, often using fiber optics and video equipment.

endotracheal tube: A tube placed in the throat past the vocal cords used by an anesthesiologist to protect and guarantee good ventilation and breathing during deep anesthesia.

endplates: The portion of the cortical bone of the vertebral body that is immediately adjacent to the intervertebral disc.

entubulation: A method of repairing nerves involving the use of biosynthetic tube materials to connect the severed nerve elements and promote nerve regrowth.

enzyme: A type of protein that acts to increase the speed of a chemical reaction.

EOB: Explanation of benefits. A notice from an insurance company explaining the payment or lack of payment for a medical insurance claim.

epicondyle, medial: The bony prominence on the inner part of the elbow at the end of the humerus. The ulnar nerve passes posterior to it as it curves through the cubital tunnel

epidural abscess: An infection in the area outside the dura membranes.

epidural catheter: A catheter used to administer pain medication in the area outside the dura.

epidural injection: A generalized type of treatment for spinal pain in which typically steroid medication is spread over an area of dura.

epidural stimulator: A type of electronic device for applying a distracting stimulus to the low spinal cord or nerves with involving the placement of an electrode pad over the dura.

epidural: In the space just outside the dura.

epiduroscopy: The use of a video-based visualization system to advance and move a catheter outside the dura and inside the spinal canal, typically to lyse or breakup adhesions.

ergonomics: The design of furniture, tools, and equipment to minimize undesired physical stress on the human body.

esophagus: The tube carrying food from the throat into the stomach.

euphoria: A state of elation or excitement, sometimes abnormal and associated abnormal, associated with narcotic medication.

evoked potentials: Electrical activity in the brain or nerves caused by computer controlled equipment; typically used to provide monitoring of the nervous system.

exercise-based treatments: Nonsurgical treatment for pain in involving bodily activity to produce relief of the pain.

explanation of benefits: See EOB.

exposing: A portion of a surgery during which the incision is made and retractors are advanced so that the surgeon has direct visualization of the critical part of the spine or nerve to be operated on.

extensors: Muscles that extend or straighten a joint.

extremities: The arms or legs.

extruded disc: A portion of the nucleus pulposus passes entirely through the annulus fibrosis and is free within the spinal canal.

facet block: An injection used to numb a spinal joint or facet.

facet joints: The joints on the posterior part of the spine between the lamina.

facetectomy: A surgery to remove all or part of a facet joint.

false positive: A result of a medical test that incorrectly shows a positive finding.

fascia: A dense fibrous layer within the body.

fascial sutures: Sutures used to close and repair the fascia, typically of the spine after a surgery.

fascicle: An individual internal element of a nerve.

fasciitis: Inflammation affecting the sheet-like coverings or separating layers that occur in some body regions.

FDA—Food and Drug Administration: A United States government agency that evaluates whether a manufacturer can make certain advertising claims about a medical product.

Femoral nerve: Large nerve that innervates the quadriceps muscles on the anterior surface of the thigh.

femur: The main upper leg bone from the hip to the knee.

fiber optic: A material similar to glass that transmits light. These "light wires" are used to transmit information or to deliver bright light that shines out the end of the fiber to illuminate a surgical target.

fibrocytes: Cells that produce fibrous material or scar.

fibrosis: The development of scar tissue.

fibula: A bone on the outer or lateral aspect of the lower leg between the knee and the ankle, that is much smaller than the main weight-bearing bone, the tibia.

filum terminale: A small fibrous thread extending from the low end of the spinal cord at the L1 level often as far as the sacrum.

fixation: Holding structures in place.

flexion: Bending forward.

flexion/extension X-ray: Two X-rays taken of the spine, typically one with the body or neck flexed forward and one with the body or neck extended backward.

flexor retinaculum: A ligament that forms the roof of the carpal tunnel.

fluoroscopy: X-ray imaging involving a fluorescent screen, typically observed in real-time by a video camera, for motion X-rays.

foramen magnum syndrome: A headache syndrome involved with a malformation at the base of the brain and skull, with the cerebellar tonsils, or the low end of the cerebellum, passing through the foramen magnum and compressing the spinal cord and blocking spinal fluid flow.

foramen magnum: The opening in the base of the skull.

foramen: A passage between successive vertebrae that allows the spinal nerve to exit from the spinal canal to extend out into the body.

foraminotomy: Surgery to open or expand the spinal foramen to increase the space for a nerve root to pass from the spinal canal out to the body.

fusion: Causing two bones to grow together into one.

gadolinium: An element used to provide image contrast during MRI scanning, typically held by a carrier, or chelate molecule, called DTPA.

ganglion: A group of nerve cell bodies.

gastrointestinal tract: Referring to the throat, esophagus, stomach, and intestines.

gene therapy: The use of techniques that change the genetic makeup of a cell or which otherwise introduce a functioning gene into a cell for the purpose of causing the cell to produce proteins that are helpful to correcting a disorder.

general anesthesia: A type of sleep induced during surgery in which the patient is not awake and does not experience pain, typically involving intubation and control of respiration by the anesthesiologist.

general risks: Risks common to many type of surgery.

genito-femoral nerve: A nerve originating at the L2 and L3 levels of the spine that travels along the inguinal region and provides some sensation in the genital area.

gluteal crease: The fold of skin between the base of the buttock and top of the thigh.

gluteus maximus: A large muscle in the posterior pelvis that originates along the iliac crest and inserts into the femur. It is innervated by the inferior gluteal nerve and helps extend the thigh backwards relative to the pelvis.

gluteus medius: A muscle that originates on the ilium and inserts on the greater trochanter of the femur. It is innervated by the superior gluteal nerve and is a powerful abductor that holds the body up when the opposite leg is off the ground during walking.

glycosaminoglycan— A complex biomolecule in the carbohydrate family including both sugar-like and protein-like components—hyaluronan—a lubricant material in joints and around nerves is in this chemical family.

gray matter: The areas of the brain or spinal cord that have neural connections and nerve cells within them.

greater trochanter: A bony prominence on the upper end of the femur that on which the gluteus medius inserts along with the piriformis muscle and the obturator internus muscle. A bursa on the outer surface—the trochanteric bursa—may become irritated in patients with piriformis syndrome.

guidelines: Recommendations generated by the major medical societies that suggest how physicians should practice based on high quality published research reports—these constitute a major component of evidence based medicine.

Guyon's Canal: A passage in the wrist through which the ulnar nerve reaches the palm of the hand. This is distinct from the carpal tunnel that carries the median nerve.

hamstring attachment: An area on the ischial tuberosity that has the origin point for the biceps femoris, semi-membranosus and semi-tendinosus muscles.

Harrington rod: An old type of spinal instrumentation used to correct scoliosis.

health maintenance organization: A type of insurance coverage for medical care in which all care is given by a group of doctors who are under contract to provide services at a reduced fee often referred to by the acronym HMO.

herbal medicine: Non-regulated medications made directly from plant parts.

herniated disc: A lumbar intervertebral disc in which a portion of the nucleus pulposus has moved to an abnormal position.

hologram: A three-dimensional image projection.

humerus: The bone extending from the scapula (shoulder blade) to the elbow.

hyaluronic acid: A natural lubricant material found in the joints and around the nerves. The monomers (single units) of this compound can polymerize (join together and form cross links), thus turning into a type of scar tissue.

hyaluronidase: An enzyme capable of dissolving polymerized hyaluronic acid to return it to its lubricating monomeric state.

ICD-9 (*International Classification of Disease, Ninth Revision*): A coding system that provides a number for each type of medical diagnosis.

IDET: Intradiscal electrothermy. A process in which a wire is placed into the intervertebral disc to attempt to melt and repair an annular tear.

iliac arteries: The large arteries in the pelvis that start at the low end of the aorta and become the major arteries leading into each leg.

iliac crest: The upper edge of the ilium bone of the pelvis.

iliac crest bone graft: A bone graft taken from the hipbone, or iliac crest.

iliac veins: The two large veins that feed from each of the legs into the inferior vena cava in the low abdomen, the largest vein of the body.

ilioinguinal nerve: A nerve originating at the L2 and L3 levels of the spine that travels in the inguinal region innervating skin and muscle in the low abdomen and uppermost thigh.

image guidance: The use of real time imaging—such as X-ray fluoroscopy, ultrasound or MRI—to guide the performance of an interventional procedure or surgery.

impar ganglion: A collection of neurons involved in the sympathetic portion of the autonomic nervous system. It is located at the sacro-coccygeal joint on its deep surface. If plays a role in sphincter and genital function.

impingement: An abnormal contact between two tissues including types of pressure on nerves often called a "pinched" nerve.

impingement syndrome: Abnormal joint function, such as in the shoulder or knee.

in situ ulnar nerve release: A decompression of an entrapped or impinged ulnar nerve at the elbow in with the cubital tunnel is opened up or released, but wherein the nerve is not moved or "transposed" to a new location.

incentive spirometer: A device used by a patient after surgery to exercise and expand the lungs to prevent pneumonia and treat atelectasis (collapse of lung tissue).

indemnity plan: A type of medical insurance in which payment is made for individual medical charges as they arise.

inferior: Lower in the body, toward the feet.

inflammation: A natural process in the body in which there is local irritation, heat, redness, and typically pain.

informed consent: An agreement by a patient to allow a practitioner to perform a procedure in which the patient understands what is to be done to the best reasonable level.

innervate: Effect of a nerve reaching muscle or skin that provides movement or sensation.

instrumentation, spinal: Screws, rods, plates, and other devices used to hold spinal elements in place during or after surgery.

interbody fusion: A surgical procedure in which two vertebral bodies are caused to fuse together.

interbody implant: Device, made either of bone, metal or synthetic materials, that is used to replace an intervertebral disc.

intercostal nerves: Nerves that run along the lower margin of the ribs and whose branches innervate much of the skin of the back, flank, anterior chest and abdomen.

interspace: The space between two successive vertebral bodies.

inter-spinous spacer: A type of implanted device used for treatment of spinal stenosis and neurogenic claudication. It is placed between the spinous processes of two successive vertebrae to they are angled in a fashion simulating the effect of the patient leaning forward.

intradiscal Electrothermy: See IDET.

intradiscal injection: See discogram.

intradural: Inside the dura membranes.

intraoperative X-rays: X-rays taken during surgery.

intravenous sedation: Sedating medication given through the blood stream to allow a patient to tolerate a procedure but without producing a full general anesthesia requiring intubation.

iodine: An element used for intravenous contrast and X-ray studies.

ischial tuberosity: The lowest point of the pelvis. It provides the origin for the hamstring tendon. The sciatic nerve passes just lateral to it in the ischial tunnel and the obturator internus has part of its origin on the medial aspect of it.

isometric: Maintaining the length of a muscle while the tension changes.

jugular vein: a large vein in the neck, draining the brain and face toward the heart.

kyphoplasty: Procedure to correct the alignment of vertebra in a patient whose spine is angled forward.

kyphosis: Forward angulation of the spine.

lamina: The posterior portion of a vertebra, behind the spinal canal.

laminectomy: Removal of all or part of the posterior part of the vertebra.

laminoplasty: Reshaping of the posterior part of the vertebra.

laryngeal mask: A type of general anesthesia in which the tube does not pass through the vocal cords; this reduces the risk of vocal cord injury and it is useful for some shorter operations.

larynx: The voice box.

laser discoplasty: Reduction of the size of a disc by placement of a laser into the disc and evaporation of disc tissue.

lateral mass screws: Instrumentation for the cervical spine, that is directed through the lateral posterior part of the vertebra.

lateral recess stenosis: Narrowing of the lateral corner of the spinal canal, typically in the lumbar spine causing nerve root entrapment inside the spinal canal.

lateral X-ray: An X-ray taken from the side, showing the vertebrae in profile.

lateral: To the side.

ligamentum flavum: A yellow elastic ligament between the lamina of the vertebrae.

light emitting diode (LED): An electronic component that emits light when current is passed through it.

lipomyelomeningocele: A fatty collection at the base of the spinal canal, associated with a congenital abnormality.

listhesis: Slippage.

load bearing: A construction of screws and rods used to fixate vertebrae for a spinal fusion in which the components are capable of supporting much of the weight of the body.

load sharing: A construction of screws and rods used to fixate vertebrae for a spinal fusion in which the components are flexible enough to allow part of the weight of the body to be supported by the vertebral fusion implant.

local anesthetic: A medication of that stops all sensation at the site where it is injected.

long tracts: The axon fibers of nerve cells running from the cerebral cortex to the parts of the spinal cord.

lumbar drain: A catheter placed into the dural sac in the lumbar region to divert or drain cerebrospinal fluid.

lumbar puncture: Passing a needle into the dural sac in the lumbar region to drain or remove fluid or to introduce dye for a myelogram.

lumbar: The low back between the thoracic region and the sacral region.

lumbosacral plexus: The collection of nerve elements in the pelvis situated between the lumbar and sacral spine that feed into it and the sciatic, femoral and other leg nerves that lead away from it.

lysis: Separation or destruction, depending on its use in the medical term.

Magnetic Resonance Imaging: a way of visualizing the interior of the body using magnetic and radiofrequency fields.

malleolus, medial: The bony prominence on the inner side of the ankle. The tibial nerve passes posterior to it as it curves through the tarsal tunnel.

marrow: Tissue within bone that helps form new blood cells.

medial: Toward the midline or the opposite of lateral.

median nerve: A nerve that starts in the shoulder area and then runs into the hand. It carries sensory fibers to the thumb and first two fingers and motor nerves to the upper arm and to the base of the thumb to enable flexion of the fingers.

Medicare: Health care financing provided for individuals over 65 and for those who are disabled, under supervision of the Federal Government—also Health Care Financing Administration (HCFA) and Centers for Medicare and Medicaid Services (CMS).

meninges: The various membranes that line the spinal cord and brain.

meningioma: A tumor that derives from the membranes around the spinal cord or brain.

meningitis: An infection in the spinal fluid and in the membranes around the spinal cord and brain.

meralgia paresthetica: A pain syndrome affecting the anterior and lateral portion of the thigh due to a problem with the lateral femoral cutaneous nerve.

metastatic: A tumor that spreads to various locations within the body.

microdiscectomy: The removal of lumbar disc material under microscope magnification.

microplates: Small titanium plates, used to hold the bones in position after repair, closure or fusion.

minimally invasive surgery: A surgical incision and approach modified to reduce the amount of tissue that must be disrupted to accomplish the surgical objective.

modalities: Different types of physical therapy treatment such as ultrasound, stretching and strengthening.

modulus of elasticity: The degree to which a structure can be bent and returned to its previous shape.

Morton's neuroma: A painful swelling in a nerve between the toes.

motor evoked potentials: Activation of the movement system, which is induced with magnetic fields applied over the surface of the brain.

motor neurons: Nerve cells in the spinal cord that operate muscles.

motor units: Groups of muscle cells operated by the branches of a single motor nerve cell.

MR angiography: An image of the blood vessels, obtained using MRI scanning without any requirement for injection of contrast into the blood system.

MR neurography: a method for imaging nerves with specialized MRI scanning.

multidisciplinary pain management: An approach to pain management that involves psychology, psychiatry, anesthesia, and nursing as a multi-specialty team.

muscle spasm: A condition of increased muscle tone that may be chronic—or continuously present. It can result in stiffening of a muscle in a way that places pressure on nerves adjacent to the muscle and may be directly painful.

musculocutaneous nerve: A nerve originating in the shoulder that activates the biceps muscle.

musculoskeletal: Anything pertaining to the bones, muscles, tendons and ligaments.

myelin: A fatty material that surrounds and insulates the nerve cells and allows them to conduct their electrical signals optimally.

myelogram: An X-ray and CT image of the spinal cord and nerve roots, produced by injecting contrast dye into the spinal fluid. Magnetic resonance (MR) myelograms do not require any injections

myelomeningocele: A birth defect affecting the spine, in which the spinal cord may be exposed through the skin.

myelopathy: Symptoms that arise when the spinal cord is compressed.

narcotic: Opiate medication used for treatment of pain.

necrosis: The death of some cells or parts of a tissue in a person or animal in which the surrounding tissue remains alive and in which the person or animal overall remains alive. Examples include strokes and heart attacks in which there is cell death called an infarction.

nerve block: An injection that causes numbness and weakness by preventing function of a nerve.

nerve conduction velocity (NCV): The speed at which an electrical signal travels along a nerve. This may be abnormal when a nerve is compressed or injured.

nerve cone: The growing tip of a severed nerve that it is trying to re-establish its connection after injury.

nerve entrapment: A location at which a nerve is squeezed or trapped in such a way as to cause pain, numbness, and/or weakness in tissues innervated by that nerve and also—often pain at the site of the entrapment.

nerve graft: A segment of nerve—often taken from the sural nerve—used to bride a gap when a severed nerve is surgically repaired.

nerve release: Surgical removal of an adhesion, entrapment or impingement that is causing dysfunction in a nerve.

nerve root: A structure that carries axons between the spinal cord and the starting point of the spinal nerve. The nerve root crosses the spinal fluid space and has the internal structure of spinal cord tissue. The spinal nerve has fascicles and Schwann cell linings that do not occur in the nerve root.

nerve tube: A synthetic tube used to help in repair and reconnection of nerves.

nerve nervorum: Small nerve fi bers that innervate larger nerve bundles. Th ey allow us to feel pressure on the nerve itself.

neuralgia: Pain originating in a nerve.

neuritis: Inflammation of in a nerve.

neurofibroma: A tumor arising within a nerve.

neuroma: A clump of tissue, not necessarily a tumor, that can arise at the site of nerve injury.

neurons: Nerve cells.

neuropathic pain: Pain that derives in nerves and may not be responsive to routine pain medications.

neuropathy: Malfunction in a nerve due to a medical disease of nerves or to compression of the nerve.

neuroplasty: Technical term for a nerve release surgery—replacing the older term "neurolysis."

neuroprotective agents: Medications that are intended to help limit the damage suffered by a nerve or neural tissue such as spinal cord, brain or nerve, when the blood supply is cut off or there is a traumatic injury.

neurosurgeons: Surgeons with specialty training for operations involving the brain, spine and nerves.

nociceptor: A type of nerve ending that produces a sensation of pain when it is stimulated.

non-ferrous: A type of metal without iron in it.

Nonsteroidal anti-inflammatory drugs (NSAIDs): medications that reduce swelling, inflammation, and pain without the use of steroids, e.g. Tylenol or Motrin.

notocord: A primitive part of the body plan in evolution that has remnants in humans in the form of the nucleus pulposus of the intervertebral discs.

nuclear medicine: Diagnostic tests that involve the use of radioactivity administered to the body.

nucleus pulposus: The soft spongy material surrounded by the annular ring that makes up the center of an intervertebral disc.

obex: Opening in the floor of the fourth cerebral ventricle through which spinal fluid enters the center of the spinal canal.

oblique X-ray: X-rays taken from an angle that allows for a direct view through the nerve canal or foramina.

obturator: An opening in the low pelvis.

obturator internus: A muscle on the internal surface of the pelvic bone whose tendon reaches to the external surface of the pelvis, crossing the sciatic nerve to reach the greater trochanter of the femur. It is a hip abductor innervated by the nerve to the obturator internus. The pudendal nerve travels in the medial wall of the muscle for part of its course.

occipital condyle: The joint at the base of the skull that articulates with the upper part of the first cervical vertebra.

occipital muscles: Muscles behind the back of the neck that reach the back of the skull.

occiput: The back of the skull.

off-label: The use of a medication of device by a physician in a manner that differs from what the FDA has allowed to appear on the label.

operating microscope: A type of microscope that is used for surgery, typically spinal surgery, that provides a 3-dimensional magnified view with superior lighting.

opiates: Narcotic medications.

OPLL (ossification of the posterior longitudinal ligament): An abnormal bone formation within the spinal canal, along the dura that is anterior to the spinal cord and posterior to the vertebrae.

orthopedic surgeons: Surgeons with specialty training for operations involving bones who may have sub-specialty training for spinal surgery.

osteoblast: A type of cell that generates new bone.

osteoclast: A type of cell that can digest or destroy bone.

osteoconductive: Material that helps provide a medium for bone formation.

osteocyte: a bone cell.

osteogenesis: The formation of new bone.

osteogenic proteins: Proteins that promote the formation of new bone.

osteoinductive: Proteins and materials that encourage the body to produce osteogenic proteins.

osteomyelitis: An infection of bone.

osteophyte: An abnormal prominence or projection from a bone that is also called a "bone spur."

osteoporosis: Softening of bone due to loss of calcium, typically with age.

pain fibers: Axons of pain sensitive nerve cells.

pain generator: A site in the body that is thought to be the cause of a particular pain symptom.

paralysis: Loss of the ability to move a part of the body caused by a neurologic problem. This may be due to a problem in the brain, spinal cord or nerve.

parasympathetic nerves: part of the autonomic nervous system.

pars interarticularis: The part of a vertebra between the lamina and the superior facet; this may be abnormal in the condition called spondylolysis.

PCA (patient controlled analgesia): Method of pain treatment after surgery that allows the patient to self-administer pain medication under a controlled regimen.

pedicle screws: Fixation screws that are placed through the pedicle of the vertebra.

pedicle: Portion of the vertebra that connects the lamina (posterior part of the vertebra) to the body anteriorly and helps forms the walls of the spinal canal.

PEEK (polyethyletherketone): A plastic-like material used for spinal implants because it has elasticity and strength in compression that is similar to bone.

peptides: Small proteins.

percutaneous Treatment: A interventional treatment done inside the body without a formal surgical incision.

percutaneous: Procedure done through a puncture in the skin, typically by a needle or through a very narrow cannula.

perineum: The area between the legs.

periosteum: The lining of the bone. It has sensation and it helps control the shape and growth of bone.

peripheral nerves: The nerves after the departure from the spinal canal, proceeding out to their end point in the skin and muscles.

periphery: The parts of the body furthest away from the spinal cord and brain.

peritoneum: The internal lining of the abdominal cavity.

peroneal Nerve: A nerve that commences just above the knee, passes along the lateral aspect of the lower leg and helps activate muscles that lift the foot.

phased-array coils: Equipment used in MRI scanning to improve the signal to noise or image quality of the MRI scan.

phrenic nerve: A nerve originating at the C3, C4, and C5 levels of the spine that travels along the front of the anterior scalene muscle then descends through the chest to innervate the diaphragm muscle for respiration.

Pilates: An exercise based treatment for the spine and for overall body maintenance.

pinched nerve: A nerve that is involved in pain, numbness or weakness due to some mechanical interference or pressure at some point along its course.

piriformis muscle: A muscle that runs from the sacrum to the top of the femur, that can cause buttock pain and entrap the sciatic nerve and other nerves.

piriformis-pudendal syndrome: A sub-type of pudendal pain in which the pudendal nerve or its S2 and S3 spinal nerve contributors suffers impingement by the piriformis muscle as a cause for the syndrome.

placebo effect: Improvement of a condition experienced by a patient who believes a treatment has been administered even if the treatment was not actually done.

placebo: A pill that carries no actual medicine.

plantar fasciitis: Pain syndrome affecting the bottom of the foot due to irritation of fascia and ligaments in the foot. It needs to be distinguished from nerve based causes of foot pain such as tarsal tunnel syndrome or entrapment of the medial plantar nerve.

plasticity: It is adaptation of the nervous system to new connection patterns.

PLDLA: A polymerized form of lactic acid (poly L-lactic acid and poly D/L-lactic acid) which is used to make spine implants that dissolve over time.

pleural lining: A thin lining of the lungs.

pneumonia: An infection of the lungs.

point based treatments: Acupuncture or acupressure for a nonsurgical treatment of back pain.

Point of service (POS) insurance: A plan in which the patient can enter either an HMO plan, a PPO (a preferred provider) or a non-contracted plan depending on how they commenced care for any given condition they experience.

polymers: Complex molecules with many individual parts, typically such as plastics or other complex absorbable molecules used in surgical treatment and implants.

posterior longitudinal ligament: A ligament behind the vertebral bodies and anterior to the spinal dura and spinal cord.

posterior-anterior X-rays: Images obtained with the X-ray source behind the spine and the film in front of the spine.

posterior: Toward the back of.

posterolateral fusion: A lumbar fusion done from a posterior approach and incorporating the transverse processes of the lumbar vertebrae.

PPO (preferred provider organization): Type of health insurance in which patients may choose from a physician from a list of providers who have agreed to offer care at a discount.

preemptive anesthesia: The administration of pain medication before surgery in an attempt to prevent the pain from becoming intense as the surgery progresses.

prognosis: Expectation of the outcome of a condition.

prophylactic: Something administered to prevent the development of a problem such as antibiotics given to prevent the possibility of an infection.

prospective cooperative study: test to evaluate the efficacy of a treatment, typically done by determining the clinical plan before any of the patients commence treatment and involving many different hospitals.

provocative discogram: A test to evaluate whether an intervertebral disc is a pain generator. Fluid is injected into the disc to learn whether the resulting pain is similar to the patient's usual pain.

pseudoarthrosis: Literally "false joint," a painful contact between two bones that develops at the site of a failed fusion.

psoas muscle: A long muscle that originates along the sides of the vertebrae and attaches to the proximal femur. It is innervated by anterior branches of the L1 through L4 spinal nerves and acts to flex the leg at the hip.

pudendal nerve: A nerve that provides motor and sensory functions for the perineal region between the legs as well as for the urinary sphincter, rectal sphincter, bladder and structures involved in sexual function.

pus: A reactive material produced in an infection by the accumulation of the body's white cells attempting to digest bacteria.

quadrangular space: A space bounded by the teres major above, the teres minor below, the triceps long head medially and the triceps lateral head laterally. The axillary nerve departs from the posterior cord of the brachial plexus and passes through this space to reach the deltoid muscle. The axillary nerve is sometimes entrapped in this location.

quadriceps femoris muscle: The muscle group made up of the vastus lateralis, vastus medialis, vastus intermedius, and rectus femoris muscles. They are innervated by the femoral nerve and act to extend the lower leg at the knee.

radial: On the side of the radius which is the arm bone nearest the thumb.

radial nerve: A nerve that is formed when the posterior cord of the brachial plexus divides into the axillary nerve and the radial nerve. It innervates the triceps, as well as the extensors of the wrist and hand and it provides sensation for the back of the arm and hand.

radiculopathy: Pain, numbness, and weakness in the distribution of a spinal nerve.

radiofrequency lesion: A lesion of the nerve carried out with the controlled heat that is actuated by the administration of radiofrequency energy down a specialized needle.

radius: A bone extending from the elbow that has the major portion of the surface of the joint with the wrist, and which rotates around the other forearm bone, the ulna, when the wrist is pronated (turned palm down) or supinated (turned palm up).

RBRVS: Resource-based relative value scale. A federal-government-based method of assessing the work and training involved in a medical procedure for the purpose of proposing an appropriate relative charge or a price for the medical procedure.

recombinant protein: A protein manufactured from DNA that has been reassembled for purposes of optimizing pharmaceutical production. Hylenex is a recombinant version of the hyaluronidase enzyme generated from a modified human gene. Hylenex is used to dissolve some adhesions. Some BMPs (bone morphogenetic proteins) are also manufactured by recombinant gene technology.

rectus abdominis: A muscle originating on the lower end of the sternum and inserting on the pubis. It is innervated by branches of multiple different spinal nerves.

referred pain: Pain experienced at a location different from the injury causing the pain, usually due to neurologic relationships in the spinal cord.

reflex sympathetic dystrophy: Abnormality of the autonomic nervous system causing burning pain, temperature and color changes in the skin, often associated with nerve irritation and nerve injury—see also Complex Regional Pain Syndrome.

reinnervation: The arrival of a new nerves to replace damaged nerves for the supply of muscle and skin.

rejection, immune: An attack by the body on an implant.

relative value units (RVUs): A numerical system for describing the value of a medical procedure for the purpose of assigning a price or charge.

resorbable suture or implant: Meant to be dissolved naturally by the body.

retroperitoneal: Tissues in the space between the posterior body wall and the peritoneal cavity (containing the intestines).

retrospective review: An analysis of outcome or success with a medical treatment based on reviewing medical records that were prepared without prior plan for carrying out research or a study.

Rolfing: A type of treatment for health of musculo-skeletal pains involving manipulation of the patient's muscles and fasciae by the practitioner.

rootlets: The small initial branches of nerves arising in the spinal cord that join together to form nerve roots and ultimately peripheral nerves.

sacro-iliac ligament: A ligament forming the posterior border of the sciatic notch.

sacro-spinous ligament: A ligament extending from the ischial spine to the sacrum. In many individuals, the pudendal nerve cross over this ligament.

sacro-tuberous ligament: A ligament extending from the sacro-iliac ligament to the ischial tuberosity. The pudendal nerve travels on the deep surface of this ligament in some individuals.

sacrum: The vertebrae between the lumbar and caudal region, that are fused together and that also connect through the sacroiliac joint to the iliac blades of the pelvis.

salicylates: Various medications related to aspirin which derive from salicylic acid. The original form of this medication came from the bark of the willow tree.

scalene muscles: Muscles that run between the vertebrae of the cervical spine and the first rib. The major nerves of the brachial plexus between the spine and the arm pass between the anterior and middle scalene muscles. They may become involved in a pain syndrome called a thoracic outlet syndrome.

scapula: The bone of the shoulder blade.

scar tissue: Abnormal tissue formed by the body in an attempt to repair damage to connective tissues. It may be loosely formed from polymerized hyaluronate or it may have more firm collagenous components. New symptoms can arise when scar tissue causes pressure on a nerve or limits natural movement of a nerve.

Schwann cell: A type of cell that wraps around a nerve and is filled with a fatty material called myelin. These cells provides the insulation allowing the nerve to rapidly conduct electrical signals.

schwannoma: A usually benign nerve tumor arising in the Schwann cells.

sciatic nerve: A large nerve carrying motor and sensory fibers to the posterior thigh and the leg below the knee.

sciatic notch: An opening in the pelvis through which the sciatic nerve passes from the lower abdomen out into the buttock and upper leg.

sciatica: Pain in the distribution of the sciatic nerve that may involve L4, L5, S1, or S2 dermatomal components.

scoliosis: Curvature of the spine.

secondary injury: Additional injury of brain or spinal cord, after a primary vascular or traumatic injury. The secondary injury is due to natural destructive factors released within the neural tissue.

segmentation: The forming of the various body segments during embryological development, including the differentiation that distinguishes cervical from thoracic from lumbar and from sacral types of vertebrae.

semispinalis muscle: A muscle in the posterior neck that acts to extend the neck in looking upwards. It is innervated by the greater occipital nerve.

sensory neurons: Nerve cells that carry signals from the skin and muscle and special sensory organs back toward the central nervous system.

shiatsu: A type of manual physical treatment for maintaining general health and relaxation, as well as for treatment of pain.

shimmed: Fine tuning of the performance of a magnet, such as an MRI scanner.

shunt: A catheter or tube that carries fluid to bypass it from one body space to another.

somatic nerves: The nerves that carry out movements and deliver conscious sensation, as distinguished from the autonomic nervous system.

somatic pain: A pain arising in the body tissues, typically associated with injury or trauma to the body tissues.

somatosensory evoked potentials: Electrical signals produced along the nerves and in the cerebral cortex that can be detected with electrodes, the potentials having been evoked or triggered by repeated stimulation actuated by a computer.

spasticity: Increased muscle tone that causes an increased hardness or instability of muscles.

specific risks: Risks of surgery that are particular to the individual type of surgery being done.

spina bifida aperta: Open spina bifida in which a congenital malformation leaves a deep part of the spinal cord, such as the cord itself, exposed through the skin.

spina bifida occulta: Abnormal closure of the spine or spinal membranes that is concealed within normal intact skin.

spinal canal: The space between the vertebral body and the lamina through which the spinal dura and spinal cord and nerves pass.

spinal cord: The portion of the central nervous system extending from the base of the brain down to the L1 or L2 level in most individuals, that includes both the gray matter for the neuron connections and the white matter of the long tracts running from the brain to the final connections that feed the nerves of the body.

spinal gray matter: The area of the spinal cord that has the connections between neurons.

spinal nerves: Nerves that original at the spinal foramina and continue outward to either become intercostal nerves or join the lumbar, sacral, or brachial plexuses.

spinal tap: The passage of a needle into the spinal fluid inside the dura to drain fluid.

spinal white matter: Long tracts of axons reaching from the brain down to the lower portions of the spinal cord.

spine series: A series of X-rays in a defined set of the views that provides an assessment of the spine.

spinous process. A portion of a vertebra that is in the midline and directed posteriorly toward the skin.

splenius muscle: A muscle in the posterior neck that acts to extend the neck in looking upwards. It is innervated by posterior branches of several cervical spinal nerves.

spondylo-: A word root used to mean a vertebra.

spondylolisthesis: Slippage between two vertebrae.

spondylolysis: A separation or break between the lamina and the articular process of vertebra.

SSEP: Somatosensory evoked potentials.

stem cells: Cells in the body that have the potential to develop into various different types of tissue.

stenosis: Narrowing of the spinal canal or foramina.

stent: An implanted device that is expanded inside a blood vessel or other tubular structure in the body for purposes of re-establishing and maintaining the open space inside the vessel.

sternocleidomastoid: A muscle originating from the mastoid process on the base of the occiput and inserting on the clavicle and sternum. It is innervated by the accessory nerve (eleventh cranial nerve).

sternotomy: A surgery involving cutting the sternum from top to bottom in order to gain access to the anterior chest and heart.

sternum: The large bony structure in the anterior chest to which many of the ribs connect.

steroid: A type of medication that mimics a natural body material and reduces inflammation.

stroke: A damage to an area of neural tissue caused by abnormal function in a nearby blood vessel. The term includes both damage from bleeding and damage from insufficient blood supply.

subclavian artery: The major artery carrying blood into the arm. It can be pinched by the anterior scalene muscle in some cases of thoracic outlet syndrome.

subcuticular stitches: Buried stitches placed below the skin to achieve a cosmetic skin closure.

subdural empyema: The accumulation of infection and pus between the dura membrane and the arachnoid membrane just outside the spinal fluid space.

sublaminar wires: An instrumentation in which wires are passed below the lamina to secure a rod or screw to the lamina.

subluxation: Slippage between two vertebrae.

superficial: Toward the skin. Opposite of deep.

superior: Toward the top or upper portion of the structure.

supraclavicular approach: A surgical method of reaching the brachial plexus and scalene muscles that involves an incision just above the clavicle (collarbone).

sural nerve: A nerve on the lateral surface of the leg beginning behind the knee and reaching to the lateral surface of the foot. The nerve is sometimes subject to biopsy to test for nerve disease or is taken to be used as a graft for nerve repairs.

surgical series: A series of surgeries that are evaluated and subjected to statistical analysis to evaluate outcome.

surgicenter: An outpatient facility that offers a full range of anesthesia to carry out surgical procedures.

sympathectomy: The removal of sympathetic ganglia in order to attempt to treat abnormal function of the sympathetic nervous system.

sympathetic ganglia: Collections of nerve connections, usually on the outer or lateral surface of the vertebral body, that help moderate and drive the autonomic nervous system.

sympathetic nerves: A portion of the autonomic nervous system that travels to the skin and helps control skin temperature and color by adjusting the constriction or dilation of blood vessels.

syringomyelia: The accumulation of fluid within the center of the spinal cord.

syrinx: A cavity within the spinal cord typically caused by the accumulation of fluid.

tai chi: An exercise-based treatment for general body health or treatment of pain.

tarsal tunnel syndrome: Pain in the foot due to entrapment of the tibial nerve in the tarsal tunnel—a space in the medial aspect of the ankle that carries the tibial nerve into the foot.

tensor fascia lata: A muscle extending from the greater trochanter of the femur and inserting on the knee. It is innervated by the superior gluteal nerve.

tethered cord: A developmental embryological abnormality in which the spinal cord remains attached abnormally to the sacrum and does not ascend to the L1 or L2 level during the course of growth but remains trapped and under tension in the low lumbar spine.

thermistor: Temperature monitor used in the radiofrequency lesioning system to control the temperature of the tip of the radiofrequency probe.

thoracic outlet syndrome: Pain in the neck, shoulders, arms, and hands due to nerve entrapments affecting the brachial plexus.

thoracic spine: The rib-bearing portion of the spine between the cervical and the lumbar regions.

thoracostomy tube (or chest tube): A catheter or drain placed in the pleural space of the lung to help reinflate a collapsed lung.

thoracotomy: A surgery in which the chest is opened by making an incision between the ribs. This is used in order to gain access to the thoracic spine in some surgeries.

tibia: The major leg bone between the knee and ankle.

tissue glue: A biological adhesive or sealing material made from natural human blood proteins that are normally involved in clotting.

titanium: An element or type of metal that is nonmagnetic and hence compatible with MRI scanning and is the major component of many alloys used for surgical implants.

TNF (tumor necrosis factor): A natural protein in the body that functions to identify newly forming tumor cells and then activates the inflammatory system to attack and destroy the abnormal target cell. In some cases the TNF becomes mis-directed leading to inflammation of normal tissues such as nerve, joints or intestines.

tolerance: The requirement of the body for higher and higher doses of narcotic medication in order to achieve the same amount of pain relief.

topical: Medication for application directly to the skin.

torques: Twisting forces applied, such as to the body or spine.

trachea: The tube between the mouth and lungs that carries the air that we breathe.

traction: The application of tension or pulling to the spine.

transabdominal: A surgical approach that goes through the abdomen.

transarticular: A type of screw or instrumentation that crosses between the facet surface to attempt to prevent movement across the joint that it crosses.

transaxillary: A surgical approach through the axilla, or underarm.

transcutaneous electrical nerve stimulator (TENS): A device used for pain treatment in which pulsing electrical currents are applied to the skin to provide a distracting stimulus, making pain more tolerable.

transforaminal epidural: A type of injection in which the needle is passed through the neural foramen to apply a steroid and/or anesthetic medication. This provides treatment to an individual selected spinal nerve, as well as to the general spinal dura nearby.

transfusion: The administration of blood products to replace lost blood.

transgluteal approach: A surgical method for reaching the structures of the sciatic notch (piriformis muscle, sciatic, pudendal and superior gluteal nerves). It differs from older methods in that a non-destructive path is made through the gluteal muscles as oppose to older methods where the gluteal muscles are cut.

transorally: A surgical approach carried out through the back of the mouth to reach the dens or other portions of the C1 or C2 vertebra.

transpedicular: A surgical approach carried out through and inside the pedicle of a thoracic vertebra to reach a thoracic disc without requiring retraction of the spinal cord.

transposition: The repositioning of a nerve into a modified position. This is often done in the treatment of ulnar nerve entrapment in the cubital tunnel. The nerve can be moved to a location under skin anterior to the medical epicondyle (subcutaneous transposition) or some of the flexor muscle origin can be temporarily detached so the nerve can be placed under the muscle (submuscular transposition).

triceps: A muscle in the forearm, originating on the clavicle, scapula and humerus that attaches on the posterior surface of the ulna. It acts to extend (straighten) the forearm at the elbow.

triplicate prescription: A specialized type of medical secure prescription used for controlled-substance narcotics and are closely monitored by the DEA (Drug Enforcement Administration). These must be delivered to the pharmacist within 14 days of being written, are not subject to refills, and cannot be faxed or called in to a pharmacy.

trochanteric bursa: A fluid filled pocket of tissue on the lateral surface of the greater trochanter of the femur.

trophins: Natural compounds or proteins that promote growth of tissue, such as nerve tissue.

tubular retractor: A surgical device that provides a fixed access or view through the body tissues for use by a surgeon during a procedure.

tumors: Abnormal growth of tissues.

ulceration: Breakdown of tissue usually due to pressure or infection.

ulna: A bone in the forearm extending from elbow to wrist along with the radius.

ulnar nerve: A nerve arising in the shoulder area, passing around the elbow, and entering the hand on the side of the small finger. It is responsible for sensory innervation of the fourth and fifth fingers, as well as for movement of most of the small muscles of the hand.

ultrasound: A type of imaging system that uses sound and echoes to produce a picture of deep tissues.

uncovertebral joint: A joint surface between the vertebral bodies of cervical vertebrae.

urinary tract infection (UTI): An infection that develops within the bladder or urethra.

vena cava: A large vein that runs toward the heart. The superior vena cava descends from the base of the neck and inferior vena cava ascends from the pelvis.

ventilator: A machine that provides controlled breathing to a person under general anesthesia or otherwise deeply unconscious.

ventricle: A fluid-containing space within the brain.

vertebra: A bony element of the spine.

vertebral artery: An artery arising at the base of the neck and extending up to the posterior parts of the brain. It passes through small canals in several of the cervical vertebrae.

vertebral body: The anterior or front of the vertebra that carries most of the weight and that contacts directly with the intervertebral discs.

vertebrectomy: The removal of a vertebral body.

whiplash: A syndrome of neck pain—typically after a motor vehicle accident—in which there is a soft tissue injury such as pain in the scalene muscles as opposed to a primarily spinal injury.

white matter: A portion of the brain or spinal cord containing mostly fiber tracts (communicating "wires") rather than any nerve cell bodies.

X-ray: An image obtained by shining high-energy electrons through a tissue.

X-ray myelogram: An image of the spinal canal obtained with an X-ray machine after first injecting dye into the spinal fluid.

xenograft: A graft of tissue from a different species.

XLIF: A lateral approach for a lumbar fusion (Extreme Lateral Interbody Fusion).

yoga: An exercise-based treatment in use for thousands of years for general health and well being. It is also used for the treatment of some types of spinal pain.

» Index «